**Rita Arditti** came to the United States in 1965 to do research in molecular biology. Born in Argentina, in a Jewish Sephardic family, she studied biology in Italy where she got her doctorate at the University of Rome. She has co-edited *Science and Liberation* (South End Press, 1980) and is on the faculty of Union Graduate School. She is one of the founders of New Words, a women's bookstore in Cambridge, Massachusetts. She is currently one of the editors of *Reproductive and Genetic Engineering: A Journal of International Feminist Analysis*.

**Renate D Klein** has a biology degree from Zurich University and degrees in Women's Studies from the University of California and London University. She is the editor of *Infertility: Women Speak Out About Their Experiences of Reproductive Medicine* (Pandora Press, 1989) and co-author with Gena Corea et al of *Man-Made Women* (1985). In 1986 she was awarded the Georgina Sweet Fellowship to research the experiences of women who drop out of test-tube baby programmes in Australia. She is currently a research fellow at Deakin University, where she is continuing her research on the new reproductive technologies and genetic engineering. Renate Klein is a founding member of the Feminist International Network of Resistance to Reproductive and Genetic Engineering (FINNRAGE).

**Shelley Minden** became concerned with the potential applications of reproductive technologies while working as a technician and as a research assistant in the field of medical genetics. She has an MS degree in biology from the University of Oregon. She has been an editor of *Genewatch*, the newsletter for the Coalition for Responsible Genetics, and an active member of the Reproductive Rights National Network. She was the 1986/87 co-ordinator of the US FINNRAGE group. Shelley Minden now works as a science writer, and she also writes fiction.

# TEST-TUBE WOMEN
# What future for motherhood?

*Edited by Rita Arditti,
Renate Duelli Klein and
Shelley Minden*

# PANDORA PRESS

London  Boston  Sydney  Wellington

First published by Pandora Press, an imprint of
Routledge and Kegan Paul in 1984
Reprinted in 1985
This edition published by Pandora Press, an imprint of the Trade
Division of Unwin Hyman, in 1989

PANDORA PRESS
Unwin Hyman Limited
15/17 Broadwick Street
London W1V 1FP

Unwin Hyman Inc
8 Winchester Place, Winchester, MA 01890

Allen & Unwin Australia Pty Ltd
P.O. Box 764, 8 Napier Street, North Sydney, NSW 2060

Allen & Unwin NZ Ltd (in association with the Port Nicholson Press)
60 Cambridge Terrace, Wellington, New Zealand

Printed in Great Britain by Cox and Wyman


British Library Cataloguing in Publication Data
Test-tube women: what future for motherhood.
  1. Man. Reproduction.    Scientific innovation.
  Social aspects
  I. Arditti, Rita, 1934–    II. Dvelli Klein,
  Renate      III. Minden, Shelley
  306.'46

ISBN 0–04–440429–8

# CONTENTS

# ACKNOWLEDGMENTS

One of the many lessons we learned from working on this collection is that the international feminist network thrives and *functions*. Women in many countries shared their information, enthusiasm and support, and we particularly thank the following: Melitta Benn, Marge Berer, Charlotte Bunch, Subhadra Butalia, Urvashi Butalia, Vienna Carroll, Jane Cholmeley, Estelle Disch, Andrea Dworkin, Cynthia Enloe, Christiane Erlemann, Kathy Freeperson, Maree Gladwin, Mona Howard, Cathy Itzin, Caeia March, Margrit Minto, Mary Brown Parlee, Ruth Richardson, Colette Ritchie, Helen Roberts, Judy Zimmet, and Christine Zmroczek.

We distributed our 'call for papers' widely in the international feminist media, and thank *Off Our Backs, Sojourner, Isis, Outwrite, Spare Rib, Big Momma Rag*, the *Science for the People Newsletter*, the *Reproductive Rights National Network Bulletin*, the *CARASA Newsletter*, and any others that may have also printed our announcement.

Judy Norsigian, Norma Swenson, and the Boston Women's Health Book Collective provided a wealth of information, including international contacts on Depo-Provera, infant mortality, and midwifery. Karen Stamm, Belita Cowan and Cheryl Heppner of the National Women's Health Network also gave us many important contacts. The Committee to Defend Reproductive Rights helped to circulate our call for papers among reproductive rights activists.

The women at New Words bookstore in Cambridge, Mass.: Mary Lowry, Gilda Bruckman, and Madge Kaplan shared their knowledge about book titles and covers, and also helped us to check up on what seemed like countless

ACKNOWLEDGMENTS

references. To the women at Routledge & Kegan Paul on both sides of the Atlantic – Philippa Brewster, Jane Hawksley, Helen Armitage, Wendy Lee, Helen Mott, Carol Taplin, Ellen Cooney, Kate Dunn, Deirdre Doran, and Cyd Smith – go our special thanks for their enthusiasm and support for our project.

We are grateful to all of the contributors, especially those who stayed with us through laborious and sometimes multiple revisions. With all of them we have developed a close working relationship. We hope to meet them in person some day, and in the meantime look forward to following their continuing work. We especially thank Genoveffa Corea, who, despite the fact that she had a deadline for her own book to meet, was incredibly generous and helpful with her advice, contacts, and encouragement. We received many other good papers which for lack of space we are sorry not to be able to include.

We also want to thank each other for the many fantastic hours we spent together on this project. Despite the difficulties of working across the ocean, the times we spent together were energizing, sisterly, and stimulating. Working collectively has reaffirmed our belief that we all have a lot to learn from and to share with each other.

Finally, our warmest thanks go to Dale Spender, who not only says there's nothing she knows she wouldn't share – but who actually shares it!

The editors and publisher are grateful to William Morrow & Co., Inc., New York, for their permission to reproduce passages from Robert Edwards and Patrick Steptoe, *A Matter of Life* (1980), which appear in Genoveffa Corea's chapter, 'Egg Snatchers'.

# PREFACE TO THE 1989 EDITION

In 1984, new reproductive technologies were just beginning to become part of the public discussion. In deciding to put together *Test-Tube Women* we wanted to take a look at new technologies such in-vitro fertilization, embryo flushing and transfer. We also wanted to investigate technologies that were not really that new, such as artificial insemination, and further developments of contraceptives. Sex selection and the use of amniocentesis in the so-called 'Third World' was a further area of concern to us. The scientists developing these technologies told us that women should be grateful for their inventions and that they had been developed because women wanted them. They also said the technologies would open up new choices for motherhood and they would help infertile women.

We were sceptical. Although we could not know at the time what the specific developments would be, nor how quickly the technologies would proliferate, affecting an increasing number of women all over the world, nevertheless, two crucial pieces of information were already obvious. The first was that a white medical and scientific establishment is in control of the technologies and that there is a long history of exploitation of women by these groups, specifically in relation to reproduction. Women of color, poor women, lesbians, disabled women, elderly and young women have all been experimented on and used by the 'technodocs' in their human trials and applications of contraceptives such as the Pill, Depo-Provera and IUDs, in particular the Dalkon shield. With these new technologies it seemed to be the turn of mainly white and middle-class women to serve as experimental guinea pigs.

The other piece of information was the recognition, emerging from feminist analyses of science, that technologies are born in a particular moment in history to a particular society, that they do not fall from heaven and that they are not 'neutral'. In other words, a technology is not 'objective': it carries embedded in it a vision of the world and of what is considered important and valuable for the particular society where the technology is developed. Thus these new technologies supposedly invented to 'assist procreation' have been developed in the western part of the world in order to control 'infertility-as-disease'. In the so-called 'Third World', however, and among poor and socially 'undesirable' women in the west, 'fertility-as disease' control continues with new types of contraceptives which make women ill (eg injectables such as NetEn and implants such as Norplant) as does coercive sterilization under abysmally unhygenic circumstances.

Since the first publication of *Test-Tube Women* what we have learned about these technologies, their rapid development and above all women's experiences with the various procedures, have all too clearly validated our initial scepticism as well as the concerns voiced by many of the contributors in this collection.

In the case of in-vitro fertilization – hailed as a 'miracle cure' for infertility – feminist research has shown clearly that IVF is a *failed* technology. It does not work: out of 100 women who enter an IVF programme only 5 to 10 have a chance of leaving with a baby. This is now internationally acknowledged (eg 8.6 per cent for Britain in 1986; 8.8 per cent for Australia for 1986/87, see Klein, 1988a). But IVF clinics in which a child has *never* been born, claim success rates as high as 25 per cent (Corea and Ince, 1987). Biased reporting of 'success' – often pregnancies rather than live births of which up to half can end in a miscarriage – also obscures the fact that IVF presents serious risks to the health of women. The 'hormonal cocktails' administered to superovulate them, that is to stimulate their ovaries so that they will produce more than one ripe egg per month, bring with them the risk of burst ovaries (as many as 47 eggs are reported to have been collected at one time; Veitch, 1987), ovarian cysts, septicaemia, tubal and ovarian adhesions and a host of other so-called 'side-effects'. Women are used as 'living test-sites' – as 'living laboratories', the term Australian critic Robyn Rowland used for the first time in her piece in this book. The adverse reactions from the drugs range from migraine, dizziness, vision problems, weight gain and depression to breast cancer and ovarian cancer (see Klein/Rowland, 1988 for a detailed overview of the dangers associated with superovulation). Also, it is feared that children who are born to women who have used clomiphene citrate (one of the drugs given to millions of women internationally both on 'conventional' infertility treatments, IVF programs or on 'egg donor' programs) might be affected in a way similar to the children of women who took DES during their pregnancy (Klein/Rowland, 1988).

Woman also die on IVF programs, but this not usually publicised by the media. Who knows about Zenaide Maria Bernardo in Brazil who died in 1982? She suffered a respiratory arrest while undergoing a laparasopy exam and 'the doctors, for reasons that could be difficult to establish, took some time to notice' (Gomez dos Reis, 1987:127). She was part of an experimental program in which Australian IVF scientists were teaching IVF in Brazil. And who knows about Aliza Eisenberg in Israel, who died whilst donating eggs, Andrea Dominquez in Spain (Corea, 1988a) or Lynette Maguire and a second, as yet unnamed, woman (Treweek, 1988) both of whom died in Perth, Australia in 1988?

Since the original publication of *Test-Tube Women*, much more has become known about the emotional and physical trauma that many women suffer after repeating the IVF procedure eight or nine times with no child at the end (Klein, 1988b). The violent and coercive nature of this procedure has been exposed, the question of 'informed consent' seriously queried. Gradually women who have undergone these procedures begin to tell their own stories, as in *Infertility: Women Speak Out About Their Experiences Of Reproductive Medicine* (Klein, ed. 1989). It is an important step forward when infertile women themselves who have undergone such unsuccessful treatment, are critical of it and expose its fallacies.

As many of the contributors of our collection had predicted, the number of women for whom the technologies were said to be 'helpful' has greatly expanded. Despite its high failure rate, IVF, originally designed for women with no fallopian tubes is now being used on women and their partners with unknown (idiopathic) infertility, which is said to account for as much as 30 per cent of infertility cases. It is also used on women with endometriosis, only one blocked tube, immunologic problems, uterine infertility and ovulatory dysfunction (Roh et al., 1987). Importantly, it is increasingly used on perfectly fertile women whose partners – mostly husbands as IVF remains a technology reserved for heterosexual couples in a stable, financially secure relationship – have a fertility problem (eg a low sperm count; low or no sperm motility). In fact, one of the 'hot' areas in IVF research, with intense international competition, is a specific technique called 'microinjection' which is designed to inject one such sperm which otherwise wouldn't make it, into an egg collected after superovulation, thus creating an embryo in the lab which will then be inserted into the woman's womb. There are a host of unknown problems and the medical ethics of such a procedure are highly questionable. Yet the research is pushed on.

Since the technologies really don't work, there is contant further experimentation – all on women's bodies with the concomitant health risks involved for them, and possibly also for their children. The new techniques are all variations of IVF, but each is hailed as the ultimate 'success': GIFT (gamete intrafallopian transfer): DIPI (direct intraperitoneal insemination); POST (peritoneal oocyte and sperm transfer) – and who knows what next. None of them works properly – but failure seems to spur the technodocs on.

The pro-technology hype pushes people, who appear not to be able to have children 'naturally', to do something about it. Increasingly quickly they find themselves on IVF without being informed that the technique continues to be experimental, dangerous and usually unsuccessful. The infertility business creates its own market. In the USA, Serono, the company that manufactures Perganol (used to stimulate the ovaries to produce multiple eggs) has increased its sales from $ 7.2 million in 1982 to $ 35 million in 1986. IVF is estimated to be a $ 30 to $ 40 million industry (Blakeslee, 1987). As insurance companies in the US begin to pick up some of the cost of IVF, the medical profession envisages even more business.

The mainstream media continues to present us with an uncritical view of the technologies. We see pictures of men in white lab coats holding babies. But usually there are no babies. And in those cases where the technologies work, there are often three or four children all at once. Medicine's miracle: at what price to the woman? The media also fosters the view that a 'technological fix' will solve the life crisis that infertility can produce. It does not publicise how much more difficult it is for people finally to adjust to a life without their own biological child (or another child) after years and years on the emotional roller-coaster of IVF: hopes up and down, and up and down . . . until, ultimately, they will have to embark on the process of grieving, of giving up . . . which after years of (dashed) hopes is often much harder. The media also does not highlight the fact that a child 'free' life can be happy and creative – not just 'second best' – and that there are plenty of opportunities in the world at large to nurture and love.

The new reproductive technologies offer the possibility of controlling the lives of women at a level previously unheard of through the patriarchy's public support, control and regulation of the technologies. New methods for genetic screening of embryos, sex-predetermination and sex selection are constantly being refined and developed further, whilst research into the causes and possible prevention of infertility remains a low priority in the scientific and medical world. The crucial role of women on IVF programmes to procure the raw materials necessary for such experimentation – eggs and embryos – becomes more and more obvious. The latest feat, 'preimplantation diagnosis', enables the scientists to check the embryos produced by IVF – or flushed out of a woman's body after 'natural' conception. A single cell is taken from an early embryo and while the rest-embryo is frozen and stored, the removed cell is grown in the lab and screened for chromosomal damage. This method brings us dangerously close to human germ-line gene 'therapy' by which is meant the practice of genetic engineering by eliminating a 'defect' gene or inserting a new one. Our concerns about sex selection and eugenics expressed in *Test-Tube Women* in 1984 have been validated by these recent developments (Marchant, 1987).

And the technological development forges ahead. For all the genetic engineering experiments, what is needed are lots of embryos. Women are born with approximately 400,000 immature eggs, and now a major international research project is trying to develop techniques to mature these immature eggs *in vitro*; i.e. in the lab. (Scientists are investigating this is England, Australia and the USA; see Klein, 1989.) A wedge of an ovary is removed (any ovary – from a young or old woman will do), the eggs are matured in the lab and then fertilised with sperm (any sperm will do). If the research on cattle is any indication (as it usually is) we are not too far away from seeing the first 'real' test-tube baby: one whose production is entirely in the hands of the babymakers. The consequences of such mixing and matching are frightening – the technologies are at the scientists' fingertips and it is only a question of time until they are put into practice.

The development of the artificial womb is another impending technology that, as some people continue to reassure us, is the subject of science fiction. Yet in May 1988, the US journal *Fertility and Sterility* reported a 'first' from Italy: in Bologna, researchers had connected a living womb (extracted from a woman in a hysterectomy) to a so-called perfusion machine which provided it with oxygen and nutrients similar to the conditions of an early pregnancy. They then injected a spare embryo from a woman on IVF. The embryo developed normally for 52 hours (Bulletti et al., 1988). This experiment represents the officially published beginning of ectogenesis – a further step in the removal of the making of life from women?

The use and development of all these technologies are intimately connected with one another. This is clearly indicated by what is going on in the US with the so-called 'surrogate' industry: yet another case in which *fertile* women are exploited under the guise of alleviating some oneelse's pain of infertility. (We put 'surrogate' in quotes because we want to point out that it is a misnomer: 'surrogate mothers' are mothers in every sense of the word. The use of this term is one more example of the male take-over of language to create a false reality.)

The case of Mary Beth Whitehead and her child, Baby M – or S for Sarah as Whitehead continues to call her – attracted widespread attention and put the issue of commercial surrogacy squarely in the public eye. From January through to March 1987, Baby M was front page news in *The New York Times* and other newspapers and made the cover of magazines like *Newsweek*. In the US, more than 500 babies have been born through commercial surrogacy contracts and more than 20 surrogacy business agencies have sprung up across the countries. Clearly commercial surrogacy can thrive because of class differences and the exploitation of poor women. Surrogacy produces children *for men*, and creates a new type of family where the father is both the biological and social parent from the beginning, while motherhood is split into the 'natural' and the social mother. A partial victory was won for women when in February 1988, the New Jersey Supreme Court ruled that commercial surrogate motherhood contracts are illegal, and restored parental rights to Mary Beth Whitehead. The Court, however, allowed custody of the child to remain with the sperm donor, William Stern, and his wife Elizabeth (Arditti, 1987; 1988).

IVF and other reproductive technologies are increasingly combined with surrogacy. We know of:

- Surrogacy combined with sex predetermination: Patricia Foster was inseminated only with male sperm – the sperm donor wanted a *son*;
- Surrogacy combined with amniocentesis: Mary Beth Whitehead was required to submit to amniocentesis, even though she was under 30. This was to ensure 'quality control' over the product baby;
- Surrogacy combined with superovulation: Laurie Yates

and 'Jane Doe' were given superovulatory drugs, to get them to ovulate 'on time' and to increase the probability of fertilization;

- Surrogacy with *in-vitro* fertilization. Shannon Boff in the US, Pat Anthony in South Africa and Maggie Kirkman in Australia were all implanted with embryos produced through an IVF procedure. In the case of Pat Anthony, she was implanted with four eggs removed from her daughter and fertilized in vitro with the sperm of her son-in-law.

- Surrogacy combined with embryo flushing: Alejandra Munoz, a 21 year old woman from Mexico was brought illegally to the US to produce a child for her cousin's husband. She was told that the embryo would be flushed out and implanted into the womb of her cousin. But once she was pregnant, the procedure was not carried out and she was ordered to carry the pregnancy to term. After the birth of her child she fought in court and obtained joint custody of her child. But because she is an illegal alien, her situation is very precarious: she can be deported any moment and so lose her connection with her daughter (Corea, 1988b).

The developments and the increased use of the new reproductive technologies have spurred governments and social policy makers to pay more attention to these technologies. Unfortunately, as Ruth Hubbard notes in *Test-Tube Women*, the patriarchal policy-makers have focused their attention on the welfare of embryos and on abstract social values without paying any attention to the needs and concerns of women. Reports from government sponsored inquiries in Britain, West-Germany, Australia and Canada, though sometimes differing in their judgment about a particular issue, reveal similar perspectives on the technologies: implicitly, they all approve of the medical and social control of women and they all support the interests of the patriarchal nuclear family and of the scientists (Spallone, 1987).

Because the separation between mother and fetus is

such a central feature of the new conception technologies, they have far reaching implications for the status and rights of pregnant women. In the US, there is an attempt by the state to extend child support statutes and to create a new crime: 'fetal neglect'. In 1986, criminal charges were brought against Pamela Rae Stewart 'for acts and omissions during pregnancy'. Stewart, who had a condition known as placenta abruptio (a tendency for the placenta to separate from the uterine wall), was told by her physician that if she began to haemorrhage she should go to hospital immediately. Instead, she waited for twelve hours. By the time she got to the hospital the baby was in fetal distress. It was born with massive brain damage and subsequently died. Someone in the hospital notified the child protective services; someone there notified the police; they in turn notified the DA's office. Pamela Rae Stewart was arrested for disobeying her doctor's orders (Goodman, 1986).

Again in the US, the most recently well-publicized case of abuse of pregnant women's rights is the case of Angela C., a 28-year old pregnant woman with terminal cancer. In this case, a judge with a police escort was rushed to the hospital. In her 26th week of pregnancy – against her clearly expressed wishes – she was ordered to have a cesarean. The operation was performed and the fetus died within two hours. Angela C. died two days later, knowing that her child was dead. Court-ordered cesareans on healthy women have also occurred, despite the fact that this is an area of obstetrical care with a wide array of different opinion about its safety and efficacy (Annan, 1988).

On the positive side, what has emerged since 1984 is a feminist network of international resistance, critique and analysis of the new technologies – FINNRET – as suggested by Jalna Hanmer in the first edition of *Test-Tube Women*. In April 1985, West German women organized the largest feminist conference against the technologies up to the present time: the 2,000 women who participated passed a resolution strongly condemning gene and reproductive engineering as a violation of women's dignity, and emphasised the fundamentally eugenicist and racist ideology of the technologies. It is significant that this historical occasion took place in Germany and the movement of concerned women has been growing ever since.

In July 1985, the Women's Emergency Conference on the new Reproductive Technologies was held in Sweden. Women from 20 countries met to exchange information and to devise strategies against the technologies. FINNRET became FINRRAGE (Feminist International Network of Resistance to Reproductive and Genetic Engineering) in order to express not just concern about, but resistance to these developments.

In March 1986, women from GRAEL (the Women's Bureau of the European Parliament's Green Alternative Alliance) and FINRRAGE held 'alternative' feminist hearings in Brussels after the European Parliament's planned hearing on the technologies failed to include women's perspectives. In May 1986 Australia had its first national conference in Canberra: 'Liberation or Loss: Women Act On the New Reproductive Technologies'. In June 1986, there was a conference in Vienna, Austria. In 1987 another international conference was organized by the Office of the Status of Women in Montreal, Canada.

A number of conference proceedings have been published (including *Made To Order* edited by Patricia Spallone and Deborah L. Steinberg, 1987) and 1988 saw the first issue of *Reproductive and Genetic Engineering: A Journal of International Feminist Analysis*: further channels of distributing and exchanging information about the new technologies, and of trying to stop them.

In 1984 we were sceptical – and we knew a great deal less than we know now. In 1988 we are angry and outraged about the continued experimentation on women's bodies, about the infliction of violence and pain, about the perpetuation of lies, about the increasing control of our reproduction. Opposition to the technologies, however, is growing and expanding. The many women from an increasing number of countries who have decided not to put up with this latest control of women's lives are a source of strength and hope. As we go to press for this third edition of *Test-Tube Women*, we look forward to yet another German

Conference Against Gene and Reproductive Technologies in October, 1988 and the next international FINRRAGE Conference in Bangladesh in March 1989. This choice of the location is significant: we want to make it very clear that the 'old' and the 'new' technologies are but two sides of the same coin and that in order to ensure a better future, *all* women must be free from dangerous and inhuman interference in their lives and be given the resources to live with dignity.

It is not too late to say 'no' to these technologies. As the German women said at their conference in 1985, 'We did not ask for these technologies. We do not need them. They are produced at our expense'. We therefore put aside that sort of liberalism that says 'anything goes'. And to those who brand us as 'Luddites', as 'back-to-nature freaks', as naive creatures opposing 'progress', we respond with the last paragraph of the Resolution passed at the FINRRAGE conference in Sweden (Spallone and Steinberg, 1987:212):

> We seek a different kind of science and technology that respects the dignity of womankind and all life on earth. We call upon women and men to break the fatal link between mechanistic science and vested industrial interests and to take part with us in the development of a new unity of knowledge and life.

Rita Arditti, Renate D. Klein, Shelley Minden
Boston and Melbourne, September 1988

## REFERENCES

Annas, George, J. 1988. She Is Going To Die: The Case of Angela C. *Hastings Center Report 18* (1), February/March: 23–25.

Arditti, Rita. 1987. The Surrogacy Business. *Social Policy 16* (2), Fall 1987: 42–46.

Arditti, Rita. 1988. A Summary of Some Recent Developments on Surrogacy in the United States. *Reproductive and Genetic Engineering: Journal of International Feminist Analysis* 1 (1): 51–64.

Blakeslee, Sandra, 1987. Trying to make money making 'test-tube' babies. *The New York Times*. May 17.

Bulletti, Carlo et al., 1988. Early human pregnancy in vitro utilizing an artificially perfused uterus. *Fertility and Sterility* *49* (6): 991–996.

Corea Gena. 1988a. *The Mother Machine: From Artificial Insemination to Artificial Wombs*. Harper and Row, New York, 1985; rpt. with a new Afterword The Women's Press, London, 1988.

Corea, Gena. 1988b. Opening Speech at the Forum International Sur les Nouvelles Technologies de la Reproduction Humaine, published in *Sortir la Maternite du Laboratoire*. Gouvernement du Quebec, Conseil du statut de la femme, Montreal.

Corea, Gena, and Susan Ince. 1987. Report of a Survey of IVF clinics in the US. In *Made to Order: The Myth of Reproductive and Genetic Progress*, edited by Patricia Spallone and Deborah L. Steinberg. Pergamon Press, Oxford and New York.

Klein, Renate D. 1988a. Biotechnology and the Future of Humanity: An Investigation of the New Reproductive Technologies and Their Impact on Women. *Women's Worlds ISIS – Wicce 17* (March: Part I) and *18* (June:Part II). Geneva.

Klein, Renate D. 1988b. *The Exploitation of a Desire: Women's Experiences with IVF*. Report Deakin University.

Klein, Renate D. ed. 1989. *Infertility: Women Speak Out About Their Experiences of Reproductive Medicine*. Pandora Press, London.

Klein. Renate/Rowland Robyn. 1988. Women as Test-Sites for Fertility Drugs: Clomiphene Citrate and Hormonal Cocktails. *Reproductive and Genetic Engineering: Journal of International Feminist Analysis*. 1 (3): 251–73

Gomez Dos Reis, Ana Regina. 1987. IVF in Brazil: The Story Told by the Newspapers. In *Made to Order*. op. cit. eds. Spallone and Steinberg: 120–132.

Goodman, Ellen. 1986. A California case tests the rights, obligations of pregnant women. *The Boston Globe*. October 7:17.

Marchant, Gary. 1987. New developments in embryo research. *GENEwatch*. May/June.

Roh, Sung. I. et al. 1987. In vitro fertilization and embryo transfer: treatment dependent versus independent pregnancies. *Fertility and Sterility* 48 (6), December: 982–986.

Spallone, Patricia. 1987. Reproductive Technology and the State: The Warnock Report and its Clones. In *Made to Order*. op. cit. eds. Spallone and Steinberg: 160–183.

Spallone, Patricia and Deborah L. Steinberg. 1987. *Made to Order. The Myth of Reproductive and Genetic Progress*. The Athene Series. Pergamon Press. Oxford and New York.

Treweek, Ann. 1988. Coroner investigates IVF patient deaths. *Australian Dr. Weekly*. May 5.

Veitch, Andrew. 1987. Doctors fear world trade in stockpiled embryos. *The Guardian*, London, October 5: 4.

# INTRODUCTION

'Test tube babies,' 'frozen embryos,' 'artificial insemination,' 'sex selection,' 'surrogate motherhood,' 'prenatal screening' – these were some of the keywords that started us off, a year ago, to compile this anthology. We were curious to know the meaning of all these new technologies for a woman's decision to have a child – or to remain childfree. Will they, as Shulamith Firestone suggested in 1970 in *The Dialectic of Sex*, contribute to women's liberation and freedom? Should we as feminists endorse them? Or are they just one more way to keep women subordinated to men's control? To make us comply with yet another set of rules and regulations, all, of course, for our 'own good'? What are we to make of all these male scientists and doctors who seem so keen – and so dedicated – to, for instance, help 'infertile' women to have children of their own?

Women's power to procreate – men's attempts to remain in control over women's bodies. Of women's lives. We decided to take a close look at reproductive technologies, which we define as all forms of biomedical interventions and 'help' a woman may encounter when she considers having — or not having — a child. At first glance these technologies seem to offer women – some women, at least – freedom of choice: the choice of having a 'wanted' child, a 'normal' child (whatever that is), a child, perhaps, of the preferred sex. It might become a woman's 'choice' in the future to provide her planned child with the kind of 'superman' genes the sperm banks advertize. A surrogate mother might 'free' some of us from the burden of pregnancy and let us get on with our professional interests. And the prospect of making babies outside a woman's womb could bring with it the potential to

1

free women and children from the exclusiveness of the 'sacred' mother-child bond.

We as feminists are pro-choice, of course. We support women's right to choose in all areas of our lives. But how can women choose freely in a society where the right to choose must be bought? Where people of color are systematically exploited and discriminated against and population 'control' is blatantly racist and in the service of the white minority worldwide who wants to remain in power? Where women are taught to subordinate their interests to those of men? Where a woman isn't 'real' without husband and child, and where a 'real' man treats his wife and children as property?

Each time a new technological development is hailed the same question arises: is this liberation, or oppression in a new guise? To answer this we need to know more about reproductive technologies than the newscasters tell us. Who are the developers, the promoters, the 'experts'? Who benefits – which sex, which class, which race? How much does it cost, and who is going to pay? Why is it so hard to get accurate information?

WOMEN are the targets of all this manipulation, but we are not in control; neither at the professional level as scientists or doctors, nor at the personal level as consumers. It is women who are sterilized by the thousands, made infertile by Depo-Provera or IUDs, women who are exploited as surrogate mothers. It is women who are the disappointed test-tube candidates, the unhappy biological mothers who were socially coerced into having a child, the targets of guilt hurled by anti-abortionists, the victims of back alley abortions . . . and yes, as well, the happy mothers of wanted children. At the mercy of 'benevolent' male experts. At the mercy of technologies developed by men who see women as something 'other,' 'strange,' 'not-the-norm.' Technologies that were not made by us. We doubt that they are in women's interests.

Why is it that men are so interested in tampering with women's reproductive biology? The question is intriguing. Why is the old boy's network spending millions to fund research on every aspect of the *female* reproductive system (why not the male?)? How sincere is this concern to help infertile women to *have* children?

A case in point: in vitro fertilization. Why don't the television documentaries ever tell us that only a fraction of all female infertility problems (specifically, blocked oviducts that cannot be treated surgically) can even potentially be helped by this treatment? And why do they call the babies that result from it 'test-tube babies', implying that the babies emerged from a laboratory instead of a woman's body?

Why is so little attention paid to the social and iatrogenic (medically induced) causes of infertility, and why is it so important for women to have our own 'biological' children, why this focusing on female biology as the only path to mothering?

At the same time as the new technologies make the news headlines worldwide, abortion rights – worldwide too – are under attack. In the United States, since 1976 the Hyde Amendment has restricted federal Medicaid funding for abortions. As we go to press, there are new efforts in Congress to tighten this amendment so that even when women's lives are endangered, free abortions cannot be obtained. Abortions are made less and less accessible to those most economically vulnerable: poor women, women of color and teenage women. The right of teenagers to have an abortion without parental consent is continually being threatened or denied.

The same women who are denied access to abortions are also threatened by sterilization abuse. And, in the name of 'population control,' millions of women in so-called Third World countries are injected with the contraceptive Depo-Provera, despite short and long-term side effects. 'Easy to handle,' we are told by scientists, medics, and the marketing representatives of the drug companies: 'a shot every three months will do' – and it doesn't even require the woman's consent.

So while 'man' knows how to fly to the moon and produce the nuclear bomb, we still have no safe contraceptive: the most important and needed technology for women's reproductive health. And how come contraception is still the burden of females? Apart from the condom (and vasectomy) there is no other contraceptive available for men, and this perpetuates the unequal responsibilities between men and women with respect to sexual intercourse.

And why, if the new technologies reflect a concern for children, are infant mortality rates so high in many parts of Western society and throughout the Third World? Among the poor, women and children suffer most; the 'feminization of poverty,' long a bitter reality in the Third World, is today hitting hard in industrialized Western societies. Why isn't more money spent to help the children already among us, the women who are mothers *now*?

Thus each new technology is born in a mire of complex social issues – issues the technologists, apparently, never stop to debate. They believe that their work is entirely objective; this conviction, in fact, is one of the cornerstones of science and technology. For every human problem there is a 'technological fix,' and the technologists guarantee that they'll find it if we don't contaminate their rational thinking with messy feelings. Technological fixes have already brought us to the point where we're wondering if the world will be around for the next generation. No matter. Scientists and technocrats still believe that a pill, a test, a computer, or whatever their next invention, can magically set us right.

But new technologies do not fall from heaven. Technology is a social institution, and its developments reflect the social and political system of which it is a part. How can a small group of white men based in industrialized countries, who support, fund, and control science and technology worldwide, convince us that they are 'objective,' that their work is politically neutral? A separation between technological developments and the world in which they are applied is unreal. It is but one world.

At this point one may ask why don't we advocate 'feminist scientists' to take an active part in developing reproductive technologies: perhaps because we feel that at this point such an attempt would be a contradiction in terms. Science, we believe, mirrors the power relations in society, and to try to add on feminist values to its current structure could only result in a superficial, if any, change. Only in a feminist society would a truly feminist science develop. So what then could we ask of feminists who work in projects related to reproductive technologies? We think what can be done is to monitor and, if possible, expose blatant anti-woman research and actions. And above all to distribute what they learn as widely as possible to the feminist media worldwide.

When we voice doubts and remain skeptical about the new technologies, we are often thought to be siding with the conservatives. In the United States, specifically, we are seen as siding with the New Right, a wealthy coalition of groups that attack women's rights, and also support racist segregation, attacks on homosexuals, increased militarism and the suppression of trade unions. The New Right has become the champion of the most oppressive aspects of the nuclear family, and the Right to Life groups – one of its most active branches – is consistently working against all technological interference with pregnancy. They oppose in vitro fertilization and all experimentation with human eggs on the grounds that the fertilized egg is a 'person' and deserves full legal rights. They are also afraid that these technologies will destroy the 'American' family. We don't think they need to worry. The new technologies are promoted in ways that support the most conservative ideas about families. For example, in the case of in vitro fertilization, women who are eligible for the procedure have to be in a heterosexual relationship, preferably married, and must provide guarantees to the scientific fathers that they will raise their children with a father, biological or not, in residence. In vitro fertilization seems unlikely to serve the needs of single women, lesbians, poor women, etc.

As feminists, where do we stand with respect to clashes between conservative groups and biomedical research? Can we side with either group knowing that what they both share is to dismiss the *women* involved in these technologies . . . calling us 'the fetal environment'? What is the *real* message for women in all this?

When we began our research in 1982, we approached all these questions with a great deal of caution. But as we hasten to get this collection to press, we are no longer merely curious or cautious. What we have learned in the process of compiling these papers has shocked us. Profoundly. We believe these essays should be read as widely as possible, and *soon*. They are not the 'definitive' words on the subject, but they are a beginning of what could become an international exposure by women of the politics of reproductive technologies.

This book includes the words of women who have all been in contact with reproductive technologies in one way or another—and with the 'new' ones as well as with the 'old' – be it through choice or coercion. They all care deeply about the implications of these developments for women's economic, physical, and emotional well-being. They come from the USA, Britain, India, Australia, New Zealand and Germany.

The three of us who have worked together on this collection come from different places to this project. One of us, at 49, is the mother of a grown son, the others, at 38 and 31, have chosen to remain childfree. All of us have a background in the biological sciences. One of us is South American, one is Swiss, and one is North American, and we live in the United States and in England.

Working across the ocean has not always been easy but it has provided us with the benefit of meeting with women from different countries and cultures who are every bit as concerned about these issues as we are and who work very hard in their environments for women's well-being. Many of the authors have been working for years on the issue of reproductive technology and reproductive rights. Betty B. Hoskins and Helen B. Holmes edited a two-volume collection on this topic in 1981 (*The Custom-Made Child* and *Birth Control and Controlling Birth*); two others, Genoveffa Corea and Barbara Katz Rothman have forthcoming books on these topics, both due in 1984 (*The Mother Machine* and *The Products of Conception*, respectively). Some of our contributors are 'experts' in the field, others write for the first time as 'laywomen' but all of us speak out of our personal concerns and experiences.

We believe that the issues raised in this collection are important for *all* women. Because female biology is exploited in *all* spheres of *all* women's lives. Whether we want children or decide to remain childfree, or are beyond our childbearing years, and whatever is our sexual preference, we are *all* at risk of becoming *TEST-TUBE WOMEN* – at risk of being subjugated to a variety of controls: from technological interference when we are pregnant, to legal regulations that declare the fetus and the woman bearing it to be two separate 'patients', to workplace policies that pressure women employees to become sterilized.

Despair, hopelessness, and paralysis are not, however, the message of our book. We believe that knowledge is power. Making available women's opinions, experiences and information on these pages – and they reflect many of the contradictions and difficulties of the issues – will hopefully lead women to be wary and skeptical. Maybe the next time we are faced with a male 'expert' we will pause a moment and think what it is that we ourselves want and need, rather than this person who represents the interests of a special and privileged segment of society. But individual action is not enough. We need to pool our efforts and build an international feminist network that will monitor, raise consciousness and organize around the new developments in reproductive technologies and their implications for women's lives. Hopefully this book will contribute to the creation of such a network.

Can we stop this time-bomb silently ticking into a future that – should the 'other' bomb not fall – might intensify women's oppression and increase the exploitation and domination of women to an unimaginable degree? We think there is hope. In countries all over the world, feminists are organizing against sterilization abuse, demanding the development of good contraceptives, defending a woman's choice to remain childfree, to live whatever lifestyle we choose. Without a partner if we wish so. With a man – on equal terms if we desire so. With a woman – without being harassed. Life as self-determined, full human beings.

We hope this book will contribute to women's active *resistance*. We are determined not to accept – once again – subordination on the grounds of our biology. Biology need not be destiny. Female biology, one day, might mean choice – real choice – in a world in which women's different needs, interests, and experiences are recognized and validated. Let us support each other to attain our diverse life choices, and to take the control in our own hands.

Rita Arditti                                   Renate Duelli Klein
Shelley Minden               Cambridge, Mass., September 1983

# IN THE BEGINNING

# A YENGA TALE

BarbaraNeely

'A Yenga Tale' is a story about our prehistoric ancestors,
beings who had the ultimate reproductive right —
parthenogenesis. The heart of the tale is our ancestors'
attempt to pass along this ability to the women of today, as a
means of ending reproductive tyranny. 'A Yenga Tale' is
part of BarbaraNeely's series of black feminist myths.

This is a story told among the Yenga women of West Africa.
The women say the story is as old as truth. It is told to all
young girls at the onset of their menses, as part of their
legacy of adulthood.

I will tell you the story as it was told to me:

Before the dawn of what is called time, our ancestors
were but one — not mother and father, female and male, but
one single being, neither woman nor man but both, though
they looked much as our women look today.

These people, these ones, possessed all the ancient
powers. They could merge their minds, they could communicate with all things, and though you may laugh, it is said they
could fly and walk on water if sorely pressed.

These ancestors lived in small clans in caves along the
sea coast. Every member of the clan played an important and
honored role in the group's survival and each was called by
the name of the service performed for the group.

As was the custom among the ones, on the first night of
the red season, when the night air was heavy with the smell
of things being born and returning to the earth to be reborn,
the clan gathered around the one called The Sayer — so called
because she alone among them had the words to speak
tomorrow.

11

It was through The Sayer that the clan had learned of the need to leave their inland valley home and seek the sea. From a nearby hill, they'd heard the earth groan, then watched the place of their birthing crumble into dust, as a huge ragged tear ripped open the belly of the valley below. It was through The Sayer that they knew to store up memories of certain creatures who had disappeared from the earth in their lifetime – like the Jyngomane, whose singing was as sweet to the ear as berries to the tongue, and the Anbrox with its healing touch. So the clan was eager to pool its spirit and learn what it was that tomorrow held so that they could prepare for its coming.

The clan squatted in a circle around The Sayer, who knelt in their midst. They inclined their kinky heads toward her. Dark arms outstretched, they held each others' hands and concentrated on the Hijicki bird. This huge and gentle creature was the doorway to tomorrow. Only with her help could The Sayer make the future known.

Soon the slow flapping of large wings was heard overhead. The Hijicki glided slowly into the circle to stand before The Sayer. They regarded each other. First with the left eye and then with the right. Then the bird stepped closer to The Sayer and enclosed her in its magnificent wings. In this way, The Sayer knew the Hijicki, felt the ripple of feathers and the strength of beak and claws. In such moments, all the world was like a flower opening beneath her gaze as she was carried into the future on the wings of the Hijicki and the spirit of the clan.

But this seeing was unlike any she had known. For the first time, The Sayer was unwilling to speak when the great bird finally spread its wings and released her. The Sayer looked beyond the circle of ones to the two half-grown strange others who slept beneath a nearby tree. It was of them that she had seen.

There had been born into the clan two others who were different from the ones. These others had no place from which the young could issue, only loose bits of skin and flesh where the birth opening should be. These were not the first strange others to be born among the ones. There had been two joined together at their fronts and three born without mouths or ears. The clan thought these strange others were somehow connected with the rains that came up from the ground and filled the night with things the clan could not name. But all the strange others, so far, had been reclaimed by the earth within days of their birthing, except these last two. They had not died. They had grown large, with heavy limbs and slow ways that made some of the ones uneasy. Still, the strange others were tolerated. It was not the way of the ones to destroy those whom the earth did not claim and the strange others played so little part in the life of the clan, no one thought to cast them out.

The Sayer looked around the circle from face to face: The Firekeeper, The Healer and Youngtender, The Cavefinder and Seedkeeper, The Forager and all her beloved ones. She wanted to draw them to her, to comfort and delight them with stories of much abundance and joy in the tomorrows, but it was not to be so.

The Sayer stood. The clan gathered in a semicircle before her. She began to raise her arms, slowly, as though the weight of the world was balanced on her limbs. Then she moved her hands in the gesture of final parting and made the parting sound, like the echo of the last heartbeat.

The clan was shocked to silence. This was a ritual that, until now, had only been used at the time of death or when some one or group split off from the birthing clan.

The Sayer spoke into the bewildered silence:

'I speak thus to you,' she said of the ritual, 'for in the far tomorrows we will be no more.'

A rumble rose from the clan but was quickly silenced by The Sayer's voice.

'I have been in the eye of the Hijicki,' she said, 'and I have seen that the strange others will be our end. At their birthing, I saw that they had no place from which the young could issue.

'These are not of us,' said the one inside. 'But I did not understand. Now it is clear. These strange others are the first of those who will call themselves men. Their beginning is the beginning of our end. In the tomorrows, there will be these men and . . . and . . . ,' she choked, as if the words burned in her throat.

'There will be these men,' she repeated, 'and those much

the same as we. The men will name these creatures women. These women will bear the young much as we do, but they will bear much, much more in the far tomorrows. And they will not be whole. For without the men, these women will be unable to bear young.'

At this, a number of the ones began to laugh and ceased to worry. The Sayer had been with the palm drink. Its headiness had set her to telling tales when she was supposed to be speaking tomorrow.

'It is not a thing of play!' The Sayer shrieked. Her eyes were wild, her face twisted by sadness.

The buzzing and chuckling ceased. A ripple of concern ran through the ones. They had never seen The Sayer so. Could she have eaten roots not meant for the ones? Had she strayed into a pool of earth rain?

'I speak tomorrow!' The Sayer cried. 'Have I not always spoken tomorrow?'

And this was true. None could dispute it.

But how could it be that the strange others, so pitifully deformed as to be unable to bear the young, could someday be needed for the making of the young? The clan pooled its concentration and tried to see the pictures in The Sayer's head. But there was only blinding white pain to be found there.

The Healer moved toward her.

'You are with us and of us and we of you,' the clan members chanted, as was their way when one of them was in deep distress.

But The Sayer would not be soothed. She cast off The Healer's hands and screamed the ones to silence.

'Listen! Hear what I have yet to tell.'

A heavy hush fell over the clan, a stillness like the moment before thunder.

'In the far tomorrows,' The Sayer said, 'such as we will be of little more account than small blades of grass in the wind. We will be but creatures for others' pleasure or work, to move to the beat of the master, the men. The daughters of the night, dark ones much as we, will be most despised because they are dark and full and knowing as the night's eye. But those such as we, of *all* shades, will do not as they wish, not as they should, but as they are told. And the men will attempt to hold all things, all creatures in the sky and ground, all clans living everywhere – not with kindness as we hold one another, but with implements of destruction, with tongues twisted into falsehoods so fine that only the mother of truth could recognize their lies! And the women will bow down before them, desire them, ape them and forsake their birthrights to be among them. Some few women will oppose the men, but mostly so that they can replace the men as owners of the world. A few others will take their pleasure and share their joy with other women. But that will not be enough to stop the world from dying.

In the far tomorrows, those much like us, those women, will stand by while great hunger continues in the midst of great abundance and The Seedkeepers are rewarded for allowing the land to lay fallow. The women will stand silent as the young are locked away for learning what they have been taught in that man's land and practicing it. The women will pretend they do not know that the rain has begun to kill the fish, that. . . .'

'Then what are we to do?' cried The Forager, unable to stand the anguish that wracked her as she felt The Sayer's words.

'Always there has been something to be done before the coming of the tomorrows – to move or hide, to plant or dig. What is it that we must do for a tomorrow that is so far from us yet foretells our end?'

No one spoke. No one had any idea what it was they should do. In the past, what must be done was so clear that all could see it. But this time, the horror of what lay ahead blocked out all other thought.

That night, The Sayer wandered to a far cave where she lay shrieking and crying out her grief and helplessness for two openings of the night's eye. She wept and keened so that wolves and pythons, cockroaches and fan birds were drawn to her side. They heard and knew her truth and joined in her lamentations till she slept. They they gave her dreams. When she woke, she knew what must be done and all that was needed to accomplish it.

The Sayer gathered the clan around her and told them of

her plan. Then some went in search of a certain system of caves: deep, dry and light, with smooth walls, big enough inside to hold the horror of the world to come. Other ones began gathering, pounding, and simmering barberry and madder root, indigo, ironwood, sedge and many other plants and roots long gone out of this world. To these they added mordants and gums until they had pot on pot of brightly-colored and thickened dyes.

Then, once again, they squatted in a circle around The Sayer. Arms linked and eyes closed, they concentrated on the Hijicki bird. When the great creature appeared, The Sayer spoke to her without words. The plan The Sayer found in her dream was not without cost to this gentle creature. It would cause the Hijicki some effort to carry the whole clan into the future. But, of course, if she did not agree, there would not be much future.

The Hijicki hovered over the circled clan like a multi-colored cloud as the clan members made the sound of one mind. The sound rose in the air and enfolded the Hijicki and the clan, just as the Hijicki's wings enfolded The Sayer. And they were all made to see into the tomorrows.

They clung to each others' hands and moaned aloud as the vision coursed through their mind. It nearly broke their spirits to see such a woebegone world – hardly more than a string of battlefields littered with disease.

But they were struck dumb to see what would happen in this place where they now dwelled and what would become of those who looked most like them. How it grieved them to see the beautiful dark ones kidnapped from their land and taken off to toil and die in degradation on behalf of those whose only color was blinding white hate of all who had color, in a country whose heart would grow so rotten and infested with greed and injustice that it would someday collapse under the weight of its own cruelty.

Worst of all for the clan to see was the sight of the children of these dark captives, denying their real heritage and forsaking their birthright, while bowing and scraping before the colorless idol that was used to enslave their parents.

When the Hijicki released them, the clan continued to

squat, like stones in a field, unable to move, to feel anything other than the weight of the dying world the Hijicki had taken them to.

The Seedkeeper was the first to move. She rose from her squat and urged the ones on either side of her to rise as well.

'It is time for the sowing,' she said.

'Yes, we must make the light,' The Firekeeper said and also rose.

All the clan followed suit and began to carry the calabashes of dye to the newly-found system of caves far above and in from the sea.

Once all of the calabashes, as well as leaves of various sizes and sticks of differing widths were assembled, the clan once again assumed the seeing squat and locked themselves into a vision of what they were about to do. Then each one moved to a separate wall and began to paint the warning — the future as it has been seen by them.

They painted a world in which the few most willing to kill ruled over the many less able to defend themselves.

The painted women weeping for the babies they could not afford to bear; and others with hollow places where their wombs should be — made forever childless by grey men in white garments with mouths full of foreign words.

They painted women bound by their belief in men's right to bind them.

They painted men caught in the trap of their need for power — separated from their tears and joy, empty, frightened, totally without power in all the most important ways.

They painted air unfit to breathe and a sun clouded out by a miasma the ones could not begin to understand.

They painted cities and towns left deserted because that which men buried in the ground killed the earth and all that sprang from it or rested upon it.

They painted a world so brutal and frightening, so far from the beauty and joy they knew that the ones were sickened by it.

But they painted on, determined to leave their knowledge as a warning to the women who would follow them. It would be a great long time before it was too late. Every action altered tomorrow. It would only need for the women to find the cave, to see and understand and simply stop.

That was all that was needed. For the women to stop and say no to being objects, to stop defining happiness and well-being on the basis of men's madness; for the young to stop and refuse to carry on the life of lies their parents passed down to them; for those whose hunger was not so great to rise up and demand that the resources of the destitute be returned to them and that all be allowed to share equally in the world's bounty.

Then they were done. The system of caves that went deep into the sheltering mountain was now alive and nearly writhing with color, life and death so real they could feel its heat.

'Surely this will make them understand, bring about the change that must come!', The Sayer told the ones.

But she could see in their faces that they did not believe any more than she. What they had seen and felt in the caves had left them with little belief in the tomorrows of the women, let alone the children. And they did not care to think about the men.

But there was one among them who still dared to hope.

'Come sad ones,' The Healer said. 'As in all sickness, there is health, if only one can find the way within oneself. These women, they will be much the same as we. They can do what must be done, but they will need all of our help.

'Come,' she told them. 'There is still one last thing to be done.'

The clan members followed The Healer back inside the cave and watched as she began to draw the circle of life and the secret of its perpetuation. Inside the circle she painted the dance of the long night and the embrace of the all. The clan began to help her. They did not stop until all the herbs and seasons, the sounds and motions with which the ones were able to generate the seed of life within themselves were displayed with loving care upon the farthest wall of the cave.

'Now!' The Healer said. 'We have shown the women the way to make the young without these strange others, these men. Now the women can choose.'

And the clan was pleased and satisfied. They had done all

they could do for the tomorrows and the ones to follow. It would be up to the women to decide if the men could be saved.

With one mind, the clan members began to gather their belongings and pack them in their small swift boats.

'Now we will find a place,' The Cavefinder said, as they gathered by the water's edge.

'A place far from this place, a place no others have ever seen or will see.'

And so they went: The Seedkeeper with her pouch of woven grass; The Firekeeper, cradling the mother of fire in her smoldering sticks; The Healer, with the memory of cures in her hands; all the ones of the clan, with all that they possessed. No one left even a broken tool behind, except the Youngtender. On the shore, The Youngtender left the nearly grown strange others sitting idly in the sand.

Among the Yenga women, it is said that the cave of the ones still exists and will be found by the women in the time when all else fails.

# WHAT FUTURE FOR MOTHERHOOD?

# THE MEANINGS OF CHOICE IN REPRODUCTIVE TECHNOLOGY[1]

## Barbara Katz Rothman

The new reproductive technologies are heralded for their choice-giving capacity. This article looks at the negative side, the choices lost as the technologies develop. The author concludes that individual choice, while it must always be defended, must be understood in the context of the society which structures the choices available to individuals. The individual right to choice is an absolute necessity, but not alone sufficient to ensure an ethics of reproduction.

*Choice* and *information* have served as the cornerstones of the women's health and the reproductive rights movements. We are, above all, pro-choice. We support the rights of the individual woman to choose, to choose pregnancy or abortion, to choose alternative medical treatments or none at all. And choice, we claim, rests firmly on information: to choose treatment for breast cancer, for example, requires information on the full range of medical treatments, their side effects, and their probability of success.

This emphasis on choice and information all sounded very logical at the time, sounded like women were going to get more and more control as first their access to information and then their choices expanded.

I'm beginning to have second thoughts.

Technology is also about information, and about choice. More information on how things work seems to give us more choices, new and better ways of doing things. That is true of the technology of transportation, which brings us cars and jets, and of the technology of reproduction, which brings us the Pill, amniocentesis and fetal monitors.

But while technology opens up some choices, it closes down others. The new choice is often greeted with such fanfare that the silent closing of the door on the old choice goes unheeded. For example, is there any meaningful way one could now choose horses over cars as a means of transportation? The new choice of a 'horseless carriage' eventually left us 'no choice' but to live with the pollution and dangers (as well as the conveniences and speed, of course) of a car-based transportation system.

Reproductive technology is heralded for its choice-giving capacity. For those who can afford it, the enormous growth of information about reproduction does make choice newly possible: the pregnant can choose whether or not to continue the pregnancy, can even learn more about the fetus and then choose whether or not to continue; the infertile can choose new ways of attempting pregnancy; birthing women can choose alternative ways of managing their labors and births. Choices abound. I want to look a bit at the negative side, though, look to see what, if any, choices are being lost to us, going the way of the horse.

Fetal monitoring is a good place to start. Fetal monitors, belts to go around the pregnant belly and electrodes to screw into the fetal head during labor, are a piece of reproductive technology whose sole stated purpose is to bring more information, to enable more and better choices. By knowing more about the condition of the fetus during labor, more informed choice was to be possible for the management of the labor. But some strange things happened. We didn't really get all that much more information than we had before – good nursing care always provided considerable information about the fetus. It certainly did *look* like more information though, with those long strips of print-out. But more importantly, the information came in a new context. Instead of having to approach the woman, to rest your head near her belly, to smell her skin, to feel her breathing, you could now read the information on the fetus from across the room, from down the hall. While still one being on the bed, medical personnel came to see the woman and fetus as separate, as *two different patients*. And indeed more choices could be made: the fetal heart rate indicates mild distress – should the mother be sectioned?

When a woman *chooses* to have a cesarean section because she is *informed* that the fetal monitor indicates some distress, is she gaining or losing control? In part, the answer is going to depend on the accuracy of the information. If medical practitioners are overly quick to read fetal distress, as they have been, then the loss of control is clear. The woman is having major surgery, with all of its attendant risks to her health and life, making herself sick, weak and dependent as she enters motherhood. But if the information is correct, and the fetus, her baby, is at risk and the section could ensure its greater health, then she is gaining control over her motherhood, as she makes this short-term sacrifice for the long-term health of her child.

What happens when the woman and her medical practitioners disagree, disagree either about the accuracy of the information, or about the choice which should be made based on the information? What if a pregnant woman does not want to make this sacrifice? Has all this new information expanded her choices? It seems not: medicine is once again turning to the state, as it has so many times in the past, to put medical choice ahead of women's choices. In several bedside Juvenile Court hearings, with a lawyer appointed to represent the unborn fetus, another representing the pregnant woman, and yet others representing the hospital, women have lost the right to choose, and have been ordered to submit to cesarean sections, the fetus within them claimed by the state as a 'dependent and neglected child'. (Hubbard, 1982)

Thus information may expand the opportunity for choices, but it certainly does not guarantee whose choices will be honored.

In 1981 the journal *Obstetrics and Gynecology*, writing to an audience of obstetricians, carried an article reporting on one such case, in which the woman, although found to be psychiatrically competent, was forced to undergo a cesarean section very much against her will. The article quotes the current edition of one of the classic obstetrics textbooks, *Williams* (Pritchard and McDonald, 1980, 6th edition), which states that the fetus has 'rightfully achieved the status of the second patient, a patient who usually faces much greater risk of serious morbidity and mortality than does the mother'. Then, referring to the Supreme Court decision which allowed abortion in the first and second trimesters of pregnancy, the authors state:

> Roe v. Wade allows the state to assert an interest in the protection of potential life in the fetus once it has reached a stage of viability. It is put forth in this case that it is also proper, even necessary, for the health professionals involved to assert the same interest. (Bowes and Selgestad, p. 213)

Most women, of course, do not carry their objections this far. Most women, given the *information* that they 'need' a cesarean section *choose* to have the section. They do not ask *who* needs the section, do not raise the two-separate-patients issue: most women, it seems, either do not question that the fetus is a part of themselves, accept medical judgment as to what is necessary, or both.

We thought that information would give us power. What we perhaps overlooked is that it is *power* which gives one control over both information and choice.

Let us take another example from the wealth of reproductive technologies, and examine its impact on the choices women have. We can take as our example one of the oldest and most basic, the technology of fertility limitation. Self-imposed limits on fertility, through contraception or abortion, are the *sine qua non* of the reproductive rights movement. Without such control

> women cannot gain access to or participate effectively in the political and social processes which shape every aspect of their lives. The degree of control women are able to exercise over their reproductive lives directly affects their educational and job opportunities, income level, physical and emotional well being, as well as the economic and social conditions the children they do bear will experience. (quoted by Taub, 1982: 169)

Nina Taub, professor of law at Rutgers University, quoted this as an 'understood premise' of a Reproductive

Rights Symposium at Rutgers in 1982. I think it is a statement with which most feminists and most liberals would
agree. It is a statement of choice and control: to be free,
women must be able to choose to control their fertility.

Wait a minute. Did I say that to be free women we must
be able to choose to control our fertility? Then what of the
choice NOT to control fertility? At that same symposium, in a
related but different context, Ruth Hubbard said, 'As
"choices" become available, they all too rapidly become compulsions to "choose" the socially endorsed alternative.'
(Hubbard, 1982: 210)

I have been troubled in recent years by reactions, including my own, to unlimited fertility. A woman I see each
summer was pregnant this year. Again. It was her fourth
baby in five years. I know that she is having problems with
money (and who wouldn't be, with four kids?). I know she is
overworked and tired, trying to find affordable child care so
she can work part time. Four babies, I thought. My god. And
then we talked. She's the classic case: the woman who has
gotten pregnant with every birth control method, in place,
used correctly. This last pregnancy, the doctor said, 'C'mon,
I'll abort it right now, you can go home not pregnant and
forget it.' She was tempted, sorely tempted. But no, she chose
not to abort. She really didn't want to have an abortion. She
had had several, years ago, before her children, and she didn't
want any more. It was a choice she made, an unpopular
reproductive choice, one which is not, in her community of
friends, socially endorsed. And if her educational and job
opportunities are severely reduced, if she's physically and
emotionally exhausted, if the economic and social condition
of her children suffers, well, that's her choice, isn't it? And if
another woman in these circumstances chooses to abort, she
too is exercising her choice.

While on the one hand we worry, with very good reason,
about losing the option of legal abortions, on the other hand
we are losing the option not to abort. When women are not
allowed, or cannot afford, safe and legal abortions, that does
not mean that they can afford children: what they resort to is
their 'only choice,' abortions which may be neither legal nor
safe. This woman who kept her fourth pregnancy made a

choice, but it is a choice which may be rapidly slipping away from us. She is suffering not just the inevitable consequences of four children, but the consequences of her poverty. If she was rich, if her husband made a fortune, she would still be tired, I'm sure, but she would have many more choices in how she lives her life as the mother of four young children.

The choice of contraception simultaneously closed down some of the choices for large families. North American society is geared to small families, if indeed to any children at all. Everything from car and apartment sizes to the picture book ideal of families encourages limiting fertility. Without the provision of good medical care, day care, decent housing, children are a luxury item, fine if you can afford them. So it is a choice all right that contraception gave us, and a choice we may very well experience as being under our control, but it may be a somewhat forced choice. In its extreme, legislation has been repeatedly introduced to punish 'welfare mothers' by cutting off payments if they have more children. Sterilization abuse is the flip side of the abortion battle: the same sorry record. And, at a different place in the economy, just sometimes, when I think wistfully about another baby, a bigger family, and realize I could never 'afford' it, afford the schools, the private medical care, the trappings of middle-class life expected of, and for, and by me for my children, I almost envy my great grandmother her eight children. Does the choice not to be burdened with continual childbearing have to be paid for with the choice to have larger families?

So there may be choice brought to us by information and technology, the choices we get when we learn how to use contraception and back-up abortion for fertility control, but the choices may very well be heavily weighted for, or against, us.

Both the medical monitoring and management of labor, and the use of contraception and abortion, are very well-established aspects of reproductive technologies; it is just the specifics which keep changing, as newer techniques, machinery and chemicals get introduced. The next level of reproductive technology I want to address combines fetal monitoring with fertility control to produce something new:

'quality control,' control not just of the number of children we bear, but of the 'quality' or condition of those children.

Amniocentesis and sonography are the technologies which provide the information to make this new set of reproductive choices possible. Sonography, the use of sound waves, allows the visualization of the fetus in utero, and the detection of gross anatomical deformities. Amniocentesis is the withdrawal of a small amount of the amniotic fluid which surrounds the fetus. When done between the sixteenth and twentieth weeks of pregnancy, the fetal cells in the fluid can be cultured and examined. Other tests can also be performed on the fluid. These techniques allow the diagnosis of many (under a hundred at this writing, but increasing all the time) genetic diseases and syndromes. Test results are available by the twenty-fourth week, the legal limit on abortion in the United States. If the fetus is found to have a terminal illness (like Tay Sachs disease which invariably kills in early childhood), a severely incapacitating condition (a syndrome which leads to such profound retardation that the child would be unable to learn to walk or to talk), a moderately disabling condition (say, wheelchair-bound or unable to walk without assistance), or a socially undesirable condition (if, for example, the fetus is found to be of the 'wrong' sex, such as a third or fourth daughter), a woman can use this information to choose an abortion.

The opening up of choices and control with this technology is astounding. There is, of course, still no guarantee of a perfect baby – and even a perfect baby can be made terribly imperfect in accident or illness after birth – but one no longer need fear Down syndrome, spina bifida or a host of other diseases and unwanted conditions. This of course begs the basic question of what makes any particular condition either disabling or undesirable. Why Down syndrome, why daughters, why wheelchair-bound? But information is available, and information makes choice possible. And it is the woman's choice. There may be pressure, subtle or powerful, from genetic counselors, doctors, family members, but it is still the woman who chooses to abort or not to abort. Or is it?

When we have this information, when we make these choices for our children, are we not then accepting responsibility for their condition, responsibility without any genuine control? If we choose not to abort a 'defective' fetus, and the agonized adolescent it becomes hurls at us, as adolescents so often have, 'I didn't ask to be born!' whatever are we going to say now? Will our children be able to sue us for wrongful life, as they have successfully sued their doctors? The doctors failed to provide the information which would have given the mothers the choice of abortion. What of the mother who, given the information, chooses not to abort? Can she be held responsible for her child's condition, denied state services, insurance payments, even charged with child abuse?

And if we do choose to abort, is that truly a choice? What of the woman living in the fourth floor, walk-up apartment in a city designed without access for the disabled – is her 'choice' to abort a fetus with spina bifida an exercise in free will? What of the woman with few economic or family resources who chooses to abort a fetus with Down syndrome because she is fully and truly informed about the state services which will be available to her child after her own death?

It seems that, in gaining the choice to control the quality of our children, we may be losing the choice *not* to control the quality, the choice of simply accepting them as they are.

Another choice this technology may be losing for us is, interestingly, what we might think of as a 'right' NOT to know. In our focus on the 'right to information,' we forget that there may be some things one might rather not know. The least dramatic but most pervasive of these is fetal sex. It is not possible to test for Down syndrome or the other genetic diseases and conditions without learning sex. These are not selective tests, but rather are like reading. Can you look at the word 'test' to check if it has, say, an 'e' without also observing the presence of an 's' and two 't's? No more can you see the extra twenty-first chromosome which indicates Down syndrome without also seeing the two X chromosomes which indicate female or the presence of a Y chromosome which indicates male. One can of course ask not to be told, but, as one expectant mother explained to me, 'It's one thing not to know the unknowable. It's another to sit across from a doctor who knows, who has it written right there on your chart.'

Why does it matter? We are losing that whole second half of pregnancy where we were carrying, simply, our baby. Not a daughter, not Eleanor or Rebecca, not a son but simply a limitless, boundless, inherently abstract *baby*. In cultures with such strong gender-role expectations, we may begin to make assumptions, begin to apply sex stereotypes not just at birth, as in the past, but before birth now, weeks and months before. At its extreme, women are aborting fetuses of the unwanted sex — usually daughters. At less extreme positions, they are painting the baby's room and buying layettes in 'the right colors.' Knowing fetal sex allows people to lock in a set of expectations even before the baby is born.

There are other genetic conditions, besides sex, about which we might be better off not knowing. XYY, the genetic condition which some studies suggested may be linked to criminal behavior, is an example. The studies have been largely discredited, but my research shows there are women currently aborting XYY fetuses because, as one potential father said, 'It's hard enough to raise a normal kid. If he throws the blocks across the room will I think he's doing it because he's two, or because he's XYY?'

What will happen as we get even more information, if we can begin to predict not just retardation, but which fetuses are likely to become children of borderline ability; not just Tay Sachs, but which fetuses are likely to develop juvenile diabetes? All this information may be giving us choice, but is it coming any closer to giving us control?

And finally, briefly, what of the great expansion in the treatment of infertility, and its choices? Most discussions of the new technology for the treatment of infertility have welcomed it as giving new choices to the infertile. But here too there is a negative side to consider: all of the new treatments for infertility have also created a new burden for the infertile – the burden of not trying hard enough. Just how many dangerous experimental drugs, just how many surgical procedures, just how many months – or is it years? – of compulsive temperature-taking and obsessive sex does it take before one can now give in gracefully? When has a couple 'tried everything' and can finally stop? All of the technology still leaves many couples, about a third or more of those treated for infertility, without a pregnancy. At what point is it simply not their fault, out of their control, inevitable, inexorable fate? At what point can they get on with their lives? If there is always one more doctor to try, one more treatment around, then the social role of infertility will always be seen in some sense as chosen: they chose to give up. Did taking away the sense of inevitability of their infertility and substituting the 'choice' of giving up truly increase their choice and their control?

There are those who are successful with the new technology, those for whom the drugs and surgery are a success. Surely they have now experienced the choice of parenthood, and so their choices have expanded and they have gained control over their lives. Indeed they have, just as contraception and abortion provide us with the very real and very true experience of controlling our fertility. Choices open and choices close. For those whose choices meet the social expectations, for those who want what the society wants them to want, the experience of choice is very real.

Perhaps what we should realize is that human beings living in society have precious little choice ever. There may really be no such thing as individual choice in a social structure, not in any absolute way. The social structure creates needs – the needs for women to be mothers, the needs for small families, the needs for 'perfect' children – and creates the technology which enables people to make the needed choices. The question is not whether choices are constructed, but *how* they are constructed. Society, in its ultimate meaning, may be nothing more and nothing less than the structuring of choices.[2]

The question then for feminism is not only to address the individual level of 'a woman's right to choose' but also to examine the social level, where her choices are structured. Yes, we will have to continue to fight the good fight for information and for choice, the rights of the individual woman to choose contraception, abortion, amniocentesis, pregnancy by in vitro fertilization, pregnancy by donor insemination, labors with and labors without electronic fetal monitoring, to have no children or to have one child or to have many children. We must not get caught into discussions of which reproductive technologies are 'politically correct,' which empower and which enslave women. They ALL empower and they ALL enslave, they all can be used by, for, or against us. We will have to lift our eyes from the choices of the individual woman, and focus on the control of the social system which structures her choices, which rewards some choices and punishes others, which distributes the rewards and punishments for reproductive choices along class and race lines.

There will never be 'free' choice, unstructured reproductive choice. But the structure in which choices are made should, and I believe ultimately can, be made fair, ethical, moral. Individual rights to information and to choice are an absolute necessity for such a system, but are not alone sufficient to ensure an ethics of reproduction.

The next step in the politics of reproductive control is the politics of social control.

## NOTES

1  The author expresses her appreciation to Maren Lockwood Carden, Betty Leyerle, Eileen Moran, Rosalyn Weinman Schram, Janet Gallagher, and Joan Leibmann-Smith for their comments.
2  I particularly want to thank Betty Leyerle for her insights and wording on this issue.

## REFERENCES

Bowes, Watson A., Jr. and Brad Selgestad. 1981. 'Fetal Versus Maternal Rights: Medical and Legal Perspectives.' *Obstetrics and Gynecology*, August, 58: 209–14.

Hubbard, Ruth. 1982. 'Some Legal and Policy Implications of Recent Advances in Prenatal Diagnosis and Fetal Therapy.' *Women's Rights Law Reporter*, Spring, 7 (3): 201–18.

Pritchard, Jack H. and Paul McDonald. 1980, 6th edition. *Williams Obstetrics*. Appleton Century Crofts, New York.

Taub, Nina. 1982. 'Introduction: A Symposium on Reproductive Rights: The Emerging Issues.' *Women's Rights Law Reporter*, Spring, 7 (3), 169–73.

# TEST-TUBE WOMEN

# EGG SNATCHERS

Genoveffa Corea

A visit to a pioneer in reproductive technology prompts a reporter to ask disturbing questions about just how human eggs are obtained for experimentation in in vitro fertilization. Is it through 'egg-snatching'? Why, she further wonders, are men focusing their attention on woman's procreative power and dismembering motherhood into its components?

## I

I was early for my appointment with the famous experimental biologist, an expert in flushing embryos from pregnant sheep and cattle and transferring them to other animals. Embryo transfer in both animals and women had been discussed the previous month in West Germany at a world conference on reproductive technology he had attended. To help me with an article and a book I was writing on this technology, he would give me material from the conference as well as an interview, he had told me.

. Passing through corridors in search of his office, I walked quickly at first, then, as I looked at the pictures on the walls, progressively slower until finally I floated from picture to picture, stopping to stare, my body growing colder.

The halls and offices were all but empty. Occasionally I heard a voice, a door closing, a lock turning, steps fading away. Then silence. Alone again with the pictures.

There were black and white photographs of sperm, enormously magnified. Other microphotographs showed the uterus, revealing the very cells of the inner uterine wall.

Five line drawings sat quietly on the walls, small beside the giant sperm. They drew me back again and again. The drawings contained the same basic elements though each differed slightly from the others. There was a pink uterus in the center. A man's white gloved hand – unattached to any arm – grasped the top of it. A second white gloved hand plunged a syringe deeply into the womb. Two fallopian tubes led – not to the ovary – but to laboratory dishes.

When, half an hour later, the biologist and I stood at his office, I pointed to one of the drawings by his door and said, through my frozen face, how interesting I found that drawing as well as the others. He smiled as he unlocked his door. (He is a very charming man.)

'Egg collection,' he said. 'They illustrate the collection of human eggs.'


## II

I had been thinking a good deal about the collection of human eggs. As I researched a book on reproductive technology, *The Mother Machine*, I spent many days reading papers on egg fertilization in laboratory dishes, papers written well before the first in vitro fertilization clinic opened. Sometimes, after such a day, a question would wake me up in the middle of the night: where are they getting the eggs for these experiments?

On occasion, I knew, they would culture eggs from excised ovaries. They stated that the ovaries were 'superfluous,' those taken from women's bodies for 'therapeutic' reasons. But I recalled an article I had read years ago in the *Journal of the American Medical Association*. Dr James C. Doyle had written about physicians castrating women. He had examined surgical reports of private hospitals around Los Angeles for one recent year and found that 546 women had had perfectly normal ovaries removed from them. (Doyle, 1952)

Now, some doctors were openly advocating 'prophylactic' or preventive oophorectomies (ovariectomies) – the removal of healthy ovaries. Despite the fact that ovarian cancer is rare, they argued that all women past childbearing age should be castrated in order to prevent that cancer.[1]

Doctors were performing plenty of oophorectomies on women, I knew. *Ob. Gyn News* made that clear. In 1980, it reported that in the previous decade, castrations had increased by 48 per cent in women 45–64 years old, and by 23 per cent in younger women.

On those sleep-disturbed nights, I would remember a conversation I had had with physician Michelle Harrison, author of *A Woman in Residence* (1982). At the city hospital where she had served a residency in obstetrics and gynecology in 1979, she told me, doctors routinely removed healthy ovaries in hysterectomy patients over 45.

'The decision as to whether to take the ovaries of younger women always hung in a delicate balance,' she said. 'A slight suggestion might tip the balance.'

Sometimes the infertility specialist would appear right before hysterectomies were scheduled, she said. He would ask the gynecologists if they planned to take the ovaries out along with the uterus. He needed some, he would explain.

'Don't take them out just on my account,' he would say, and Harrison would freeze in fear, seeing the male bonds form across the room, knowing that the woman's ovaries were in jeopardy. She subsequently learned that this infertility specialist had been involved at that time in an in vitro fertilization program, the existence of which had not been publicly announced. It was then for experiments in fertilizing eggs that he most likely wanted the woman's ovaries, I thought.

Reading David Rorvik's account of what he alleged to be the first human cloning sharpened my uneasiness over egg collection. In one cloning method, researchers destroy the egg's nucleus and replace it with a body cell from the donor. The body cell has the full set of chromosomes, the same number an egg would have after a sperm fertilized it. Tricked into believing itself fertilized, the egg divides. It produces an offspring which is the genetic double of the cell donor.

Rorvik says the account in his book, *In His Image: The Cloning of a Man* (1978), is true. I am among the many who do not believe him.[2] Nonetheless, I take his book seriously as a vision. Rorvik, after all, had reported on reproductive

technologies for years. He had interviewed many technologists. The attitudes he attributes to his technologists were
attitudes I, too, had encountered in my interviews.

Here is how Rorvik described the first cloning:

Max, a wealthy Californian, wants a son who is the
spitting image of himself. So he hires a scientist, 'Darwin,' to
make a clone of him using one of his body cells. Darwin flies
with his team to a Third World country where rules regarding informed consent were 'much more relaxed' than in other
countries. After preliminary research on monkeys or other
primates, he is to use the women at a local health clinic as
'raw material' for his experiments.

When Rorvik visits the clinic and finds, to his surprise,
no experiments being conducted on animals, he inquires into
the status of the primate research. Darwin tells him they are
working with the best primates money can buy: women.
Darwin had skipped the animal research, he explained to
Rorvik, because it would have been costly, time-consuming
and of little value. (Darwin's attitude appears similar to that
of real researchers pioneering in human in vitro fertilization.
Dr Robert Edwards, 'co-lab parent' of the world's first test-
tube baby, also protested the necessity of primate studies. He
wrote: 'Many infertile couples and others with different
problems would forfeit their chances of a cure if medical
progress depended on verification in non-human primates.'
(Edwards, 1974))

Rorvik asked Darwin if he was informing his 'primates'
of what was going on. Most, but not all, of the women knew
that he was 'after their eggs,' he answered, or that he wanted
to use their wombs.

Darwin maintained he was helping women who were
flocking to him for sterilization operations. 'If he saw a
chance to get some eggs in the course of carrying out some
other procedure, he took it, naturally.'

Darwin 'superovulated' the women he operated on. That
is, he gave them the fertility drug Pergonal to force their
ovaries to ripen many eggs. Darwin assured Rorvik that this
artificial induction of extra eggs would not deplete the
ovaries. The typical woman, he explained, is born with about
half a million egg cells, of which only about 500 would mature.

Rorvik: 'It made you wonder, Darwin said, what the other 499,500 were for. Maybe nature foresaw something we didn't. Maybe, he joked, or at least I think he joked, nature was providing for "egg-snatchers" like himself.'

Egg-snatchers.

I thought of Dr Robert Edwards, the British pioneer in in vitro fertilization. He wrote a book with gynecologist Patrick Steptoe about their research. In it, he refers time and again to the difficulty of getting women's eggs or, as he once put it, the eggs of man.

As a graduate student, he had worked with mice. After he had 'bombed' their ovaries with hormones, he had learned a good deal about the way eggs ripen. Later, while researching in another field, 'the eggs were always there in the background beckoning me on to my real work.'

Occasionally, he dreamed of eggs.

He had learned from his experiments that the eggs of various species would ripen in a laboratory dish on their own without the stimulus of hormones.

'Surely the whole field then was in my grasp – cows, sheep, monkeys – and man, too, if I could only get their eggs?'

That proved a frustrating obstacle.

He arranged for various gynecologists to call him when they thought they might have ovarian tissues to 'bequeath' him. He would go to the hospital. While the physician cut into the woman's body, he would stand, masked and gowned, holding his sterile glass pot, 'the receptacle for the precious bit of superfluous ovarian tissue.'

I wondered: when the women consented to the surgery, did they know that as they lay anesthetized on the table, a man would be standing there waiting to collect their eggs in a glass pot? Did they know that, in at least one instance in Cambridge, he would add his sperm to their eggs in an attempt at fertilization in a dish? Did *they* ever dream of eggs – their own eggs – fertilized by a faceless man in a white laboratory coat?

Dr Edwards needed more eggs. He never had enough. He 'scouted around' for them and 'tried to rally more doctors to my cause.' He 'came away empty-handed.' His sources 'dried up.'

'Human eggs were still slow coming my way,' he wrote, 'despite the fact that I had struck up friendly relations with some of the gynecologists at Cambridge's Addenbrooke's Hospital' (Edwards and Steptoe, 1980).

So he worked more often with the eggs of cows, sheep and monkeys. Now and then, a lab threw a monkey ovary his way. He would get the ovaries of cows and sheep from the local slaughterhouse. He found his visits there unpleasant. It was 'sad,' he reports, to see the cows lining up, to hear the crack of the gun and then the soft thud of the creature falling.

At Cambridge, he wrote, 'I would have been content if only human eggs had come my way more freely.'

He set off for Johns Hopkins in Baltimore. Egg heaven. 'I was to share pieces of ovarian tissue with the pathologists,' he wrote.

Again I wondered: did the women know how their ovarian tissue was being disposed of? Did they know a man was trying to fertilize the eggs cultured from their ovaries?


# III

The biologist seats me in his office for a talk on the new reproductive technologies.

I am interested in the eggs. First they 'collect' them from women's bodies, I know. Then they fertilize them in a dish. When will they be able to freeze them?

Ten years perhaps, he tells me.

Hadn't he said it might someday be possible to open an embryo supermarket? A woman would choose a frozen embryo, genetically unrelated to herself, and bring it to an obstetrician who would implant it in her body.

Eventually that will happen, he replies, after people change their views on eugenics. (Established in 1869 by upper-class Englishmen, eugenics is an ideology which maintains that the human race can be improved through the control of breeding. Negative eugenics calls for decreasing the propagation of the 'unfit,' who invariably turn out to be members of lower classes and oppressed races, through birth control and sterilization. Positive eugenics calls for increasing the propagation of the 'fit' by encouraging large families among them. The fit turn out to be members of upper classes and the dominant race. Eugenics, which was a respectable movement led by physicians, university professors, scientists and other professionals, enjoyed its heyday in the United States from roughly 1900 to 1930. It lost its respectability in the 1930s when Adolf Hitler implemented his massive eugenics plan in Europe. It remains in disrepute today.)

Once people again look upon eugenics favorably, women in the embryo supermarket would presumably choose their embryos from among those produced by the sperm and eggs of 'superior' men and women. In this way, the eugenic theory goes, better people would be produced.

I had been intrigued by an interview the biologist had given on television a year earlier and I wanted him to expand on it. He had spoken then of quality control in the breeding of human beings. The ideal, he had explained, would be strong, healthy, disease-resistant people who were productive. Such qualities were partly genetic and partly environmental, he had said, adding:

> But if we cull down the lazy type that is not interested to contribute to society, I think we have done a great deal. We do that in race horses and in farm animals. We select the best dairy cow, we select the fastest horse, and we select sheep for their wool. I think we can do a little bit of selection at the human level. (McMullen, 1979)

I remind him of his comment. When will the selection begin?

'Eventually,' he says. 'Eventually.'

Someone will have to decide on the desirable qualities which should be selected for, he points out. He suggests that a governmental agency or major foundation might take on that task.

I ask him about embryo transfer – flushing a fertilized egg out of one woman and implanting it in the womb of another. A pioneer in this technology had just told me that once the technique was perfected, it would be possible to flush embryos out of every pregnant woman. Doctors would examine each embryo before deciding whether or not to reimplant it. 'Embryo evaluation,' the pioneer had called it.

I ask the biologist: might embryo flushing someday become a part of routine prenatal care?

Sure, he says. You can even evaluate the embryo – not just for its genetic health – but for its sex.

'There are modern techniques now to do so,' he adds.

Embryo evaluation, then, would be a method of sex predetermination. 'Right sex' embryos would be implanted; those of the 'wrong sex' discarded.

In the next twenty years, the biologist told me, artificial insemination and embryo transfer will change human reproduction. Various combinations of the techniques would result in three kinds of mothers: genetic mothers who provide the egg; surrogate mothers who provide the uterus; and social mothers who look after the child.

'This is already here,' he pointed out, referring to surrogate motherhood.

Companies commercing in reproduction will sprout up, he predicts. Some such firms exist now:

Frozen sperm banks. ('They're advertised in the newspaper,' the biologist notes.)

Banks for frozen animal eggs and embryos. (Owners of one bank in Denmark hope to freeze human, as well as animal, eggs and embryos once the technique for doing so has been developed. In Melbourne, Australia, the in vitro fertilization team at Queen Victoria Medical Centre, developing such a technique, is freezing human embryos now.)

International associations for transferring embryos in farm animals. ('Eventually this will be done in humans also,' he tells me. A clinic experimenting in human embryo transfers already operates in Chicago and the clinic owners, working with colleagues in California, achieved their first success in August 1983.)

Clinics for inseminating surrogate mothers. (At least ten such companies selling the services of breeder women exist

now in Dearborn, Michigan; Louisville, Kentucky; Philadelphia, Pennsylvania; Hollywood, Los Angeles and Malibu, California; Chevy Chase, Maryland; Denver, Colorado; Columbus, Ohio; and Tempe, Arizona. An estimated seventy-five to one hundred babies have been born to breeder women nationwide.)
Sex predetermination clinics for choosing the gender of a baby. (Gametrics Limited operates its main branch in Sausalito. Clinics around the country and the world provide Gametrics' technique for clients.)[3]

The biologist gives me textbooks he has written and papers on reproductive technology. He seats me in an outer office to read them. I take notes. And think:

Why are men focusing all this technology on woman's generative organs – the source of her procreative power? Why are they collecting our eggs? Why do they seek to freeze them?

Why do men want to control the production of human beings? Why do they talk so often about producing 'perfect' babies?

Why are they splitting the functions of motherhood into smaller parts? Does that reduce the power of the mother and her claim to the child? ('I only gave the egg. I am not the real mother.' 'I only loaned my uterus. I am not the real mother.' 'I only raised the child. I am not the real mother.')

I watched a television news show. (NBC, 1980.) The man interviewed was Dr Richard Levine, an artificial inseminator of breeder women and founder of Surrogate Parenting Associates of Louisville, Kentucky. The woman was Elizabeth Kane (pseudonym), the first of Levine's surrogates.

'That's what I do: make babies,' said the man.

'I think of myself as a human incubator,' said the woman.

Man is possessing woman's procreative power. She is losing it. She is a thing. She is a vessel for the babies men make.

I can read no more today. I ask the biologist if I may see the animals in the laboratory.

## IV

I wanted to see the animals because I had begun to identify with them. The first time I had done so had been at a workshop in reproductive technology in 1979.[4] Almost all of us in the auditorium that day were women. We were scientists, physicians, feminist activists, ethicists and lawyers. Dr Rosalind Herlands was describing the efforts of researchers to superovulate animals.

'Eggs and embryos are collected usually after the donor female is killed and her oviducts or uterus are removed,' she explained matter-of-factly.

We gasped. Dr Herlands looked up in surprise. In the ensuing hush, one woman said: 'That gives us some idea of what they may do to us.'

The gut-level identification with laboratory animals we women shared that day deepened in me over the following year.[5] To sense a bond with animals was a surprising, increasingly welcome, feeling. Surprising because, for most of my years, animals were invisible to me. I did not like them, never thought about them. They protruded into my life only to annoy me. At a friend's house, a cat would try to settle on my lap or a dog would come sniffing up to be petted. If socially coerced into an awkward pat of a dog's head, I wanted to wash my hands immediately. Usually, I declared my allergy to fur to shield me from unwelcome intimacies.

But as I researched, animals slowly became visible to me. In the neighborhood, I looked at animals with new eyes. I got to know the puppy next door. I saw, for the first time, that animals were living, sentient beings. And they were used, as women are used.

I thought of those cows and sheep in the slaughterhouse – the creatures Edwards heard fall with a soft thud. In scientific papers, I read of rabbits sacrificed, saw photographs of guinea pigs tied to tables, cut open, ovaries exposed. I thought of those mice, mated after men had 'bombed' their ovaries with hormones to superovulate them.

'Large mice, average mice, small mice – it was unbelievable – were all visibly pregnant,' Edwards wrote. 'Excited, we autopsied some of them immediately.'

Soon, I knew, describing his actions in therapeutic terms, he would be bombing the ovaries of women.

I read Kathleen Barry's *Female Sexual Slavery* (1979), an account of the traffic in women, and thought: just as man has a perfect right to probe, puncture and irradiate the bodies of laboratory animals, so may he violate the bodies of women. Both women and animals are objects to be bought, seized, used and discarded.

Men procure women for a pimp's stable. They procure animals for a researcher's lab. They pick up women – often runaway teenagers – at train and bus stations. They get dogs at the pound.

Sometimes they can treat the same women as both laboratory animals *and* sexual servants. Take Rorvik's science fiction account of cloning. In the course of 'therapeutic' surgery, Darwin, the reproductive engineer, feels free to remove eggs from the women. When he tries to implant embryos in the women and get them pregnant, he does not inform them of his attempts nor of his successes. Why should he give a lab animal a progress report?

Max, 67, insisted that the host for his cloned son be an attractive virgin. He might want to have intercourse with her. So teenage girls came into the clinic, were given physicals, had their medical histories and photographs taken for dossiers:

> Max, for whom women of this particular region held a special attraction, would examine these dossiers himself, discarding some, retaining others. He was being the more fussy, Darwin said, because the woman or girl who was selected as surrogate might become Max's mistress, or at least his principal mistress, and in that way would also be the 'mother' or at least the maternal influence in the rearing of the clone.

According to the biologist's sketch of dismembered motherhood, this woman would then be both a surrogate and social mother. She would function under the man's control. The child belonged to him. She merely provided services for it. She would be a reproductive and sexual servant.

I could envision women being sold into surrogacy. I could

see lawyers hanging around train stations competing with pimps for the teenage runaways who could bear babies for 'clients.' Hadn't it been reported in 1980 that lawyers were, even then, standing outside high schools looking for pregnant girls and, once finding them, offering them inducements to turn over their babies for private adoption? (Donahue, 1980.) And in England, a married couple had already hired a teenage prostitute to be inseminated with the husband's sperm, bear the baby, and then give it to them. (She did indeed bear the child but could not part with it. For this reason, the case came to court.)[6]

Enough thinking.

I wanted to see the animals. The biologist stepped into the adjacent laboratory, made arrangements for a research technician to show me around, and returned to his office.

I entered the laboratory. Passing through three or four rooms, I saw rabbits, mice, rats, monkeys in stainless steel cages. I felt like an imposter. The biologist and the technician spoke to me as though I were one of them. But I was one of the animals.

The technician was explaining to me how dangerous it could be to handle animals. Some animals would bite you if they got a chance. Here, I'll show you, he said, leading me back into the monkey room.

In one cage, two baby monkeys, looking fearful, clung to each other. The technician opened the cage. The adult monkeys watching from their separate cages screamed. The babies ran to the back of the cage, still clinging together as they fled. The technician pretended to reach for them. Screeches filled the room. The adults rattled the bars of their cages.

'That's a warning to the babies,' the technician explained to me. 'If they had been out of their cages, they'd have attacked me. They all protect the babies.'

I have often thought of that scene. Sitting at my typewriter night after night, I see my writing on the new reproductive technologies as a scream of warning to other women.

## NOTES

1  For example, Skelton (1973) notes:

> The time has come for us as members of this College (of
> Obstetricians and Gynecologists) to recognize and recommend
> prophylactic elective total hysterectomy and bilateral
> salpingo-oophorectomy (removal of uterus, fallopian tubes and
> both ovaries) after completion of childbearing as proper
> preventive medicine in obstetrics and gynecology.

Also, Dr Frederick J. Hofmeister, a former president of the
American College of Obstetricians and Gynecologists, writes:

> While it may not be an established procedure with some
> gynecologists, my experience points to the removal of the
> ovaries in the hysterectomy patient over 40. I point out that
> such a procedure is advisable because of the hazard of cancer of
> the ovaries. (Ayerst, 1979)

2  The authenticity of Rorvik's account was thoroughly discredited
at Congressional hearings on cloning. (Developments, 1978.) For
example, Dr Beatrice Mintz of the Institute for Cancer Research,
Fox Chase Cancer Center, points out the following: Rorvik states
that the adult cells 'Darwin' was working with to donate the
nucleus to the egg were erythrocytes, red blood cells. 'This is a
particularly amusing boner,' she said, 'inasmuch as the mature
red blood cells of man are the only cells in the body that are totally
devoid of nuclei.'

3  For a listing of frozen sperm banks in the United States, see
Frankel, 1975–76, pp. 290–1.

For a listing of companies which provide embryo transfer and
embryo freezing services, send for the 'Directory of Members' of
the International Embryo Transfer Society, 3101 Arrowhead
Road, La Porte, Colorado 80535.

*Surrogate Parenting News* provides information on
companies formed to sell the services of breeder women and on
clinics which perform in vitro fertilization. Write: Third Wave
Publications, Inc., 120 North 4th Avenue, Ann Arbor, Michigan
48104.

A list of centers which offer the male sex predetermination
technique developed by Dr Ronald Ericsson is available from
Gametrics Limited, 180 Harbor Drive, Sausalito, Ca. 94965.

4  The conference, held at Hampshire College in Amherst,
Massachusetts, was entitled: 'Ethical Issues in Reproductive
Technology: Analysis by Women.'

5  Two years after that conference, immediately following time
spent on farms watching the new reproductive technologies used

on cows, I became a vegetarian. As a feminist who sees the connection between the way the patriarchy views and treats women and animals, I feel a growing imperative to end my complicity in the oppression of animals.

For those who would like to think more about animal liberation, these books will be helpful: Fisher (1979); Mason and Singer (1980); Godlovitch and Harris (1971); Singer (1975).

Some addresses for further information on animal liberation:

*Agenda: News Magazine of the Animal Rights Network*, P.O. Box 5234, Westport, Ct 06881. Subscription $15/year in US, $25 abroad.

The Farm Animal Reform Movement (FARM) is a national, non-profit, educational organization dedicated to alleviating and eliminating animal abuse and other adverse effects of animal agriculture. It publishes the *Farm Report* bi-monthly. Write FARM, Inc., P.O. Box 70123, Washington, DC 20088.

People for the Ethical Treatment of Animals (PETA) is an educational and activist group opposed to all forms of animal oppression. It holds weekly activist workshops, lectures on factory farming, slaughterhouses, leghold trapping, etc. It attracts public attention to animal abuse by picketing, street theater and other actions. Write PETA, P.O. Box 56272, Washington, DC 20011.

World Women for Animal Rights is a vegetarian feminist network of individuals and of autonomous local chapters. For a literature packet, send $3 to Vegetarian Feminists NYC, 616 6th Street, Brooklyn, NY 11215.

6   She kept the child but the court gave the sperm donor limited visitation rights. (Scott, 1981, p. 217.)

# REFERENCES

Ayerst Laboratories pamphlet. 1979. *The Female Climacteric*, V (4): 4–5.

Barry, Kathleen. 1979. *Female Sexual Slavery*. Prentice-Hall, Englewood Cliffs, New Jersey.

Developments in Cell Biology and Genetics. 1978. Hearings before the Subcommittee on Health and the Environment of the Committee on Interstate and Foreign Commerce. House of Representatives. May 31. Serial no. 95–105. US Government Printing Office, Washington.

Donahue Transcript No. 02260. 1980. Multimedia Program Productions. 140 West Ninth Street, Cincinnati, Ohio 45202.

(Testimony on lawyers hanging around outside high schools was presented on the *Donahue* television program February 26.)

Doyle, James C. 1952. 'Unnecessary Ovariectomies', *Journal of the American Medical Association*, 148, no. 13: 1105–11.

Edwards, R. G. 1974. 'Fertilization of Human Eggs in Vitro: Morals, Ethics and the Law.' *Quarterly Review of Biology.* **49**. March.

Edwards, Robert and Patrick Steptoe. 1980. *A Matter of Life.* William Morrow, New York.

Fisher, Elizabeth. 1979. *Woman's Creation.* McGraw-Hill, New York.

Frankel, Mark S. 1975–6. 'Human-Semen Banking: Social and Public Policy Issues.' *Man and Medicine*, 1.

Godlovitch, Stanley and Roslind and John Harris. 1971. *Animals, Men and Morals.* Grove Press, New York.

Harrison, Michelle. 1972. *A Woman in Residence.* Random House, New York.

Mason, Jim and Peter Singer. 1980. *Animal Factories.* Crown Publishers, New York.

McMullen, Jay (producer/writer). 1979. Transcript of *CBS Reports, The Baby Makers.* As broadcast October 30. Produced by CBS News.

NBC. 1980. *NBC Magazine.* Broadcast November 8.

*Ob. Gyn. News.* 1980. March 1.

Rorvik, David. 1978. *In His Image: The Cloning of a Man.* J. P. Lippincott, Philadelphia.

Scott, Russell. 1981. *The Body as Property.* Viking Press, New York: 217.

Singer, Peter. 1975. *Animal Liberation.* Avon Books, New York.

Skelton, J. B. 1973. 'Prophylactic Hysterectomy and Salpingo-Oophorectomy – Is It or Is It Not Good Preventive Medicine?' *Audio Digest of Ob and Gyn*, 20.

# TEST-TUBE BABIES AND CLINICS: WHERE ARE THEY?[1]

Since the birth of Louise Brown – the world's first test-tube baby – in 1978 in Britain, more than seventy in vitro fertilization clinics have been established worldwide. About 130 children have been born, eighty of them in Britain. Currently, Australia seems to have the largest success rate with one test-tube child born every month. It appears that on average every fourth pregnancy of an implanted in vitro embryo results in the successful birth of a child (see Glossary, p. 457, for explanation of technical terms).

Durga Agarwal was the second in vitro baby. She was born in India, Calcutta, in 1978 and followed by James Montgomery in Scotland, Edinburgh, in 1979. Australia saw its first test-tube child in 1980 (Elizabeth Reed in Melbourne). The US lagged behind in the production of test-tube babies due to a 1975 ban on all experiments on human IVF research which was lifted only in 1979. Elizabeth Carr, the first US test-tube child, was born in Virginia in 1981. The same year saw the first French IVF baby (René Frydtman, Paris) and in 1982 West Germany had its first test-tube child: Oliver Wimmelbacher, Erlangen. Since then, test-tube babies have been born in Sweden, Austria, Switzerland, the Soviet Union and Japan.

Despite the considerable expenses of IVF (not to speak of the lengthy, emotionally and often physically painful procedure), there is an enormous demand for test-tube babies and the waiting lists in the US seem to be full for the next five years. Average costs for IVF treatment are: £1,600–2,000 in Britain, DM 9,000 in West Germany, $4,000 in the US). Britain and Australia seem to be leading in the field. Some of the clinics which perform IVF are:

*Britain*: Bourn Hall, Cambridge (private clinic of Patrick Steptoe and Robert Edwards, Louise Brown's 'fathers'); St Thomas's Hospital, London (Ronald Taylor); The Royal Free Hospital, London (Ian Craft); King's College Hospital, London (B. Collings); Hammersmith Hospital, London and St. Mary's Hospital, Manchester.

*Australia*: The Royal Women's Hospital, Melbourne (Alexander Lopata, Ian Johnston); The Queen Victoria Medical Centre, Monash University, Melbourne (Carl Wood, Alan Trounson).

*USA*: Over fifty clinics perform in vitro fertilization in the US. Some of them are Norfolk General Hospital, Virginia; Northridge Hospital, Northridge, CA 91328; Yale University Medical School, New Haven, CT 06510; Vanderbilt University Medical Center, Nashville, TN 37232; Mount Sinai Hospital, Chicago, IL 60608; Union Memorial Hospital, Baltimore, MD 21218; Beth Israel Hospital, Boston, MA 02215; William Beaumont Hospital, Royal Oak, MI 48072; University of Medicine and Dentistry of New Jersey, Rutgers Medical School, New Brunswick, NJ 08903; Columbia Presbyterian Medical Center, New York, NY 10032; North Carolina Memorial Hospital, Chapel Hill, NC 27514; Ohio State University of Columbus, Columbus, Ohio 43210; Baylor College of Medicine, Houston, TX 77030; University of Wisconsin Medical School, Madison, WI 53706.

*West Germany*: The women's clinics of the universities of Erlangen (Sigfried Trotnow); Kiel (Liselotte Mettler) and Lübeck (Dieter Krebs).

This is an incomplete list. At the time of writing (September 1983) new IVF clinics are virtually popping up overnight worldwide.

## NOTE

1 Based on information compiled by the editors from 'Retorten-babies. Zeugung im Glas' (Test-tube babies. In vitro fertilization), with permission by its author, Christiane Erlemann.

# WHO OWNS THE EMBRYO?[1]

## Rebecca Albury

The same range of issues are involved in the discussions of the use of IVF as in the debate about abortion: the role of medical technology, the power of the medical profession, the needs of society, the function of the law and the relations between women and men. An examination of the common assumptions about the position of women in society in relation to the two points of intervention into the reproductive process leads to the conclusion that feminists must break the silence about the unequal power relations between women and men that are reproduced by scientists and law reformers in their development and practice on the new reproductive technologies.

Biological reproduction, that most 'natural' of human activities, has become the subject of major technological intervention during the past thirty years.[2] Although scientific understanding of the processes of reproduction is still underdeveloped, it is possible to apply technology at several stages in the process, at least in the female body – contraception, abortion, pregnancy, childbirth, and now conception. Today the new technologies of in vitro fertilisation (IVF) and embryo transfer are receiving considerable scientific, moral and legal examination. It is striking how the discussion about the use of IVF has much in common with the now familiar debate about abortion.

The same range of issues is involved: the role of medical technology, the power of the medical profession, the needs of society, the desires of the woman in question, the place of her partner and the function of the law. The similarities and differences in the way questions and answers about these two points of intervention in the process of human reproduction suggests that what is at stake is not the often repeated issue of the 'sanctity of life'. Throughout both debates run a set of related but unspoken assumptions about the role of women in the 'family'. Through a discussion of those assumptions it is possible to point to the likely outcome of the numerous government-sponsored inquiries about law reform to meet the challenge of the new technologies. Giving voice to the unspoken may also open the debate about technologies of human reproduction to questions that have been excluded.

To begin the task of examining possible directions for discussion and action about the technologies I will place current technical and legal developments in their social and political context. Then I will look at some of the social practices surrounding the use of IVF. A consideration of the process of law reform about reproduction then leads to an examination of some concepts that are at the centre of contemporary political thought – rights and needs. Through this discussion the practice of IVF emerges as a political rather than technical problem with ambiguous consequences for the lives of women.

The debates about human reproduction take place within the boundaries set by the definitions and categories of liberal democratic political theory.[3] At one level it is assumed that society is made up of individuals who share equally the responsibilities and benefits of their common life. This assumption is, however, a myth that denies a multitude of inequalities of race, class and sex. These rest on a deeper assumption of inequality: the profound separation of public and private (or personal life) that supported the exclusion of all but certain white males from political life. This division has served as the model for the division of many human experiences and relations; thus it has provided ways of viewing the world and acting in it. Public life is the location of politics and the institutions of liberal democracy – parties, parliaments, legal systems. In classical liberalism (now called conservatism) even the economy, trade unions and popular movements were not a part of the public sphere of politics. Even today the whole range of affective relations is located outside the public sphere in private life, by definition.

The separation of public and private life has been accompanied by the division of various areas of action and concern between men and women. Thus, women are commonly defined by their biological function as child bearers and then assigned the social function of child rearers. Men, on the other hand, are defined by their capacity for rational thought and their ability to go beyond the purely biological (Okin, 1979). This separation of public and private has served to confine women in the private realm of the family and isolated them from the main arenas of political and social debate. It has also disguised the unequal power relations between women and men. Liberal theorists claim to discuss equal genderless individuals but it is clear that those individuals are, in fact, white, property-owning, male heads of households. The interests of all family members are assumed to be the same without any argument. At the same time, even women's potential to take part in public life is denied on the grounds that their biological functions make them ill-suited to the harsh competitive public world. Yet the personal qualities said to come from female biology – emotional tenderness, empathy, nurturance, and altruism are all assumed to be necessary to the survival of the human race. The rich and varied feminist criticism of the contemporary social order has received little serious attention, except from social commentators who defend a gender-based division of human capacities and labour as a means of returning to a happier past when conflicts of interest in the family were not said to be at the base of social conflict nor described with such skill and passion. In most social commentary the family is treated as a 'natural' and unproblematic, universal feature of society, instead of being recognised as a vague term that covers a variety of specific living arrangements. Therefore, in policy debates the basic premises of liberalism remain unchallenged and women remain securely positioned in male-headed families in the private sphere.

The prescribed role of women in those families is central to the opposition to abortion and the justification of technological conception. In a family defined as a heterosexual, male-headed, child-rearing institution, women gain their status from their relationship to men; they are daughters, wives, mothers. There are no widely accepted words to describe autonomous women, instead the phrases suggest a woman's deviance from the role as appendage of a man – childless women, single mothers. Pregnancy and birth, or at least motherhood, are a part of the conventional definition of women. Motherhood is the foremost institutional structure in the lives of women (Rich, 1976)); women who resist institutionalisation, even briefly, are regarded with suspicion and contempt. One needs only to remember the terms of the abortion debate or the charge of selfishness levelled at women who remain child-free by choice. It is no surprise that infertile women in an Australian IVF programme speak of their childlessness in strong terms.

> I went through all those feelings about how unfair it was that women who don't really want kids can have them when I can't. It really felt I had a disability.

> I don't see how being infertile is so different to being deaf or blind. You just aren't complete.

> It was probably silly but I felt that Len might not love me as much if I couldn't have a baby. Perhaps he wouldn't consider me as feminine. (Tedeschi, 1982)

> Stephen is the child I have been attempting to conceive for the past seventeen years. Stephen is why Toby and I are involved in the IVF programme. Stephen is waiting inside my mind. His spirit lives inside me and waits for nature or my doctors to form his body – the body that will set him free to live.

> Stephen and I are the survivors of a tragedy in which I lost my fertility and the body of my child. (Walters and Singer, 1982: 120–2)

The desperation of these women who cannot meet the cultural definition of feminine womanhood by becoming mothers is accepted by medical researchers, ethicists and law reformers as unproblematic. One Australian medical team describes their work as the 'result of intense public demand' (*Sun-Herald*, 28 March 1982: 61), but does not discuss the responsibility of the medical profession for establishing that demand. Both of the women quoted above lost their fallopian tubes as a result of misdiagnosed pelvic infections, of repeated complaints of pain that were ignored or dismissed as an excuse to get out of work (Walters and Singer, 1982: 14, 121). Today women who were defined as malingering teenagers by medical professionals must rely on members of the same profession for a technical solution to the infertility caused by the earlier definition. They are also likely to be defined as incomplete women because of their infertility. Those two are not alone, but joined by thousands of women made sterile by contraceptives as well as misdiagnosis (Seaman and Seaman, 1978). Further, the role of the medical profession in the definition of women's sexuality and life experiences is never raised, nor is the increasing literature analysing that role ever acknowledged, much less discussed. It seems as if the medical technologists and their apologists remain purposively ignorant of the most systematic critique of their practices.

Although the social practices surrounding IVF and other technologies of reproduction do not formally articulate assumptions about female sexuality and women's place in society, they certainly reproduce them. Medical practitioners are acknowledged as experts about the functioning of female bodies and thus occupy a privileged place in defining the standards of normality and deviance (Ehrenreich and English, 1979). The laws of most countries grant doctors, not women, the power to authorise abortion. A woman must demonstrate her worthiness to become a part of a techno-logical conception programme; she must fit the practitioner's notion of a 'good mother'. First she must be married (Walters and Singer, 1982); the technical solution to the inability to give birth and fulfill the total definition of 'woman' is reserved for those who have indicated their willingness to accept this definition by getting married. While some official inquiries are willing to accept *de facto* marriages, others are not.[4] In addition a woman must demonstrate the suitability of her skills and motives for parenting. A woman also must be a 'good patient'. While each programme and set of procedures is different in its requirements, all consist of a formidable battery of physical and psychological tests as well as a rigorous 'treatment' schedule for those accepted (e.g. Wood and Westmore, 1983).[5] The medical profession has added a new technique to its practice of social control of women; a control that remains unacknowledged either by the practitioners and their supporters or by the critics they recognise.

In the debate on IVF the feminist critiques of social attitudes and medical practices are dismissed as inappropriate to the questions at hand. One writer, in an article highly critical of technological conception, nevertheless says when discussing the desire of an individual woman to have a baby:

> An extreme feminist might take umbrage at such a feeling, and claim that the cure for it is not IVF but a change in the attitudes of society. I doubt if the woman in question would be much helped by this approach. Her need is real enough to her, and the object of it, surely is a good one: the having of a baby.
>
> I propose we accept that the desire of a childless couple to have a child of their own is a reasonable one. (Walters and Singer, 1982: 73)

Father William Daniel, SJ, seems to be saying that because some infertile women want babies, neither he nor anyone else needs to think about the mechanisms of social control that made them feel 'that somehow you weren't a real woman unless you were fertile' (ibid: 73). He uses the word 'reasonable' in a way that suggests that any investigation into the social origin of the couple's desire for a child will call their rationality (sanity?) into question. It is also unlikely that anyone so unwilling to question the equation of 'woman' with 'mother' would notice the shift from a woman's personal need to her inclusion as a part of a couple's desire, much less examine the distribution of social power in a society in which that shift can be made.

A brief examination of the rhetoric of the abortion debate provides a useful comparison with the IVF discussion, for it raises a number of questions about the claim that medical services are delivered according to public demand and the desires of women. The laws and judicial interpretation give the decision-making power to doctors not to women. Women are exhorted to be responsible and unselfish, to use high technology contraception regardless of their personal evaluation of its dangers, to think of the moral fibre of the nation, and to support the hierarchy of authority in the family by submitting to the will of men or the inevitability of biology. In the polemics, fatherhood is reduced to an act of fertilisation and childhood is extended to before birth. The Right to Life Movement has achieved such success with this language that a recent court case in Australia was reported with the headline: 'Father Fights For His Unborn Child!' even though the story made clear that the man did not want to care for a living infant but only to prevent an abortion and then force an adoption (*Daily Telegraph*, 24 March 1983: 1).[6]

What would happen if the terms of the abortion debate included the sympathy towards women's needs expressed by William Daniel when he opposed IVF? A simple alteration in his original argument reveals that his sympathy rests on the same assumptions of the social role of women as the practices he opposes. For when the discussion is changed to that of a woman who wants to terminate an unwanted pregnancy his basic argument can be used to answer one of the major assertions of many Right to Life arguments – abortion is no solution to the social problems of women with unwanted pregnancies.

> An extreme anti-feminist might take umbrage at such a feeling, and claim that the cure for it is not abortion but a change in the attitudes of society. I doubt if the woman in question would be much helped by this approach. Her need is real enough to her, and the object of it surely, is a good one: the avoidance of a child she does not want.
>
> I propose we accept that the desire of a woman [couple] to terminate an unwanted pregnancy is a reasonable one. (My paraphrase)

The assumption of 'reasonableness' of the desire to terminate as well as the desire to achieve a pregnancy indeed changes the position of the various parties in the abortion debate. Women seeking abortions are no longer distressed or misguided but rational, capable decision-makers. Those with moral objections to abortion could counsel women to avoid abortion but would find it difficult to demand laws to outlaw abortion or to deny women their decision-making power. There might then be pressure on governments to decriminalise abortion from the same influential legal and medical bodies that today press for laws to clarify the practices of technological conception. While such an outcome would be welcome, it is highly unlikely to happen because decriminalised abortion challenges the unspoken assumption that women are mothers and belong in families.

The law, like other liberal institutions, supports the assumption that women are not a part of public life. Its function as an enforcer of the dominant sexual politics can be seen in studies of judicial decisions in cases involving protective or exclusionary legislation (Sachs and Wilson, 1978). Mary Eastwood suggests that many United States Supreme Court decisions have been based on the relatively unsophisticated formulation: 'Men are in power; they have established their control, and it should stay that way' (Eastwood, 1971: 285). Similar beliefs inform the law reform process even though reformers recognise the injustice of some old laws.

Abortion law reform has been the focus of both feminist and anti-feminist organisation. In English-speaking countries abortion laws were changed to give women more access to legal abortion during the years between 1967 and 1973.[7] Subsequent changes have been in the opposite direction. In Australia the process has occurred, state by state, in formal legislative or judicial ways and informal changes in the practice of law enforcement. As a result medically safe abortions are available to most women, but based on the right of a doctor to make decisions about medical treatment, rather than the right of a woman to control her own fertility. Support for the changes has been based on the notion that unwanted pregnancy is an individual problem: ignorance of contraception, irresponsible sexual activity, psychological disturbance, temporary or permanent social deprivation, extreme youth, or medical unfitness. All of these are special cases that justify the doctor's decision, and it was assumed that 'normal' women do not seek abortions (Greenwood and Young, 1976). Thus the reforms achieved the transfer of women from the control of individual men in families to the control of state sanctioned groups of specialist men. Liberal abortion reform laws have given 'women more rights without giving them a right to themselves' (Kickbusch, 1981: 153). The liberal reformist position that allows this transfer of authority is not so very different from the anti-abortion position. Advocates of both positions are unwilling to acknowledge women as autonomous political and moral agents; though they differ on how best to enforce their views. Without a doubt, the gender-based hierarchy is supported by both groups in their advocacy of legal changes.

Law reform discussions in Australia about human reproduction have been largely technical examinations of how the accepted structure of law and legal practice can assimilate new technologies, rather than how the new technologies reinforce the social relations already encoded in the law. This is no surprise, since such discussions fall into the categories implied by the separation of public and private life, categories that reinforce the male-headed family as the basic unit in a hierarchical society, and that hold up a vision of a progressive and rational science. Although the debate about reproductive technologies like IVF includes a variety of legal and ethical questions, the law reformers see questions of property as their particular brief, with the custody of the child as an area of considerable concern (Mason, 1982). To what extent does the contribution of genetic material to the biological process of reproduction entail legal and economic responsibilities? The apparent problems in cases of AID (see Glossary) are multiplied when a woman is engaged to gestate a pregnancy (so-called surrogate motherhood; see Ince, this volume). The naming of the hired woman a surrogate 'mother' raises a different primary question than one of simple custody. What constitutes motherhood, a biological or a social relationship with a child? The separation of pregnancy from child rearing has the potential to raise questions about the role of women in new ways, but only if the assumptions behind the use of the term 'mother' for both pregnant women and child rearing women are subjected to searching examination.

In vitro fertilisation seems simple by comparison, but only in terms of custody of the living child. Who owns the components of the biological processes that are assisted by technology; the sperm, the ova, the embryo? The ownership of the embryo has profound implications beyond the often-raised questions of frozen embryos in laboratories. If the ownership of an embryo in vitro is legally established, what will be the status of an embryo *in vivo?* Will a man be able to prevent an abortion because he is the joint *owner* of the implanted embryo regardless of whether a woman consents to continuing the pregnancy? Could a man take out an injunction to enforce a particular diet, non-smoking, or regular exercise on a pregnant woman as an expression of his concern for the care of his property – his share of the fetus? Such speculations reduce women to little more than ambulatory incubators, but are not as far-fetched as they might seem, for men have already gone to court in attempts to deny women abortions in several countries. There is also pressure to provide legal protection for doctors against various charges of malpractice. The legal solution to the challenge of technical change could reinforce the social control of women by men. In the absence of the searching examination suggested above, technical developments and the legal responses to them may only serve to place further aspects of human reproduction under the control of specialist men and further deny the different experiences of women and men in the process of reproduction. The unquestioned availability of technological conception could provide increased pressure on women to conform to the definition of femininity that requires motherhood.

The failure to examine the assumptions that uphold the concept 'family' in the debates about reproductive technologies (regardless of whether the technologies would prevent or allow conception or childbirth) has led to a confusing repetition in the use of language. The same terms are used by both sides in the debates about the use of the technologies, often with very different meanings. Thus the abortion debate explores the opposition of the 'right to choose' for women and the 'right to life' and lack of 'choice' for fetuses. In the Australian parliament there was considerable debate about whether fetuses were humans within the intention of the Human Rights Commission Bill (enacted 1981). While the claim that such a reading of the International Covenant on Civil and Political Rights and the Declaration of the

Rights of the Child was specifically ruled out by the drafting committees (UNESCO, 1977: 19), the Covenant does privilege the family. 'The family is the natural and fundamental unit of society and is entitled to protection by society and the State.' (Article 23, Section 1). The family is assumed to be unitary rather than an association of individuals with unequal power and the possibility of conflicts of interest and conflicts of rights. The nineteenth-century 'legal fiction' of the unity of the wife within the husband is the immediate antecedent of this kind of formulation in use by liberals and conservatives alike.

One outcome of new technologies of human reproduction may be the provision of further dimensions to the definition of women as mothers by providing new opportunities for state intervention. Already commentators have asserted that the state has an obligation to provide IVF services because childless couples have a 'right' to bear children (*Daily Telegraph*, 12 May 1982). To use the term 'right' here is to expand the conventional thinking about rights beyond the requirement that states do not stand in the way of an individual's exercise of her capacities as long as her activities do not cause harm. The right to bear children only makes sense as a demand against a government that has outlawed childbirth, not as a call for services to reverse physical infertility. Childbearing, as a 'right' in a family perceived as a 'natural and fundamental unit of society', could become a symbol of adult good citizenship rather than a biological consequence of heterosexual intercourse or a socially valued option for young adults, especially women. If the state provided the means for achieving conception, it would allow 'good' citizens to be distinguished from 'bad' anti-social childless couples and individuals and a framework for state-defined criteria of good motherhood. This is but a step beyond the state intervention in the fertility decisions of many women, who 'choose' abortion or sterilisation in the face of inadequate child care facilities, low welfare benefits, high unemployment, and personal isolation. The public sector is reluctant to provide financial support for the private realm on which it depends.

Rights and needs are used to attack and defend technical intervention in the biological process of reproduction. The demands of women for abortions are labelled selfish or even anti-social by some, while the IVF programmes are justified by the demands of women as a recognition of their 'need' to have children. Both arguments involve a reinforcement of the definition of women as mothers either by compelling or enabling motherhood. Sterility is indeed a social problem when childbearing is the only acceptable activity for women in a world divided into public and private realms. Human rights can be interpreted as excluding women's rights to abortion and perhaps contraception, while including the right to give birth, even if sterile, only from a political perspective in which the existence of rights depends on a division of society and the assumption that male-headed families constitute a 'fundamental unit'. In such a society the power relation upheld by the law and by medical technology is taken as given, not critically examined as the context in which changes are taking place.

The demands of women that their lived experience be incorporated in medical research and technology cannot be heard, much less met, while priorities are set according to the 'needs' of scientists to do exciting frontier research and their 'right' to be funded for those priorities. The priorities are hard to change when critics are accused of ignoring the pain of infertile women or denying the value of a highly reliable contraceptive, and when feminist turns of phrase are used to restructure the control of women (e.g. IVF offers the 'choice' to give birth). Laws that criminalise abortion cannot be altered to acknowledge the control women have always sought to exercise over their fertility, but only to hand control to a group of male-oriented specialists. The growing orthodox literature on reproductive technology is silent about the social relations that structure human reproduction. The consequences of the changes during the past thirty years that have led to the development of IVF and other new technologies will be better understood once those silences are broken and the network of power relations in which they are embedded is exposed. Until then any changes are likely to reinforce the familiar relations of power and control. With sufficient knowledge, feminists can avoid the empty polemic that closes discussion and engage in a passionate and informed examination of the concerns of 'private' life. Yes, it will be hard, but, with women's lives at stake, can anything less be attempted?

## NOTES

1  This essay has appeared in different versions: first as a conference paper at the 1982 Australasian Political Studies Association Conference in Perth, Western Australia, then in a collection of articles by members of the APSA Women's Caucus (Simms, 1984). No ideas fall from the sky; this article is no exception. Barbara Blackadder and Kay Fielden forced me to see the connections between their work on IVF and mine on fertility control, and conversations with Lynne Hutton-Williams and Terri Jackson have made significant contributions to the development of those connections.

2  The widespread use of the 'pill', IUD, AID, fetal monitors during labor, and instrumental or surgical deliveries have been instituted within this time. They are different from earlier interventions because they are now seen as routine, not reserved for 'problem' cases.

3  Liberal democratic theory was a product of the struggles to overthrow absolute monarchical regimes. John Locke, Jean Jacques Rousseau and John Stuart Mill were prominent in its development. Feminist accounts of their work can be found in Okin (1979) and Eisenstein (1981).

4  For example: yes, in the Royal College of Obstetricians and Gynaecologists Ethics Committee Report in Britain; no, in the state government inquiry in Victoria, Australia.

5  Pfeffer and Woollett (1983) provide a welcome feminist account of the experiences of women during the process of diagnosing infertility in addition to a description of the range of tests and treatments for infertility.

6  The woman had an abortion after winning cases in three different courts.

7  1967 Abortion Act, United Kingdom.
   1969 Revision of Section 237 Criminal Code, Canada.
   1969 Menhennitt Ruling in *R*. v. *Davidson*, Victoria, Australia.
   1970 Cook-Leichter Bill, New York State was the most radical legislation in the USA during this period.
   1971 Criminal Law Consolidation Act 1935–1971, South Australia, Australia.
   1971 Levine Ruling in *R*. v. *Wald* et al., New South Wales, Australia.

1973 Supreme Court ruling in *Roe* v. *Wade*, United States of America.

# REFERENCES

Eastwood, Mary. 1971. 'The Double Standard of Justice: Women's Rights under the Constitution'. *Valparaiso University Law Review*, vol. 5.

Ehrenreich, Barbara and Deirdre English. 1979. *For Her Own Good: 150 Years of the Experts' Advice to Women*. Pluto Press, London.

Eisenstein, Zillah. 1981. *The Radical Future of Liberal Feminism*. Longman, New York.

Greenwood, Victoria and Jock Young. 1976. *Abortion in Demand*. Pluto Press, London.

Kickbusch, Ilona. 1981. 'A Hard Day's Night: Women, Reproduction and Service Society' in Rendel, Margherita, ed. *Women, Power and Political Systems*. Croom Helm, London.

Mason, Stephen. 1982. 'Abnormal Conception'. *Australian Law Journal*, vol. 56, no. 7.

Okin, Susan Moller. 1979. *Women in Western Political Thought*. Princeton University Press, Princeton, NJ.

Pfeffer, Naomi and Anne Wollett. 1983. *The Experience of Infertility*. Virago, London.

Rendel, Margherita, ed. 1981. *Women, Power and Political Systems*. Croom Helm, London.

Rich, Adrienne. 1976. *Of Woman Born*, Norton, New York.

Sachs, Albie and Joan Hoff Wilson. 1978. *Sexism and the Law: A Study of Male Beliefs and Legal Bias in Britain and the United States*. Martin Robertson, Oxford.

Seaman, Barbara and Gideon Seaman. 1978. *Women and the Crisis in Sex Hormones: An Investigation of the Dangerous Uses of Hormones from Birth Control to Menopause and the Safe Alternatives*. Harvester Press, Sussex.

Simms, Marian. 1984. *Australian Women and the Political System*. Longman Cheshire, Melbourne.

*Sun-Herald*, Sydney. March 28, 1982.

Tedeschi, Claire. 1982. ' "Love-child" Pippin'. *Sun-Herald*, 28 March.

*Daily Telegraph*, Sydney. May 12, 1982 and March 24, 1983.

UNESCO. 1977. *Human Rights Aspects of Population Programmes with Special Reference to Human Rights Law*. Paris.

Walters, William and Peter Singer, eds. 1982. *Test-Tube Babies*. Oxford University Press, Melbourne.

Wood, Carl and Ann Westmore. 1983. *Test-Tube Conception*. Hill of Content, Melbourne.

# EGG FARMING AND WOMEN'S FUTURE

Julie Murphy

To scientists, it's an early procedure of in vitro fertilization, but to feminist Julie Murphy, the patriarchal practice of removing eggs from women's bodies is more aptly described as 'egg farming.' In this paper, Julie Murphy describes how, through reproductive technologies, women's eggs have become a sought-after commodity. She discusses the implications of egg farming for women's lives and women's future.

Women are defined in patriarchy as 'reproductive bodies.' Our bodies are regarded as potential carriers of unborn generations. Our bodies (we are told) exist for the production of the species. We are constantly discouraged, forbidden to use our bodies for ourselves.

Reproductive technology offers new methods for more complete control of our 'reproductive bodies.' There are technological methods for removing eggs from women's bodies, fertilizing eggs in laboratories with sperm, and returning fertilized eggs back into women's bodies. There are techniques for experimenting on human eggs, freezing and thawing eggs, and manipulating the contents of eggs. Scientific advances in egg research could be exciting, even liberating, for women in non-patriarchal cultures. In patriarchy, however, we have so little control of our lives that such reproductive techniques threaten our very survival.

Reproductive technology, in the service of patriarchy, assumes that women's bodies are fertile fields to be farmed. Women are regarded as commodities with vital products to harvest: eggs. Egg-farming thereby limits female bodies to reproductive bodies, more systematically than ever before.

I will use the term 'egg farming' to designate the entire scope of patriarchal reproductive techniques that remove our bodies from our control by separating our bodies from our lives. Egg farmers are patriarchal scientists who sustain the field of reproductive research by developing the stereotype of women as egg farms. Egg farmers include egg removers, egg fertilizers, embryo transplanters, otherwise known as fertility specialists, clinicians, biological researchers, and hospital technicians. All of these reproductive workers engage in egg farming to the degree that they perform their tasks without questioning the implications of reproductive technology for women's lives. The historical role of reproduction in the oppression of women suggests that any new reproductive technology warrants examination. Feminist analysis of egg farming is crucial for safeguarding ourselves from yet another even more dangerous patriarchal ploy.

Egg farming first began on female animals. In the 1920s, scientists developed methods for successfully removing eggs from rabbits. By 1959, methods were developed enabling rabbit eggs to be removed, fertilized and returned to a uterus of a live rabbit for normal growth and birth. Before the end of 1965, similar techniques were successful in mice, rats, hamsters, pigs, cows, sheep and monkeys.

Techniques for human egg farming have been developing for the past twenty years. Thousands of women in several countries have donated eggs and ovaries and have received embryos fertilized by reproductive scientists. By 1982, over one hundred children around the world had been born from eggs that reproductive scientists had successfully removed from women's bodies, fertilized, and returned to women's bodies for growth and birth. (Wallach, 1982)

Egg farming might be seen as helping women by helping 'barren' women bear children. After all, many women who experience egg farming seek reproductive techniques to solve fertility difficulties. A feminist analysis of egg farming must, however, examine how egg farming affects the total situation of women in patriarchy. Does egg farming further reinforce the assumption that women must bear children? Does egg farming give patriarchal scientists more complete control of 'child-bearing'? What shape would women's lives take if egg farming were practiced on a massive scale?

## 1  EGG TECHNOLOGY

The two processes of egg technology that directly affect women's bodies are egg 'recovery' and embryo replacement or transfer. (If the embryo is implanted in the same woman from which the egg was removed, the procedure is termed 'embryo replacement'; if in another woman's womb it is called 'embryo transfer'.) Since feminists have yet to trust patriarchy to look after our welfare, it is important to examine both of these steps in egg technology.

Egg 'recovery' marks the initial separation of women from our eggs. In the most popular method, women receive local anesthetic, gonadotropin injections, and ultrasound monitoring of the ovaries. The reproductive technologist punctures through a woman's abdominal wall, filled bladder, and ovary to obtain an enlarged follicle containing an egg. (Lenz and Lauritsen, 1982) The scientific term, 'egg recovery,' refers to the removal of eggs from women's bodies. Yet for women, 'egg recovery' is a misnomer. 'Recovery' implies prior attachment or ownership. One recovers something one once lost control of or misplaced. When eggs are taken out of women's bodies, however, women do not recover anything. Women lose something, namely, eggs. It is patriarchy that 'recovers' or possesses the eggs.

Patriarchal scientists engaged in egg 'recovery' debate the 'best' size of a harvest, the 'best' conditions for harvesting, and the 'best' women to be farmed. The egg farmer's central concern is the quantity and quality of the harvest itself, and not the life situations of the women who are farmed.

Embryo replacement and transfer, a second central use of women's bodies by egg farmers, occurs in the final step of egg farming. The egg, removed from a female body and fertilized in a laboratory, is, at this stage, an embryo ready to be implanted in a uterus for further growth. A catheter is loaded with one or more embryos and expelled into a woman's uterus. The reproductive scientist leaves the catheter inside the uterus for sixty seconds to ensure that the embryo has been expelled completely. If the embryo replacement transfer is successful, the embryo attaches to the wall of the women's uterus and is birthed by the woman's body. (Trouson et al. 1980)

The scientific terms, 'embryo replacement' or 'embryo transfer' suggest the primacy of the harvest itself. Women's bodies, the beginning and end points of the transfer, are entirely absent from the technical term.

The implications of egg technology for women's lives deserve serious consideration. Women are so necessary to egg farming research, and yet so peripheral to the egg farmers' concerns, that there is no record of exactly how many women in the world have received embryos by embryo replacement or transfer or the total number who have been egg farmed 'unsuccessfully.'[1] Egg farmers count only the number of successful harvests: one hundred as of this writing.

The primacy of the harvest marks a shift in patriarchy's perception of women, from seeing women as 'baby makers' to seeing women as 'egg storers.' Egg farmers view women as vast sources of eggs. At birth, a woman has over two million egg cells, all the egg cells she will ever have. Scientific researchers are fascinated by this huge supply of genetic material. They (Edwards, Bavister and Steptoe, 1969) describe the ovaries of a mature woman as 'a production line' of eggs.

Once egg farmers revision women's bodies as egg-storers, as housing the reproduction line of eggs, egg farmers assume, as well, the right to direct and control women's egg production. Patriarchal egg technologists approach women's bodies with the urgency of efficiency experts. The millions and millions of eggs present in women's bodies are seen by the technologists as millions and millions of unborn people. The high number of unused eggs, an average of 1,999,550 of the original two million eggs per woman, are judged as excessive 'egg wastage.' Embryos are seen as 'wasted' too. Three-quarters of all the eggs that are fertilized in women's bodies by copulation are automatically aborted. (Austin, 1972) The high rate of spontaneous abortion in women is termed 'embryonic wastage.' The terms 'egg wastage' and 'embryonic wastage' strongly indicate that, for egg farmers, women are ineffective, wasteful, storers of eggs. How can reproductive technologists remove 'waste' in reproductive practices? Egg farmers propose ways to employ new methods of egg storage that do not lead to egg wastage, and to thereby maximize the number of eggs in each harvest. Such methods include inducing superovulation in women, freezing eggs taken from women's bodies, freezing embryos outside of women's bodies, and transferring multiple embryos into a woman's uterus during embryo transfer. (Edwards and Purdy, 1982; Wallace, 1982; Biggers, 1981) Reproductive technologists use new techniques to take over and improve egg storage, leaving women to be merely the suppliers of eggs and the recipients of embryos.

Egg farming separates women from our bodies as it takes more and more control of our bodies. Advances in the removal and storage of eggs give patriarchy more immediate access to the whole of any woman's egg supply: the genetic material for creating a future population.

## 2  EGG FARMING AND WOMEN'S LIVES

How will egg farming affect women's lives in the near future? The benefits egg farming will offer women in terms of options in reproduction are far outweighed by the losses women will incur from patriarchy's technological control of our eggs.

At a glance, egg farming could be viewed as beneficial to women, or even as a sign of patriarchy's liberation of women. Through egg farming, many women who have not been able to reproduce can be involved in reproduction. Egg removal could function as a form of birth control, giving women more freedom in sexuality. Embryo transfer could enable women friends to exchange eggs and share pregnancies. Better storage techniques, egg freezing, can offer women the possibility of safeguarding eggs from environmental hazards. Embryo freezing might enable women to interrupt unwanted pregnancies temporarily by transferring embryos to other recipients. Women need not engage in all aspects of reproduction, but could be either egg donors or embryo recipients.

The benefits that reproductive technology extend to women in terms of ways to reproduce become suspicious when we realize that egg farming does not enable women to refuse to be reproductive bodies. What looks like personal fulfillment and occasional convenience for women, has, when placed in a patriarchal context, devastating implications for women.

The advantages that egg farming offers women within a patriarchal context must be seen in light of our losses. Through egg farming, women can be divided into two groups: egg donors and embryo recipients. In an entire society, all women could be engaged in reproduction, either as egg layers or egg hatchers. Both egg layers and egg hatchers would be controlled in terms of food, travel, work, and stress to ensure optimal conditions for the embryo. Women as egg layers are already in demand. I. D. Cooke announces the need for female ovum donors in the next decade. (Cooke, 1980) Women as egg layers and egg hatchers would be seen by patriarchy as the means to a vital commodity – eggs.

Women will be forbidden to keep our eggs out of circulation in patriarchy. Birth, administered by reproductive technology, will be the rule and abortion the exception. Women will not be allowed to not use, to destroy, our eggs.

Eggs, so small, so seemingly inconsequential, are prime matter for genetic engineering. Patriarchy sees our eggs as work tables for genetic manipulation.

In patriarchy's hunt for eggs, egg farming makes possible more complete control of reproduction. By dividing women into 'two classes' – layers and hatchers, our reproductive functions are further used to enforce reproduction as our *essential* being. Two reproductive classes of women can degrade women as 'parts' of 'reproductive bodies' and diminish our chances of obtaining reproductive rights for all women. As long as women are not free, as long as men determine the methods and ends of reproduction, choices in egg farming are choices for men.


## 3 EGGS AND ACTION

Our bodies are not 'reproductive bodies' in the service of patriarchy. Our bodies sustain our lives. Outside patriarchy, our bodies could even be used for our own enjoyment, for a multiplicity of purposes and pleasures we might choose. In patriarchy, we are 'reproductive bodies.' It is for reproductive ends that our bodies are sustained by patriarchal society and that we are allowed to survive.

We are not baby makers, egg layers, egg hatchers, egg storers, or egg suppliers. Our eggs do not constitute our value. In fact, until egg farming, our eggs went uncounted and unnoticed. Egg farming technology makes eggs a commodity, a scarce resource. Just as a country suddenly discovers that its minerals are necessary for the growth and expansion of a country that exploits it, we find that our eggs are suddenly of great value to patriarchy.

Reproductive technology challenges women's biological connection to our eggs by seizing control of the release, fertilization, and reimplantation of eggs in women's bodies. Women challenge reproductive technology by asserting our biological claim to eggs in order to prevent further exploitation of our bodies by patriarchal egg harvesting. In another system, not built upon the oppression of women, we might not need to lay claim to eggs found in our bodies at birth. We might even develop egg removal and egg transfer techniques that would be useful to us. Yet, since the egg farming of women's bodies currently exists within patriarchy, and is carried out for patriarchal ends, we must establish control over our eggs. We must challenge egg farming by establishing our bodies as other than 'reproductive bodies.'

We establish our bodies for ourselves by critically evaluating our function in patriarchal reproduction. We select actions that produce ways of existing that sustain us. We confront patriarchy by refusing to place our hopes for autonomy in future generations. We actively farm our present resources for concrete strategies that stop patriarchy. We separate ourselves, our eggs, our women's lives from the plans of patriarchal technologists.

## NOTE

1 In one study alone, 114 women were 'farmed' for eggs at the University of Kiel between January 1979 and October 1980. Given the incredibly high failure rate of new techniques and the long progression of technique development at major medical schools in the United States and Europe, one can speculate vast numbers of women have been 'unsuccessfully' farmed in addition to the 'successes.' For the above study, see: Mettler, Liselotte, Seki, Maritoshi and Bauklah, Vera, 1982.

## REFERENCES

Austin, C. R. 1972. *Reproduction in Mammals*, vol. 11: 134.
Biggers, J. D. 1981. 'In vitro fertilization and embryo transfer in human beings.' *New England Journal of Medicine*, 304 (February): 336.
Cooke, I. D. 'Targets for the Next Decade.' In D. W. Richardson, D. Joyce and E. M. Symonds, eds. 1980. *Frozen Human Semen*, Martinus Nijhoff, The Hague: 132.
Edwards, R. G., B. Bavister, and P. Steptoe. 1969. 'Early stages of fertilization in vitro of human oocytes matured in vitro.' *Nature*, 221: 635.
Edwards, R. G. and Jean M. Purdy, eds. 1982. *Human Conception in vitro*. Academic Press, New York: 67.
Lenz, S. and J. G. Lauritsen. 1982. 'Ultrasonically guided percutaneous aspiration of human follicles under local anesthesia: a new method of collecting oocytes for in vitro fertilization.' *Fertility and Sterility*, 38 (December): 673.
Mettler, Liselotte, Maritoshi Seki, and Vera Bauklah. 1982. 'Human ovum recovery via operative laparoscopy and in vitro fertilization,' *Fertility and Sterility*, vol. 38: 30.
Takagi, N. and M. Sasaki. 1976. 'Digynic Triploidy after superovulation in mice.' *Nature*, 264: 278.
Trouson, A. O., J. F. Leeton, C. Wood, et al. 1980. 'The investigation of idiopathic infertility by in vitro fertilization.' *Fertility and Sterility*, 34: 431.
Wallach, E. 1982. 'In vitro fertilization and embryo transfer in 1982.' *Fertility and Sterility*, 38 (December): 657.

# FROM MICE TO MEN? IMPLICATIONS OF PROGRESS IN CLONING RESEARCH

## Jane Murphy

'From mice to men? Implications of progress in cloning research' contrasts the idea that human cloning is simply science fiction material with the actual status of cloning research in mammals and the published documentation of an experiment in human cloning.

The setting of an interview with one cloning researcher (which includes several wall-poster advertisements using women's bodies to sell products to men) raises the question of whether scientists can avoid bringing society's dehumanizing attitudes toward women into their research when they surround themselves with physical reminders of these attitudes in the office or laboratory. Finally, the article discusses the implications that clonal reproduction would have for women, both as sources of 'materials' (eggs, uteri, etc.) for this technology, and as a group in a society which has a history of 'eugenics' thought and reproductive policy.

When did I first know what a 'clone' was? When I heard my first 'clone joke'? The summer I worked in the San Francisco Bay area and watched the young men wearing 'clone' t-shirts? When I noticed science fiction books incorporating cloning? During the 1980 presidential campaign when Ted Kennedy labelled Jimmy Carter a 'Reagan clone?'

Even if we have an idea of what cloning is in the back of our minds, it is easy to let it remain there, unexamined, because we are told that human cloning is no more than a science fiction fantasy or a humorous analogy for someone who is just like someone else. We picture laboratories like those depicted in Aldous Huxley's *Brave New World* (1932).

In recent years, cloning has been sensationalized in Ira Levin's novel and subsequent film, *The Boys From Brazil* (1976), in which Levin terrorized us with the threat of ninety-four Hitler clones established in families worldwide. Other science fiction novels – *Clone* (1972), *Joshua, Son of None* (1973), *Cloned Lives* (1976) – have explored the 'what ifs' of clonal reproduction.

'Science fiction.' This label has made it difficult to connect cloning with reality and to seriously consider what would be the implications of that reality. However, research is progressing and technology, such as that necessary for in vitro fertilization ('test-tube babies') is being developed. This technology may make clonal reproduction a possibility in the not-too-distant future. We must recognize that cloning is clearly more than a science fiction fantasy.

The word 'clone' is derived from the Greek word *klōn*, meaning twig or slip. As houseplants, for example, can be reproduced asexually through cuttings, cloning is a word for a form of asexual reproduction. Clonal reproduction does not involve sexual intercourse or even the union of egg and sperm. The theory behind cloning is that each body cell contains in its nucleus all of the genetic information (in the form of chromosomes) necessary to create a whole new organism that is genetically identical to the existing organism. It is only through the process of differentiation that a cell acquires its identity as a liver cell, brain cell, or skin cell, etc.: each cell still contains the entire genetic code for the organism.[1]

Each sex cell[2] has only half the genetic complement – in human beings this amounts to twenty-three chromosomes. When egg and sperm cells unite, the resulting zygote has the necessary forty-six chromosomes to develop as a human being. In cloning, egg and sperm nuclei are replaced by a somatic cell nucleus (somatic cells are body tissue cells with the full set of forty-six chromosomes) which is inserted into an 'enucleated egg.'

There are cloned frogs, cloned mice, and there is documentation of at least one experiment with human cloning.[3] Were it technically possible, the human cloning process, in very simple terms, would go like this: remove one or more eggs from a woman's ovaries. Enucleate an egg – that is, remove its nucleus (and, thus, all of the genetic information encoded in the chromosomes) so that all that remains is the egg cytoplasm (which is all of the cell material surrounding the nucleus). Remove the nucleus from the somatic cell of the clone donor and insert this nucleus into the enucleated egg.[4] Implant the egg, re-nucleated with a foreign nucleus, into a woman's uterus, where its growth will be nurtured and it will be fed for nine months until the cloned infant is 'delivered' in labor.

My immediate response to descriptions of the cloning process was a sense of horror; how perfect a metaphor the 'enucleated egg' is and has been for so many women's lives. Throughout history our accomplishments have been denied, ignored, and attributed to men. We have been prevented from passing our selves on to future generations. Men have claimed children as their 'heirs,' and women's art, writing, mathematical and scientific theories, etc., as their own. Like the enucleated egg, we are used as material in male enterprises and are prevented from expressing our identities and passing on knowledge of our selves.

I pursued the topic of cloning because of my sense that it and other genetic technologies are modern methods for patriarchy[5] to address ancient issues, i.e., the creation of life, the establishment of one's identity, and the inevitability of mortality. The popular literature on cloning is full of wonder at the possibility of immortality through the reproduction of one's genes and the promise of control over whose genes may or may not be reproduced.

My study of cloning research and literature began as an undergraduate thesis and was later supported by grant funding.[6] In August 1981, I visited a scientist who had been recently acclaimed for an accomplishment in the field of mammalian cloning.

He is younger than I expect, short and wiry. He greets me with bright eyes and animated gestures. We walk into the small cubicle that is his office. My eyes move beyond his sharply-featured face to the wall. A woman's buttocks in black-and-white-striped 'hot pants' straddle the seat of a motorcycle. For an instant, I am disoriented. The poster advertises Honda motorcycles.

'Personal touches,' I remember, 'this is his office.' I look around: prints of Oriental women dot the walls, a print of a woman who looks like a young Elizabeth Taylor. Above his desk, a row of snapshots: a middle-aged woman, young children, the family photos.

At first he is uncomfortable with my tape recorder – he is wary of being quoted in print. I explain that I will be able to concentrate better on the details of the experiments we are discussing if I am freed from note-taking. We talk for a while then, beginning with the very technical aspects of his recent experiments in 'nuclear transplantation' – a term he prefers to 'cloning,' which he considers sensationalized.[7]

We walk across the hall to use the blackboard in a small laboratory: brown light, dull grey cabinets, racks of test tubes on black formica counters, shiny steel equipment. On the wall next to the cabinets, five women in bathing suits stand on round pedestals, striking seductive poses. This poster, advertising a scientific supply company, reads: 'Brand X from any angle.'

Surrounded by these women, I feel estranged from myself. I feel him watch me, watch my responses as he illustrates an experiment in nuclear transplantation on the blackboard, and explains the ways that it may further understanding of a healthy cell's transformation to a cancerous cell. Does he see me as student, academic, writer, scientist? Or does he see me as the stereotype of my sex depicted in his posters?

I realized that his perception of me strongly affected the outcome of the interview. When we spoke over the telephone, he hesitated about giving an interview. He had declined to speak with the news media because he felt they sensationalized cloning and his recent experiments. Eventually, though, he seemed to reassure himself with my academic affiliations: the college from which I had recently received my degree, the grant supporting my study of cloning research. I suppose it was his sense of our shared academic bond that allowed him to feel comfortable sharing some ideas and fantasies that were not strictly 'straight science.'

He wanted to know what I would do with my research. It was obvious to me that I could not admit to the feminist critique of cloning that was developing as my work progressed. I explained that I felt that many people were only aware of the 'popular' notion of cloning – jokes, science fiction, etc. – and were unaware of the actual status of cloning research. I told him that I wanted to understand, and then explain, through my writing, the applications that scientists foresee for cloning research and, more generally, what the status of that research is – what can and cannot be done.

Because our interview was marked by exclamations such as 'But don't print that!' after comments that I considered important and interesting, the scientist that I interviewed will remain anonymous. He describes himself as a scientist who uses the technique of cloning or nuclear transplantation for studying 'development, differentiation, cancer. That's what I'm interested in doing. I want to gain information.' The most pressing questions he'd like to see his work address regard the cell nucleus's capacities: 'How far out in development can we go and still have that (cell) nucleus remain totipotent?'[8]

He is reluctant to state a specific goal for his research, but of all the applications suggested for cloning research, he puts understanding cancer first.

'What causes (a) cell to become cancerous?[9] The basic question (is): is that cell cancerous because of changes in the cytoplasm, or is it cancerous because of a change in the nucleus or did something happen to both the cytoplasm and the nucleus? . . . So I suppose you'd say that's my goal right now, but if you asked me a year from now my goal might be different. I may have made a discovery or I may have given up on that and done something else that looked more exciting to me.

As we discussed the idea that cloning techniques might, someday, have applications in the cure or prevention of cancer, I asked this scientist whether or not the technology to clonally reproduce an adult human being would simultaneously develop with these cancer applications. Reluctantly, he agreed that it would.

Can we take the cell from an adult mouse and reproduce that mouse? That's basically what I'm saying. But now let me say that I see no application of the technique in humans. There's no application. You still can't beat the old fertilization as the best means of producing offspring in the human population.

And yet, despite the fact that our discussion was sprinkled with vehement assertions such as the above that cloning was a research tool that had no application to human reproduction, at one point he proposed two situations in which society might *need* to use clonal reproduction:

It may be a technique that may be necessary at some time. . . . Let's say we become a population of people in outer space and, in outer space, maybe copulation cannot occur – God forbid – and so in order to have reproduction, because the population lived in space for generations, the population would have to reproduce maybe by nuclear transplantation.

I'm just saying that way out in the future that something could happen, some type of infertility could occur in the population such that normal copulation, normal fertilization could not occur . . . . who knows what the effects of irradiation[10] might be?

You might destroy the genome[11] from all germ cells.[12] But yet the individual survived the nuclear disaster, and so their (somatic cell) nuclei are possibly all right. . . . (So you might) take the nucleus from a skin cell and put it into an egg – you'd have to take the abnormal genome out of the egg and put in a healthy nucleus. That would assume that the radiation wouldn't harm a normal differentiated cell, whereas the germ cell is very sensitive to radiation.

Space colonies. Nuclear disasters. Cloning in outer space. Cloning on a devastated planet. Although this scientist takes pains to distinguish his research from what he sees as 'science fiction' – the application of cloning to human reproduction – he is able to imagine these kinds of scenarios for the implementation of clonal reproduction. How many serious 'straight science' scientists have such fantasies about the ways that their research might be used? How much do these fantasies influence the work they choose to do?

Later, as I walked to my car from the research center which housed his office, I realized how much I had been shocked by the posters – the advertising that objectifies and exploits parts of women's bodies to sell a product. I had not expected them there, neither in his office nor in the lab. I had not yet given much thought to imagining a personal context for the research that I had been reading about. But now I wondered: how can scientists help but reflect society's attitudes towards women in their work, when such objectifying and dehumanizing attitudes are a part of their own physical and mental landscapes? In these next few pages, I will explore the implications the possibility of clonal reproduction has for women, both as sources of 'materials' (eggs, uteri, etc.) for this technology, and as a 'minority' group in patriarchal society.

## FROM FROGS TO MICE: RECENT PROGRESS IN CLONING

David Rorvik's book, *In His Image: The Cloning of a Man* (1978) generated serious discussion of the possibility of human cloning, eventually provoking a House of Representatives subcommittee hearing on the subject in May 1978.

Chairman Paul Rogers's position during the hearing was that ethical questions should not precede the pursuit and realization of a technology. He closed the hearing by dismissing an ethical analysis of research in cloning because he felt that it had been proven that human cloning was impossible: 'We have learned from the scientific panel that cloning from an adult is not possible at this time. Therefore, perhaps we are premature in thinking of ethical questions that may arise.'[13]

The design of the hearing was simple: to reassure the public, through expert scientific testimony, that Rorvik's book was a hoax, that human cloning was impossible, and that it was therefore too early to ask ethical questions. The testifying scientists pointed out that research had progressed only as far as cloning frogs. The feasibility of cloning mammals was doubted because mammalian eggs are much smaller and more difficult to manipulate than those of amphibians, such as frogs.

This has proved ironic: in January 1981, Drs Peter Hoppe and Karl Illmensee published a paper in the journal *Cell*, documenting the successful transplantation of three embryonic[14] mouse cell nuclei into three enucleated mouse eggs. The three mice that resulted were each clones of the mice from which the embryonic cell nuclei were derived. Only two years after the subcommittee hearing, the 'feat' of mammalian cloning had been accomplished, providing a base for further research in cloning mice, or other mammals, at later stages in their development.[15]

A major challenge that remains to the cloning of an adult human or other mammal is to manipulate *adult* body cell nuclei (which are fully developed and differentiated) so that they 'forget' their specific identity (as skin cell, for example), and use their genetic material to direct the growth of an entire organism. The mice in the above experiment were cloned from embryonic mouse cell nuclei – which are young and relatively undifferentiated – and thus might more easily be provoked to develop into a genetically identical organism.

Dr Landrum B. Shettles,[16] a physician who has long been associated with research in sex pre-selection techniques and in vitro fertilization research, attempted to by-pass this problem with adult cell nuclei in an experiment he reported in the *American Journal of Obstetrics and Gynecology* in January 1979. Shettles used spermatogonial cells as the source for his somatic cell nuclei. Spermatogonia precede sperm in development (that is, they eventually divide and become sperm cells, with twenty-three chromosomes each) and have the full forty-six chromosomes; they also proliferate rapidly, and thus are relatively young and undifferentiated. Shettles removed the nuclei from spermatogonial cells and implanted them in enucleated eggs. These eggs underwent several cell divisions over the course of three days, before Shettles 'discontinued' the experiment. According to Shettles, 'there was every indication that each specimen was developing normally and could readily have been transferred in utero.'[17] An interesting aspect of this work is that spermatogonia are, of course, unique to men, and therefore this is a technique of clonal reproduction which could only be used to clone men.

## THE FATHER AS SOLE PARENT

*Cloning men* is exactly what much of the popular literature on cloning discusses. Rarely is the idea of a woman being cloned mentioned, and then it is to suggest the cloning of a beauty queen – Raquel Welch, for example. In an article for *Esquire*, Rorvik writes with enthusiasm that cloning 'will also make possible the birth of a child whose only parent is a male.' He continues:

> Before long, even men could, if they wished, get along by themselves. Dr. James Watson, the Nobel Prize-winning molecular biologist, predicts that clonal propagation, by which we can make identical copies of ourselves by using single body cells rather than two sex cells, can be achieved by man within twenty years.[18]

Cloning is the most extreme development along a continuum in science, religion, and other aspects of society, that attempt to immortalize men by establishing 'The Father' as the sole parent in creation. This idea runs across the patriarchal time-line from the Greek myth of Athena springing forth from Zeus' head to the Christian myth of the Virgin Mary's impregnation with a pre-formed Christ by the power of the Holy Ghost, to the creation of bodies of knowledge – 'professions,' – to the development of cloning technology.

Father of His Country. Father of Modern Science. Father of Gynecology. Father of the Industrial Revolution. Father of the Nuclear Age. Father, Son and Holy Ghost.

Patriarchy's struggle with the issues of mortality and the meaning of life are evident in this 'Father as Sole Parent' mythology. By 'creating' or 'giving birth' to *someone* – an offspring, themselves – or *something* – an invention, a profession – men somehow escape mortality and live on, into future generations.

Proponents of cloning as a reproductive technology in fact suggest that men may gain a sense of immortality by duplicating their genes in offspring. Donors of somatic cell nuclei would see themselves as sole genetic parents via clonal reproduction and, in this way, might achieve a sense of extending themselves into the next generation. 'Cloning would permit the preservation and perpetuation of the finest genotypes[19] that arise in our species – just as the invention of writing has enabled us to preserve the fruits of their life's work.'[20]

This type of thinking, which suggests that producing a clonal offspring grants the donor a certain kind of immortality, implies a belief that much of identity is tied up in one's genes. To suggest that a genetic replica will somehow *be* the donor or share in the donor's identity denies the uniqueness of personality, the differentiation of identity, that grows within a child because of her/his surroundings during early orientation to the world, and beyond, into her/his years of exchange with various kinds of people and environments.

## WHO WOULD BE CLONED?

Cloning technology promises men not only a kind of personal immortality by enabling them to view themselves as sole parent, but also a means of resolving another age-old patriarchal issue – that of the constitution and ordering of human society. Who should be reproduced? How can social hierarchy be rationalized?

> If a superior individual and presumably genotype is identified, why not copy it directly rather than suffer all the risks including those of sex determination involved in the disruptions of recombination?[21] Leave sexual reproduction for experimental purposes. When a suitable type – meaning person – is identified, take care to maintain it by clonal propagation.
>
> Dr Joshua Lederberg, Nobel Laureate

One suggestion has been to remove genetic material from each individual after birth and then promptly sterilize that individual. During the individual's lifetime, records would be kept of accomplishments and characteristics. After the individual's death a committee decides if his [sic] accomplishments are worthy of procreation. If so, some genetic material would be removed from the depository and stimulated to clone a new individual. If the committee decides the genetic material is unworthy of procreation, it is destroyed. The question indeed is not a moral one but a temporal one. When do we start?

Dr James Bonner[22]

How would cloning be used as a reproductive technology in our society? Who would determine what Dr Lederberg labels a 'superior genotype?' A committee, as Dr Bonner suggests? What would be their criteria for selection? How would they rationalize their selective process?

Perhaps the answers to these questions lie in the threads of eugenics[23] thought that are woven into the present functioning of science and society – in reproductive policies, for example, which use technologies such as in vitro fertilization to promote the fertility of married middle and upper-class white women, while encouraging the sterility of poor, black, and Third World women. Documentation of sterilization and contraceptive abuse in the US, and exported to Third World countries from the US, exposes a coalition of scientific, medical, governmental and social institutions exercising the power to control our lives and our bodies, to decide who shall give birth.[24]

Because it would allow an ultimate degree of control over reproduction – the power to decide exactly who shall reproduce – cloning is a potentially powerful tool for such a coalition with its racist, sexist and classist policies. Believing that genes determine identity, those in power could attempt to preserve the status quo by reproducing their genes exclusively or perhaps those of appropriately passive and obedient members of other groups. (Of course, the identity of these clones could not actually be pre-determined. Aside from environmental influences, there is a certain amount of genetic influence that would be exerted by the enucleated egg's cytoplasm – see note 4. I imagine that the expectations with which these clones were raised – to be a leader, an engineer, a servant, etc – would influence them as well.)

## ENUCLEATED EGGS, SURROGATE MOTHERS: IMAGES OF WOMEN IN CLONING

In order to achieve either of these goals – the ability to see males as sole parents in clonal reproduction, or to control who is reproduced through cloning – all female creativity must be extracted from the procreative process, and men (in the form of physicians, technicians, nuclear donors) must view themselves as creative agents and directors of the process. This is exactly what is expressed in the literature on cloning. Women are viewed as passive, physical material for the cloning process: ovaries, eggs, uteri. Meanwhile, men are seen as 'parents' of clonal offspring – simply by donating a set of chromosomes!

Perhaps cloning is not so appealing a technology to women[25] because we have considered mothering to be the *process* of pregnancy, of labor, of nurturance; a mutual experience involving the giving of life, the physical changes, the growth, the movement inside, the physical pushing of another being into the world, the nursing and feeding. More than the donation of a complement of chromosomes, this has been 'mothering.'

The roles that women would play in cloning technology are similar to roles that women already play in other reproductive technologies: supplying researchers with eggs from our ovaries, donating our uteri for the implantation and gestation of someone else's child – the phenomenon known as 'surrogate motherhood.'

Nobel Prize-winner James Watson expects that women would willingly volunteer our services for this male creative enterprise:

There need not exist the coercion of a totalitarian state to provide the surrogate mothers. There already are such widespread divergences regarding the sacredness of the act of human reproduction that the boring meaninglessness of the lives of many women would be sufficient cause for their willingness to participate in such experimentation.[26]

Patriarchal society has long used the institution of mother-hood to prevent women from exercising other aspects of our creativity in society. Ironically, Watson suggests that *surrogate* motherhood may provide women with an alter-native to what he considers 'boring, meaningless lives.'

In cloning, surrogate motherhood is a label used to assert the absence of a mother, to strengthen the image of father as sole parent, and therefore it serves only to diminish women's presence in reproduction.

Images of women: buttocks, breasts, and hips on the scientist's wall posters; drudges living 'boring, meaningless lives' in Watson's imagination, the 'enucleated eggs' and 'nourishing wombs' of Rorvik's cloning descriptions. A society that etches such 'pornographic' images of women into the minds of men is likely to use the technology of clonal reproduction in ways that also reduce and define us: as ovaries, enucleated eggs, and surrogate mothers to clones of 'superior genotypes.'

## NOTES

1  The process of differentiation, through which a cell develops its own particular identity (as nerve or muscle cell, for example) is not well understood. Since an organism's cells all have the same genes in their nuclei, the factors determining or triggering differentiation may be the genetic constitution of the cytoplasm, the influence of neighboring cells or perhaps other environmental influences.

2  Egg and sperm are the sex cells. They are the only body cells with one-half the human complement of chromosomes, that is, twenty-three.

3  Dr Landrum B. Shettles performed this particular experiment and described it in 'Diploid nuclear replacement in mature human ova with cleavage,' *American Journal of Obstetrics and Gynecology*, January 15, 1979, pp. 222–5.

4  The egg cytoplasm is proving to have a non-nutritive role in development of an embryo. It contains genetic information in the form of mRNA (messenger ribonucleic acid), which is derived

from the DNA (deoxyribonucleic acid) in the egg nucleus. So, although an egg's nucleus may be removed, *some* genetic information remains in the cytoplasm, which undoubtedly influences development. As Paul R. Gross wrote in *Science*, April 14, 1978, p. 128:

> There is . . . no possibility in principle of making copies identical to an individual donor by the method being discussed. All animal ova studied so far, including those of mammals, contain a population of 'maternal' messenger RNA molecules, laid down in the egg cytoplasm during oogenesis, and functioning in protein synthesis during development proper. . . . The maternal messages are not genes, to be sure, but they are immediate products of genes, and they carry an enormous amount of genetic information. . . .
>
> There is therefore no possibility that a *literal* copy of the donor individual can be produced by the insertion of a somatic nucleus into recipient cytoplasm of a conveniently available egg. A roughly similar individual, yes, but a carbon copy, no.

5  I use this word to name a tradition or society in which men dominate and are preoccupied with acquiring the power to control, manipulate and exploit others in order to establish their own identities.

6  Through the Threshold Fund, associated with Hampshire College, Amherst, Ma. In addition to expressing my gratitude to this fund, I thank David Smith, Ann Woodhull and Michael Gross, of Hampshire College, Amherst, Ma. for support and invaluable discussion and criticism.

7  As he put it,

> One of the big problems is that you get the resentment for a particular technique and this is why I didn't like the press calling it *cloning* because cloning is a term that scares people, and when you scare people it's conceivable that they would put restrictions on the funding of research such that I could not do this experiment.

8  If the nucleus is 'totipotent,' it is capable of supporting the growth and development of an entire organism, if placed in an enucleated egg; it is capable of 'forgetting' its specific identity in order to do this.

9  He is asking this at the level of the cell, rather than the environment:

> What we're looking at is the susceptibility of that cell to a carcinogen and in certain people that cell is much, much, more sensitive, more susceptible to being transformed by that

environmental factor than other people, now what accounts for that susceptibility? If we could find out, then we wouldn't have to worry about the environment. We simply prevent the susceptibility of that cell.

10  Irradiation is an assault on the body by a dose of radiation, such as would occur in a nuclear disaster.

11  All of the genes in a cell nucleus.

12  Another name for sex cells – egg and sperm.

13  Paul Rogers, speaking in *Developments in Cell Biology and Genetics*, p. 90.

14  These particular cells were taken from mice embryos four days old.

15  In *Cloning: A Biologist Reports*, Dr Robert G. McKinnell writes: 'Since nearly all mammal eggs are the same size . . . the cloning procedure ought to be applicable to most mammals, including humans.' (p. 79)

16  It is interesting to note that Shettles teamed up with David Rorvik to write *Your Baby's Sex: Now You Can Choose* and *Choose Your Baby's Sex*.

17  Landrum B. Shettles in 'Diploid nuclear replacement in mature human ova with cleavage,' *American Journal of Obstetrics and Gynecology*. p. 225.

18  David Rorvik. 'Present shock,' p. 26.

19  The complement of genes inherited from both parents.

20  Robert L. Sinsheimer. 1973. 'Prospects for Future Scientific Developments' in Bruce Hilton et al., *Ethical Issues in Human Genetics*, p. 344.

21  The merging of maternal and paternal chromosomes after conception and the subsequent reorganization of genes to create a unique individual.

22  Lederberg and Bonner are quoted by Jeremy Rifkin, testifying in *Developments in Cell Biology and Genetics*, pp. 76–7.

23  The eugenics movement dates back to the turn of the century, and sought to 'improve' society by controlling its genetic constitution.

24  For discussion of sterilization and contraceptive abuse, see Holmes et al., editors. *Birth Control and Controlling Birth: Women-Centered Perspectives*.

25  For feminist criticisms of cloning technology, see Mary Daly, 1978, *Gyn/Ecology*, pp. 101–2; Robin Morgan, 1978, 'Baby born without a mother,' *Ms.*, May 1978; Adrienne Rich, 1976, *Of Woman Born*, pp. 67–9; and Carol Rivers, 1976, 'Genetic engineers: now that they've gone too far can they stop?,' *Ms.*, June 1976.

26  James Watson, 'Moving toward the clonal man,' p. 52.

# REFERENCES

Cowper, Richard. 1972. *Clone*. Doubleday, New York.

Daly, Mary. 1978. *Gyn/Ecology*. Beacon Press, Boston.

*Developments in Cell Biology and Genetics*. 1978. Hearing before the Subcommittee on Health and the Environment. Serial no. 95–105. US Government Printing Office. Washington, DC.

Freedman, Nancy. 1973. *Joshua, Son of None*. Delacorte Press, New York.

Hilton, Bruce, et al., eds. 1973. *Ethical Issues in Human Genetics*. Plenum Press, New York.

Holmes, Helen B. et al., eds. 1981. *Birth Control and Controlling Birth: Women-Centered Perspectives*. Humana Press, Clifton, NJ.

Hoppe, Peter and Karl Illmensee. 1981. 'Nuclear transplantation in mus musculus: developmental potential of nuclei from preimplantation embryous.' *Cell*, vol. 23, January 1981: 9–18.

McKinnell, Robert G. 1979. *Cloning: A Biologist Reports*. University of Minnesota Press. Minneapolis, MN.

Morgan, Robin. 1978. 'Baby born without a mother.' *Ms.*, May.

Rich, Adrienne. 1976. *Of Woman Born*. W. W. Norton, New York.

Rivers, Carol. 1976. 'Genetic engineers: now that they've gone too far can they stop?' *Ms.*, June.

Rorvik, David. 1971. 'Present shock.' *Esquire*, August.

Rorvik, David. 1978. *In His Image: The Cloning of a Man*. J. P. Lippincott, Philadelphia.

Rorvik, David and Landrum B. Shettles. 1970. *Your Baby's Sex: Now You Can Choose*. Dodd, Mead & Co., New York.

Rorvik, David and Landrum B. Shettles. 1977. *Choose Your Baby's Sex*. Dodd, Mead & Co., New York.

Sargent, Pamela. 1976. *Cloned Lives*. Fawcett Gold Medal Books, New York.

Shettles, Landrum B. 1979. 'Diploid nuclear replacement in mature human ova with cleavage.' *American Journal of Obstetrics and Gynecology*, 133(2): 222–5.

Sinsheimer, Robert L. 1973. 'Prospects for future scientific developments.' In Bruce Hilton et al., eds. *Ethical Issues in Human Genetics*. Plenum Press, New York.

Watson, James. 1971. 'Moving toward the clonal man.' *Atlantic Monthly*, May.

# DESIGNER GENES: A VIEW FROM THE FACTORY

Shelley Minden

Working as a technician in medical genetics has made me concerned about both the inner politics of laboratories and the information they produce. Although the medical experts who 'know our genes' are primarily men, most of the actual work in labs is done by women. As the potential for abusive applications of genetic manipulations seems to be rapidly increasing, hopefully we feminists both inside and outside science can work to bring women more control over research that affects our lives.

' "The Man" is coming,' someone warns, and the white-coated women swivel their chairs away from one another and turn towards the door. The weekly meeting of the genetics laboratory is about to begin.

In 1974, when I first got a job as a technician in a genetics laboratory, I little imagined some of the experiences that were to result. For one thing, I was to become virtually an expert on the politics of 'harems', for out of the four such positions I eventually came to hold, every one involved a male medical doctor or researcher who directed a group of entirely women technicians. And for another thing – which I little expected at the time – I was about to become a first-hand observer during a dramatic burst of knowledge about human genetics. During the years since then, both the inner politics of laboratories and the information they produce have made me worried: as the potential for genetic manipulations of humans draws near, how can we expect that society's applications of that knowledge will be any less rooted in the patriarchal power structure than the laboratory workplace?

Will we witness the use in humans of what the media calls 'designer genes,' artificially created genes inserted into embryos according to someone's idea of 'improving the race'? Will women face a new battery of genetic tests and procedures – during, and perhaps even before pregnancy? Will the options that emerge be available to all women who want them, and will all women be free from the danger of being coercively subjected to them?

In working as a subordinate within the medical establishment, it's hard to ask questions about ethical and political issues. Those topics are considered best left to the 'experts,' and laboratory workers who insist on raising them are likely to be labelled as naive, disloyal, or both. Yet the experts, for the most part, are men, and, furthermore, they are an elite group with privileges and power that might be diminished if the general public was in charge of establishing and directing science policy.

## 'VALUABLE' ANIMALS

An experiment reported in *Nature* of December 1982 awakened the mass media to the possibilities inherent in genetic manipulations. The authors, a team of researchers from five laboratories, isolated a gene for growth hormone from rats. They removed eggs from female mice, and fertilized the eggs in the laboratory by in vitro fertilization. While fertilization occurred, they injected the gene for growth hormone (from rats) in to the eggs. Finally, they put the eggs back inside the mice and waited to see how the baby mice would develop.

The results were rat-sized mice, nearly twice the size of their littermates that had not been tampered with. The authors were enthusiastic about 'practical' ways in which this information could be applied to 'commercially valuable animals.' With the appropriate growth hormone, they suggested, perhaps animals could grow more rapidly, and on less food. Furthermore, they pointed out evidence which suggests that such genetic treatments may help to increase milk yields. Only a single note of caution was raised by the authors – that the quality of meat obtained from such engineered animals should be evaluated. (Palmiter et al., 1982, 614)

But what about those other 'commercially valuable animals' – people? Are we as easily subject to 'improvement'? Although no researchers have suggested that people be engineered for faster growth like farm animals, genetic manipulations have been proposed as a way to treat genetically caused diseases. Some diseases may result from complicated interactions between genes and the environment, but others have been found to be caused by single genes. These single gene disorders seem the most likely candidates for human genetic manipulations. In theory, they could be cured by 'gene therapy,' the replacement of 'faulty' genes with 'normal' ones.

So far, only one researcher has reported an attempt at gene therapy. Dr Martin Cline, once chief of hematology/ oncology at UCLA, injected genes for hemoglobin into the bone marrow of two patients with beta thalassemia, a disease caused by a single mutation within the gene for hemoglobin. The treatments were not successful, and Cline was censured for experimenting on humans before sufficient animal studies had been done. Despite his mishap, there may soon be another attempt at gene therapy, for the minutes of a meeting of a working group of the Recombinant DNA Advisory Committee of the National Institute of Health in the US includes the statement that a working group member would soon submit a proposal involving gene therapy with a human patient. (Recombinant DNA Advisory Committee, 1983)

In the day-to-day work of medical genetics laboratories, technical developments that could contribute to gene therapy are already apparent. Techniques that were developed by molecular biologists have recently come to be widely applied to human cells, with the result that it is newly possible to investigate many specific human genes. One important tool has been provided by a group of enzymes called 'restriction enzymes' that cut DNA into fragments that can then be separated from one another for detailed study. The places at which these enzymes cut DNA are determined by the sequence of the repeating molecules that make up DNA, and so variations in the pattern of cuts can reveal an abnormality within a gene.

The information gained from molecular studies of human DNA is currently being used in the development of a wide variety of diagnostic tests that can be used both pre-natally and after birth. (Orkin, 1982, reviews some recent applications of the techniques of molecular biology for prenatal diagnosis.) As it becomes increasingly possible to identify specific genes and to understand their biological function, the technical obstacles to gene therapy will be reduced.

## POLITICS AND GENES

The potential benefits of genetic manipulations are many. For example, people with Huntington's chorea carry a single gene which manifests itself during adulthood with a fatal disorder of the nervous system. If the gene could be exchanged for a normal one, then people who inherit it might be free from its effects. And if gene therapy could be practiced on embryos or fetuses, then people with the gene could have children who will not be subject to its effects.

Yet a number of crucial political issues are at stake in the treatment of genetic diseases. As activists for the rights of disabled people have asked: who will decide which genetic conditions are 'undesirable'? (See Anne Finger's paper in this collection.) What distinction can be made between attempts to reduce genetic diseases and eugenics: and what will happen if researchers attempt to associate genes with some behaviors, like schizophrenia, or depression?

Because some ethnic groups have higher frequencies than others of specific single-gene disorders, gene therapy raises the ominous possibility that specific ethnic groups may be singled out to provide subjects for the experimental development of gene therapy. For example, beta thalas-semia, the condition that Martin Cline attempted to treat with hemoglobin genes, occurs primarily in people of Mediterranean origin. Sickle cell anemia, most common among people who are Black, also involves the gene for hemoglobin. Tay Sachs disease is another single gene disorder, most common among Jews of eastern European origin. As of this writing, the Tay Sachs gene has not been identified.

The stages of life at which genetic manipulations might conceivably be applied are of crucial importance to women. Gene therapy, as it was practiced by Martin Cline, had adults as subjects, and so could presumably affect males as well as females. But if the treatments were applied to fetuses, or to fertilized eggs, as was the case with Palmiter's mouse experiment, then women would face the risk of new intervention during pregnancy, as well as the danger of being told – by medical researchers – what kind of children are 'acceptable' to give birth to. And what makes matters even more complicated is that genetic therapy could, at least in theory, be combined with any of the reproductive technologies that already exist: in vitro fertilization, embryo transfer, prenatal screening, etc.

Although the impact of genetic manipulations hasn't yet been felt, as feminists we need urgently to prepare for them. But the problem is – how do we keep informed of where the field, so dominated by men, is headed? As a technician, working in a highly compartmentalized job, it's nearly impossible to obtain crucial information, such as the areas in which the government is currently funding grants, and the ways that developments in one field might affect developments in another. But this is not to say that such information is unavailable. *Some* people know; they are the MDs and researchers who run the laboratories, travel to meetings, review each other's grant proposals, and participate in government committees that establish funding priorities and policy guidelines.

It's this imbalance of information that makes the power structure of laboratories have such dangerous implications for women. For crucial knowledge about how technologies will be developed and applied is primarily in the hands of men. And those women who do rise in the scientific hierarchy and might wish to address feminist concerns are likely to find that their positions are too precarious to permit them to do so.

The competitiveness of research is in itself a reason for much information to be confined to small groups within laboratories. Also, many researchers are afraid that public knowledge of their work could lead to reductions in funding, just as the public's concern with recombinant DNA has instilled in many scientists the fear that the public may be all too quick to curtail genetics research.

## SHARING WHAT WE KNOW

Since it is women who do much of the work in laboratories, we could, if we shared our knowledge, know as much as our male bosses do. After all, it's mainly *women* who type up grant proposals, carry out experiments, and care for laboratory animals. If we feminists in science could share what we know from all of these sources, we would no longer have to rely on the male 'experts' for all of our information.

By rejecting the notion of science as an all-male preserve, we can help to demystify its power over our lives. Hopefully, we can create channels through which feminists involved in reproductive research can connect with each other and with feminists outside of science.

Even if only a few feminists are involved in research pertaining to genetic manipulations, we could provide crucial information. Those of us in medical genetics could keep others posted on which human genes are currently being studied. Feminists who work with in vitro fertilization could share information about current research into manipulations of human eggs, and if there are feminists involved in research into cattle breeding, which now includes embryo transfer, freezing embryos, cloning, as well as genetic manipulations (see Rutledge and Seidel, 1983; and Seidel, 1981) the information they could provide would be crucial.

And if it turns out that there are more than a handful of feminists in medical research, perhaps we could organize with other women workers to make some real changes, not only in how laboratories are run, but in what it is they study.

When the mass media present ethical and political questions involved in genetics research, they address us as if there's an either/or choice to be made: either the research should continue as it is, or funding should be stopped. Yet, just as feminists have come to reject many of the dichotomous 'choices' given to us by the patriarchy, I doubt that feminists in or out of medical research are likely to agree with either of those options. There's too much potential for information that could help people's lives to justify stopping genetics research. And too much of a power imbalance is being created by things as they are now.

But what if we could change how science is practiced, and who controls the applications? Maybe it could be set up so that all of us can participate, especially those most affected – women, people with disabilities, people from different ethnic groups, and the parents of children with genetic diseases. And maybe, in a society in which all people could have input into research policies, we wouldn't have to live in dread of the applications of results from scientific laboratories.

## REFERENCES

Orkin, Stuart H. 1982. 'Genetic diagnosis of the fetus.' *Nature*, 296 (March 18): 202–3.

Palmiter, Richard D., Ralph L. Brinster, Robert E. Hammer, Myrna E. Trumbauer, Michael G. Rosenfeld, Neal C. Birngerg, and Ronald M. Evans, 1982. 'Dramatic growth of mice that develop from eggs microinjected with metallothioein-growth hormone fusion genes.' *Science*, 300 (December 16): 611–15.

Recombinant DNA Advisory Committee Working Group for Development of Response to President's Commission's Report on Ethical and Social Issues. 1983. Minutes of June 24 meeting. Department of Health and Human Services, Public Health Service, National Institutes of Health.

Rutledge, J. J., and George E. Seidel, Jr. 1983. 'Genetic engineering and animal production.' *Journal of Animal Science*, 57 (suppl. 2): 265–71.

Seidel Jr., George E. 1981. 'Superovulation and embryo transfer in cattle.' *Science*, 211 (January 23): 351–7.

# INSIDE THE SURROGATE INDUSTRY

Susan Ince

This article offers a first-hand account of a woman's experience in applying to become a surrogate mother. It exposes the lack of medical and psychological safeguards, the insensitivity to both surrogates and women with infertility, the surrogate's precarious legal and financial position, and the extensive controls over her life by the company. The essay provides a radical feminist analysis of this male-controlled 'growth industry'.

> This is not a nine-to-five job. It demands enormous commitment and understanding. It requires your total thought and consciousness, full-time, twenty-four hours a day.[1]

The job was for the key position in one of the 'growth industries' of the 1980s, and involved rigid application processes, including thorough medical examination, intelligence testing, psychological evaluation, and even genetic screening if indicated. I had just applied to become a surrogate mother.

From first reading the glowing newspaper reports and seeing the self-satisfied lawyers on television, I had been uneasy about the idea of a surrogate industry. I had played out lively and humorous 'what if' scenarios with friends, but had no substantive answers to the questions of proponents: what's wrong with it, if that's what the women want to do? Are you against them making money? Are you saying the industry should be regulated by the state? The questions were naggingly familiar, the same ones asked by apologists of the sex-buying industries, prostitution and pornography.

In order to get a first-hand look, I answered an advertisement placed in a local newspaper by a surrogate company considered reputable and established. Two weeks later, I met with the program's director and psychologist in their basement office on a street filled with small businesses and discount shops. The office looked newly occupied, and the director struggled with the unfamiliar typewriter and telephone system. Decorations included pictures of Victorian children; plump, white, and rosy-cheeked. Missing from sight were file cabinets, desks with drawers, and other standard office paraphernalia.

The director did most of the talking. I was touched by her stories of infertile couples – the woman who displayed the scars of multiple unsuccessful surgeries creating a tire-track pattern across her abdomen; the couple, now infertile, whose only biological child was killed by a drunk driver; the couples who tried in good faith to adopt an infant, and were kept on waiting lists until they passed the upper age limit and were disqualified. Stories like these, said the director, inspired her to offer a complete surrogate mother service to combine all the administrative, legal, and medical aspects of this modern reproductive alternative.

The screening and administrative procedures were outlined by the director as simple and proven successful. As a potential surrogate, I had to pass an interview with the director and psychologist, history and physical examination, and finally meet with a lawyer who would explain the contract before I signed to officially enter the program. Parents desiring surrogate services also had to pass screening by the director and psychologist, and pay $25,000 at contract-signing. Surrogate and purchasers never meet, although information about them is described so that both parties can determine if the match is acceptable. Complete anonymity is stressed as a benefit of going to this company instead of making private arrangements through a lawyer.

While pregnant, the surrogate receives approximately $200 to purchase maternity clothing, and is reimbursed 15¢/mile for transportation costs. It is her responsibility to enter the program with medical insurance that includes maternity benefits. The company will pay her medical and life insurance premiums and non-covered medical costs while she is in the program. After delivery of the baby to the father, the surrogate receives her $10,000 fee.

I tried to ask my many questions about the procedure in a curious and enthusiastic manner befitting a surrogate. The answers were not reassuring.

*What happens if you don't become pregnant?* Artificial insemination is tried twice a month for six months. If the surrogate has not conceived, she is then removed from the program and the father begins again with a different surrogate.

*And she receives no money for her participation?* 'No. Look at it this way. We pay all the fees and medical expenses. What has it cost you? Unless you start putting a value on your time.'

*What if she has a miscarriage?* Again, no money is paid to the surrogate. 'The father decides if he will take a chance again with her.' Then if the surrogate also wants to try again, there is a second attempt.

*What if the baby is born dead, or something is wrong with it and the father doesn't want it?* In this case, the surrogate has fulfilled her contract and is paid $10,000. 'We are not in the business of paying for a perfect baby. We are paying for a service rendered.' Possible fine-line distinctions between a late miscarriage (no fee to surrogate) and a stillborn premature baby (full fee paid) are made by the primary physician provided by and paid for by the company.

*What qualities are you looking for in a surrogate?* Ideally, they would like her to be married and to already have children. A healthy child provides 'a track record. It's as simple as that.' And the husband is a 'built-in support system.' They hastened to assure me, however, that there were exceptions (I am single with no children). 'Why, we just entered a single woman who had never been pregnant before. And the next couple that came in *demanded* a single donor. Things just always match up. It's a miracle!'

The director chatted on about the enthusiasm and good spirit of the 'girls' in the program so far. Many of them, it seemed, had added to the program by inventing creative ways to include the fathers more in the pregnancy and birth process. The women with infertility, who provide the basis for the industry's foundation, and who will become the adoptive mothers, are notably absent from consideration. It is expected that surrogates will 'write a nice note' to the father after conception, and many plan to follow this with a tape recording of the baby's heartbeat. One 'girl' even invited the father to be in the delivery room, and this was applauded as an altruistic gesture beyond anyone's expectations. 'But wait,' I asked wide-eyed. 'I thought everything was completely anonymous.' She looked at me as if I were a simpleminded child. 'Well, he's not going to be looking at her face! He's just there to see his baby come out.'

I was nervous two weeks later when I went to meet the psychologist who I thought would administer IQ tests and probe into my motivations to judge whether I was an acceptable surrogate. My plan was to offer no unsolicited information, but to tell the truth about all questions asked (except for my intention to become a surrogate). When I arrived, the psychologist was borrowing Kleenex from the tailor next door. I made a small wisecrack, 'What's a psychologist without Kleenex, right?', and he acted as if this was unusually clever. 'Boy, that's funny,' he said, continuing to chuckle as he returned to the office. 'You are really sharp.' Either he was attempting to put me at ease, or this was going to be easier than I thought.

We settled down for the actual interview. I was asked my name, address, phone number, eye color, hair color, whether I had any birth defects (no), whether I had children (no), whether I had relatives or friends in the area (yes, friends), whether I had a boyfriend (male friends, yes), whether I expected to someday marry, settle down, have babies and live happily ever after (no). He inquired as to my religious upbringing (Protestant) and began reminiscing about a college sweetheart ('Oh, I used to be so in love with a Protestant girl. . . .') Ten minutes later, we got back on track and I was surprised to find he had no more questions. 'I just needed to be sure you're still positive 100 per cent. You are, aren't you?' Without a nod or a word from me, he continued, 'You seem like it to me.'

Because I was 'obviously bright,' there would be no IQ testing. I was never asked whether I had been pregnant before, whether I was under medical or psychiatric treatment, or how I would feel about giving up the baby. To lower costs and save time, the medical exam would take place after I had signed the contract, while a match was being made. The psychologist pronounced me 'wonderful' and 'perfect,' and I awaited my next call.

Soon the phone rang and the director solemnly said she had two serious questions to ask me. 'It's not easy but I think it's important for us to lay our cards on the table. . . .' I gulped, thinking she was suspicious. 'I just want to ask you this straight up, right now, yes or no, are you going to have any trouble making appointments?' (I had rescheduled the last visit because of car trouble.) When I assured her that there would be no problem, she asked her second question. 'What are you going to do with the money?' This, I later heard her say, was asked of each surrogate to weed out those women who had frivolous motivations, such as 'buying designer jeans.' My answer was deemed acceptable, and screening was complete.

Although I was repeatedly assured that there had never been a problem with legal and financial arrangements made through the company, it was acknowledged by all concerned that this was a largely uncharted and confusing legal area. The contract itself repeated three times that a surrogate might seek her own legal counsel, fee to be paid by the program, to further her understanding of the concept, rules and regulations, rights and liabilities involved. After I was deemed ready to 'enter the fold,' I inquired about the independent legal consultation. There had been problems with that, the director said. Some of the 'girls' had submitted bills up to $500 for legal fees, which program members thought was exorbitant. Of even greater concern, surrogates had come back from their consultations with new doubts and questions. Because of this, I was strongly encouraged to see a nearby lawyer 'not associated' with the program, but already familiar with the contract, and selected and paid by the company to provide 'independent' consultations to all of the surrogates. When I said that I had my own lawyer in mind, she reiterated strenuously that she advised against it. As an example, she said, one girl had come back to her from an outside lawyer, saying 'He's asking me all these questions and he's really driving me crazy.' The director said, 'and after I sent her to see *our* lawyer, and he explained it *our* way, she felt much better and thanked me.'

I decided to hear how this independent company lawyer would explain the contract and our meeting was arranged. Before then, the director called to say she was eager for me to sign the contract on the same day as my consultation. A couple had been found who, after she had taken the liberty of describing me, said that they were very interested in me as a surrogate. More hesitant than I had ever heard her, she cautioned that we needed to discuss 'certain issues' which might be a problem. The father, she explained, was very bright, but Oriental, and would that be a problem? His wife was Caucasian. I said I couldn't see any problem, since the wife ought to be the one I was matching. She said that was *exactly right*, and that the couple could have easily adopted an Oriental child but they wanted a half-Caucasian. We would talk more at our next meeting.

To my surprise, the independent consultation was held within earshot of the director, who was called on by the lawyer to interpret various clauses of the contract, and who kept a record of questions I asked. The interview was held at the new corporate office, on a block filled with elegant fur and clothing shops in one of the richest counties in the United States. The move was explained as necessary for the convenience of the buying parents.

The director took me first into her office for a private chat before meeting the lawyer. A new couple was described – in the petroleum business, very wealthy, and building a new house in anticipation of my baby. She explained that this was a very common and positive sign, the parents 'inevitably building, remodeling, adding wings, buying new houses, not because they don't live in perfectly lovely homes, but because they want to be doing something for the baby during the pregnancy.' I asked if she had any plans to write a book including some of her interesting observations about the surrogate process. She nodded enthusiastically,

Oh yes, we are collecting data right now – if for nothing else than to dispel the misconceptions people have about surrogates. I'm very sorry to say it, but they don't think our surrogates are nice girls like you. When people think surrogate, they think tight black satin slacks. I don't know why, but they do.

By this time, the lawyer had arrived and we settled down with the contract. Three areas were of greatest concern to me: the extensive behavioral controls over the surrogate, her precarious legal/financial position should something go wrong, and the ill-defined responsibilities of the company itself. Each of these was broached during this interview with what I hoped were sincere and non-threatening requests for clarification. Briefly, the rules governing surrogates' behavior are as follows (quotation marks indicate exact language of contract):

*Sex:* The surrogate must abstain from sexual intercourse from two weeks before first insemination until a conception is confirmed.
The surrogate must not engage in 'sexual promiscuity.'
*Drug use:* The surrogate must not 'smoke nor drink any alcohol [*sic*] beverage from the time of initial insemination until delivery.'
The surrogate must not use illegal drugs.
*Medical:* The surrogate must keep all scheduled administrative, medical, psychological, counseling, or legal appointments arranged for her. These may be 'set by the physician in accordance with his schedule and, therefore, may not always be convenient for the surrogate mother.'
The surrogate must use the services (medical, psychological, etc.) which are chosen and provided by the program.
The surrogate must submit to all standard medical procedures and 'any additional medical precautions and/or instructions outlined by the treating physician.'

The surrogate must furnish medical and psychological records to the company and the parents.

In general, any action that 'can be deemed to be dangerous to the well-being of the unborn child' constitutes a breach of contract which means the surrogate will forfeit her fee, and be subject to legal action from the buyers.

The company lawyer responded to my questions about these restrictions by denying their importance and reiterating the good will of all concerned. On alcohol – 'You're on the honor system. No one is going to care if you have a glass of wine now and then.' On sexual promiscuity – 'Who cares? I don't know what that means. I don't know why that's in here.' When asked if there was a legal definition, he said, 'They just want to be sure who the father is. Intercourse doesn't hurt the baby, does it? Don't worry about it.'

I was worrying a lot, mostly about the company's complete control over the surrogate. There was no limit to the number of appointments that could be scheduled requiring the surrogate's participation. If she should become uncooperative, they could simply schedule more psychological visits. If they didn't want to pay her, they could schedule so many that she couldn't possibly keep them. The medical controls seemed particularly ominous: all standard procedures PLUS ANY OTHER precautions or instructions. This could include bedrest, giving up a job, etc. A medical acknowledgment attached to the main body of the contract advised that 'there are certain medical risks inherent in any pregnancy. Some of these may be surgical complications, such as, but not limited to, appendix and gall bladder.' Of course, these surgical complications would most likely arise from a cesarean delivery, major surgery which is not mentioned at all in conversation or contract. If the doctor should request one, the surrogate would have no contractual right to object.

Complications could also arise after birth. I learned that names of both surrogate and father would appear on the birth certificate, compromising promised anonymity, and that the certificate would only be destroyed several weeks, months, or years later when the child was adopted by 'the potential stepmother' (in the same way a new spouse can adopt a child if the former spouse wishes to relinquish her/his rights and responsibilities.) 'Why not right away?' I asked. The lawyer recommended a reasonable waiting period because an immediate adoption 'could be construed, by someone who wanted to construe it that way, as baby-selling.'

In fact, he elaborated, the baby-selling argument could also be used by a court to declare the entire contract illegal and void. It is acknowledged in the contract itself that its *rights and liabilities may or may not be honored in a Court of Law should a breach arise.*' The document further states that, in a lawsuit, it could be used to assist 'a court of competent jurisdiction in ascertaining the intention' of surrogate and parents.

If the surrogate breaches her contract, by abortion, by violation of rules, or by refusal to relinquish the child, the father may sue her for the $25,000 he paid into the program, plus additional costs. If the parents breach by refusal to accept delivery of the child or failure to pay medical expenses, the surrogate may sue them for her $10,000 fee, plus the expenses of child support or placing the child up for adoption. 'What about the company?' I asked. 'If something went wrong and I had to sue the parents, would they help me or pay my legal expenses?' 'No,' he replied. 'When the shit hits the fan you're on your own.' Indeed, each party is required to sign a 'hold harmless' clause which says that no matter what happens the company is not responsible. The lawyer explained this clause away as meaningless – everyone would, of course, sue everyone else if there should be a problem.

As we perused the contract, the lawyer discovered a new clause had appeared since his last consultation, the 'Amniocentesis Addendum' which stated that, should the treating physician request, the surrogate would submit to amniocentesis for prenatal diagnosis. If results were abnormal, she would consent to abortion at the parents' request. To my surprise, this clause out of the entire contract was worrisome to the lawyer. Why, he asked, should the surrogate abort at 20–4 weeks gestation and receive no fee, when she could carry the pregnancy to term and fulfill her contract regardless of the infant's condition? I was more concerned about what might be considered an abnormality sufficient to request abortion. What about a sex chromosome abnormality? What about just the 'wrong' sex? I was also concerned that this again allowed for the total discretion of the treating physician. Why was it left ambiguous in the contract when there is no legitimate indication for amniocentesis that couldn't be known before the pregnancy started? My suspicion was that it would always be requested, as an unacknowledged 'quality control' measure.

The lawyer called the director into the room, and asked about this clause's financial disadvantage to the surrogate. Any woman, she stated flatly, who would knowingly carry a defective fetus to term to cheat the parents out of $10,000 would not be acceptable to the program. Nevertheless, the lawyer suggested that I not sign until he spoke with the author of the contract, to suggest that a small fee be paid to the surrogate if there was such an unfortunate occurrence. My one request before signing was to see a copy of the parents' contract, to compare responsibilities, and to 'make sure they hadn't been promised something I couldn't fulfill.' The request was never honored.

The lawyer called the next day to say the Amniocentesis Addendum must remain as written. He paraphrased the company officials: 'The program works because it works the way it is. We cannot make big changes for the surrogate or the parents.' We arranged to meet a week later, after I had received the parents' contract, for final signing.

Before then, however, I was called by the director who had become concerned while listening in on my legal consultation. She admonished me for asking too many questions:

> The program works because it is set up to work for the couple. You have to weigh why you are participating in the program. For the money only, or to do the service of providing the couple with a baby. To be very frank, we are looking for girls with both those motivations. I felt after the last visit that this is a gal looking for every possible way to earn that money, and that concerns me. . . . We are playing with peoples' lives, with people who are desperately looking for a child. They have made an emotional investment . . . emotionally and in every other way that

baby is not yours. . . . No contract is perfect for anyone, for anything.

She urged me to take an extra week before signing, and if I was still interested to arrange to be reevaluated by the psychologist.

When I called to schedule the interview, I was informed it would not be with the original psychologist (who thought I was perfect) but with a new 'more convenient' one. I was very apprehensive about the visit, and when I knocked on the psychologist's door, about five minutes late, I expected to be confronted about my tardiness as yet another sign of my 'bad' behavior. No one answered my knock, but I could hear some-one coming down the hallway. A woman approached and let me in the unlocked door. I stood in the waiting room a few moments and the doctor arrived. As we shook hands, he said, 'I hear you've been knocking at my door.'

'Yes.'

'And you didn't even think to open it.' This was not a question but a statement: I felt my every move was open for analysis.

The doctor was in charge for the next one-and-a-half hours. It seemed he pried into every aspect of my family background. He was extremely interested in my romantic life, and my intention not to marry was considered unusual and an indication of not planning for the future. He also wondered how, with no man in town, I managed to 'feel loved and affirm my femininity.' ('By having this baby, of course!', I didn't say). As the session went on, I felt violated and bullied by this man, and too intimidated not to tell the truth. Only two of his inquiries obviously concerned becoming a surrogate mother: 'How will you feel if you aren't accepted for the program?' and 'Are you the kind of person who can start a task and complete it, or do you lose interest in the middle and abort the project?' ('Great choice of words, doctor.') He con-cluded the encounter with a short analysis of my psyche, explaining that he felt that I deserved this as payment for putting time and thought into the session. Again, I had gone through a psychological evaluation with no questions about whether I was under psychiatric care, whether I used medications or drugs, or how I would feel about carrying an anonymous man's child and giving it up after birth. He also seemed uninterested in my friends, emotional supports, living or employment situations. Only my relationships to men were probed.

About two weeks later, I received the verdict from the director: I was acceptable to the program and could start as soon as possible. I was embarrassed to find myself pleased to have 'passed' my analysis. I decided I could find out nothing further without signing the contract. Using a possible job transfer as an excuse, I asked to have my file put on hold a few months.

A few days following my last psychological evaluation, the director and lawyer for the company appeared on a holiday talk show, smiling and discussing at length the 'blessing' of this reproductive alternative. They were treated with deference by the host as they told the identical infertility stories, and outlined the tried and true professional process. At the time of my interviews, the 'tried and true' process had yet to result in even one pregnancy, so all hospital, contractual, emotional, and financial arrangements were untested.

The careful screening process was a myth. I encountered no evidence of real medical or psychological safeguards; just enough hurdles to test whether I would be obedient. The minimal questioning I did was labelled as selfish, dangerous, and unique in their experience. My impression was that there was a serious shortage of available surrogates and that any appropriate (white and compliant) woman would be rushed into contract-signing and immediately told her perfectly matched couple had been located.

Anonymity was also a myth, since the father would know the city where I lived, my name from the birth certificate, and my physical characteristics from required baby pictures, from company files and medical and psychological reports. He would have visitation rights to the hospital nursery, and perhaps to the delivery room. Company files were said to be confidential, but it was acknowledged that they would be opened upon court order.

It is a myth that women are easily making large sums of money as surrogates. The director of this program acknowledges that the woman who goes through a lengthy insemination process may end up being paid less than $1.00/hour for her participation. To earn this sum, she is completely 'on-call' for the company. She may be required to undergo invasive diagnostic procedures, forfeit her job, and perhaps undergo major surgery with its attendant morbidity and mortality risks. Of course, should there be a miscarriage or failure to conceive, the surrogate receives no compensation at all.

The flow of money is also interesting. I was told that the surrogate's $10,000 fee would be held in an escrow account until delivery, but this was not confirmed by the lawyer or contract. If the parents breach the contract, why must the surrogate sue them for her fee, which the company already holds? And if she breaches the contract, shouldn't the couple be entitled to a refund from the company without taking the surrogate to court? The company holds all of the funds, makes the profit, and attempts to take a minimum of the financial/legal risks.

Control by contract is a crucial element of this surrogate program, with power clearly in the hands of the company officials. Besides the explicit demands in the contract, an additional clause yielding staggering control to the company was brought to my attention by an unaffiliated lawyer I later consulted. She pointed out Item Nine in a list of rules for surrogates which reads: 'Surrogate mother and her husband must sign all documents provided by the (company) including but not limited to the surrogate mother agreement and contract', plus addendums listed. In essence, at any time I could be handed any new document and be obligated to sign it, no matter what its effect on my well-being or best interests.

It came as no surprise, then, when I later read in the newspaper that the first surrogate to become pregnant was to have none other that the program director as her childbirth coach. I could imagine a surrealistic scene with the director by the woman's side, the father at the foot of the bed to see 'his baby come out,' perhaps even a bag over the surrogate's head to preserve someone's anonymity. In the interest of delivering a perfect child, all birth technologies would be employed, and at the first sign of fetal distress or maternal complaint the coach could encourage or insist on a cesarean delivery.

Who is this baby for? It is clear from contract and practice that the purchasing father is the key figure of the industry. From the first phone contact, I was told 'the child is the child of the natural parents. That means the father.' The contract requires delivery of the child to the father, and every effort is made to include him in the procedures. This is in sharp contrast to the invisible woman who will become the adoptive mother of the child. She is referred to only rarely, as the 'wife' of the father, and the 'potential stepmother.' There were no plans mentioned to try and include her in the process, although it would seem she might have a greater need for company sensitivity and an active role.

The fathers, as described by the industry representatives, are largely upper middle class and well-educated. As the director explained it, 'to be able to come up with $25,000 cash, they *have* to be well-educated.' They share a desire to biologically father an infant: some have tried adoption and turn in desperation to the surrogate alternative to begin a family; others are already rearing children from their wives' previous marriages, but want a child of their own. The need to continue patriarchal lineage, to make certain the child has the sperm and name of the buyer, is primary.

The public image of the surrogate mother is important to the reputation of the companies who must distinguish their 'reproductive service' from both sexual prostitution and baby-selling. The new surrogate image is bright, altruistic, and feminine. She is a very special girl next door, a plucky pioneer in a new industry, a girl who loves being pregnant and is able to give a man what his wife can't. While company spokespersons promote the surrogate as on a par with the buyers, able to provide good genes and a clean prenatal environment, there is also an attempt to place her in a slightly different moral class from the prospective parents. They state the logical economic and convenience incentives to becoming a surrogate, then readily disclose that many have had previous abortions or have given up children for adoption. These surrogates, approximately one-third of applicants according to a Michigan psychologist, may participate in order to atone for their previous abortions (Bumiller, 1983). Such public announcements, although seemingly in contrast to the desired altruistic image, and based on spurious research citing a statistic no different than general population estimates, may have at least two positive results for the companies:

1 It may ease the conscience of liberal prospective buyers, who can more easily accept the financial misuse of the surrogate if they believe she is receiving invisible psychological/moral gains.

2 It may lure some prospective surrogates who have unresolved abortion experiences, perhaps exacerbated by new anti-abortion propaganda.

In general, surrogates may be deterred from demanding better treatment, if convinced that giving up this child is part of a moral punishment or therapeutic process.

There is a need for feminists to pay attention to the surrogate industry and to structure debate in feminist terms. There have, of course, been outspoken critics of the surrogate companies, but they have primarily questioned the industry's effect on traditional business dealings and family structure. For example, the only ethical issue raised in a lengthy *Wall Street Journal* article (Inman, 1982) was whether participants might be taking unfair advantage of insurance companies offering maternity benefits. Robert Francoeur, in his 1974 book *Utopian Motherhood*, (p. 102) envisioned a gloomy world in which so-called 'mercenary mothers' would jeopardize the traditional 'monogamous family structure.'

The metaphors of description and criticism are fascinating: Is the surrogate mother a prostitute, or is she instead a modern extension of the wet nurse? Is the surrogate arrangement like donating sperm, simply giving women the right to sell their reproductive capacity as men have done for years? Or is the arrangement more like building a house, where the father furnishes half the blueprint and materials and the labor is contracted out? Is it baby-selling? Or is it organ-selling, morally equivalent to allowing the needy to sell their kidneys to rich patients (Fletcher, 1983)? Each metaphor frames political/ethical discourse in different terms. Even the use of the term 'surrogate mothering,' or the more recently popular euphemism 'surrogate parenting,' begins by labeling the biological mother as artificial. Allowing the debate to be structured by the industry has slowed criticism from the feminist community. In California, after an educational session from an industry representative, a NOW chapter passed a resolution supporting efforts to have the surrogate contracts recognized and enforceable under California law.

Our recognition of the problems of infertile women may also be delaying a strong feminist opposition to the surrogate industry. We must not only offer support to women in the painful emotional situation of being involuntarily childless, but we must examine its broader historical basis. The infertility was largely brought to us from the manufacturers of other types of reproductive control, birth control pills and IUDs. The same laws which make it difficult for many infertile women to adopt children will make the surrogate alternative equally unavailable unless she is part of a wealthy married heterosexual couple. Older children, children of color, and those with special needs will remain unadoptable, and the traditional patriarchal family system will remain intact.

In *Right-Wing Women* (1983), Andrea Dworkin has placed surrogate motherhood in the center of her elegant model of the systematic exploitation of women. In it, she describes the brothel model and the farming model. Simply stated, in the brothel model women are used efficiently and specifically for sex by groups of men. In the farming model, women are used by individual men, not so efficiently, for reproduction. The surrogate industry provides a frightening synthesis of both which

enables women to sell their wombs within the terms of the brothel model. Motherhood is becoming a new branch of female prostitution with the help of scientists who want access to the womb for experimentation and for power. A doctor can be the agent of fertilization; he can dominate and control conception and reproduction. Women can sell reproductive capacities the same way old-time prostitutes sold sexual ones but without the stigma of whoring because there is no penile intrusion. (pp. 181–2)

This system will become increasingly efficient with the refinement of other reproductive technologies such as embryo transplanting. As Genoveffa Corea points out (forthcoming), we are not far from being able to use a combination of artificial insemination and embryo transplant to allow Third World women to become the prenatal carriers of completely white children (at the same time that Depo-Provera and other exports are compromising these women's ability to conceive their own children).

The language and process encountered in my experience within a surrogate company is consistent with the reproductive prostitution model described by Dworkin. The surrogate is paid for 'giving the man what his wife can't.' She 'loves being pregnant,' and is valued solely and temporarily for her reproductive capacity. After she 'enters the fold' she is removed from standard legal protections and is subject to a variety of abuses. She is generally considered to be mercenary, collecting large unearned fees for her services, but the terms of the system are in reality such that she may lose more permanent opportunities for employment, and may end up injured or dead with no compensation at all. Even the glowing descriptions of the surrogates sound remarkably like a happy hooker with a heart of gold.

The issue of prostitution has been a difficult one for feminists; so ancient and entrenched a part of the patriarchal system that it seems almost impossible to confront. We must not now participate in a quiet liberal complicity with the new reproductive prostitution. It is our challenge to pay attention to our feminist visionaries, and to expose the surrogate industry during its formation.

## NOTE

1  From the first telephone enquiry made by the author to the surrogate company.

# REFERENCES

Bumiller, Elisabeth. 1983. 'Mother for Others.' *Washington Post*, March 9: B1, 11–12.

Corea, Genoveffa. Forthcoming. *The Mother Machine*. Harper & Row, New York.

Dworkin, Andrea. 1983. *Right-Wing Women*. Perigee Books, New York.

Fletcher, John. 1983. Quoted in *Washington Post*. February 18: C-5.

Francoeur, Robert. 1974. *Utopian Motherhood*. A. S. Barnes, New York. p. 102.

Inman, Virginia. 1982. 'Maternity Plan'. *Wall Street Journal*. August 13: pp. 1, 8.

# TO HAVE OR NOT TO HAVE A CHILD

# AN INTERVIEW WITH MIRTHA QUINTANALES, FROM THE THIRD WORLD WOMEN'S ARCHIVES

## Rita Arditti and Shelley Minden

Mirtha Quintanales, one of the founding members of the Third World Women's Archives,[1] immigrated to the United States from Cuba with her family in 1962, when she was 13. She worked in the area of health in Chicago in the 1970s, as coordinator of a family health clinic serving mostly Latino clients, and as a volunteer worker of the Chicago Women's Health Clinic. She was one of the founders of the Chicago chapter of the Committee to End Sterilization Abuse.

In the interview that follows Mirtha describes some of her personal experiences with contraceptives and abortion and some of the community work she has done around these issues. In spite of her considerable professional experience in the health field, her personal odyssey with these technologies typifies the experience of many women whose health is constantly in jeopardy from these reproductive technologies.

I was married twice. The first time I was 22 years old and hadn't thought a whole lot about having children; motherhood was not something I had much consciousness about. Since I was 18 I had been having some serious questions about my sexual identity and even as I entered into the marriage I had at least a vague awareness that my lifestyle could potentially change in the future. I think that even entertaining the possibility of adopting a non-traditional lifestyle somehow kept me from making a conscious decision about reproduction and motherhood. I considered at the time that a life-long commitment to children was nothing to be taken lightly, and since I was obviously not prepared to make that commitment, I simply put the issue 'on the shelf.'

Several years earlier when I started college (in 1967), I had begun to be concerned about how very little information there seemed to be specifically about birth control and generally about women's sexuality. As I confronted the relative sexual freedom of college life, I discovered that I had nobody to talk to and little to read that would explain to me what I was experiencing. I felt I was in limbo when it came to sexual issues, and now, looking back, I realize that this feeling was exacerbated by the fact that I was a young Latina woman living in a completely white Northamerican environment. Since the age of 13, when I immigrated from Cuba to the United States and moved with my family to a Chicago suburb, I had had virtually no contact with other Latinos. And I was never sure about the nature of the difficulties I regularly encountered in my intimate relationships. I had no way of sorting out Cuban cultural conditioning from individual/family history; the problems associated with adolescence and young adulthood, from the problems connected to culture shock and assimilation into an alien and hostile social environment. All I knew was that since junior highschool, I seemed to have very different attitudes, expectations and needs regarding sexuality than most people with whom I got involved. There often seemed to be serious clashes between us and I didn't even have a clue as to what to do to remedy this situation. Since I was a child, 'confusion' had always led me to seek information, particularly in books. So, I began to look for books hoping to find the answers to at least some of my questions.

During my sophomore year in college I created a small library in my dorm room. It included anything and everything I could find on sexuality – from the newly published *Human Sexual Response* by Masters and Johnson (1966, Little Brown and Company) to Malinowski's *Sex and Repression in Savage Society* (1953, Humanities Press). And to my surprise, my little library was used a lot. Apparently I was not the only one looking for information. It was a bit shocking for me, though, to realize how very little the girls in my dorm (and others who soon began to drop by my room) knew about sexuality. And I mean basics: menstruation, sexual intercourse. . . . College students!

Rather rapidly, the dorm room library expanded into a referral 'center' – small-scale but effective. This small liberal arts college was located in a tiny town in central Illinois and, really, the resources available within the school and out in the community were extremely limited. No wonder people had to resort to using our 'services.'

At any rate, a friend of mine whose father was a physician had joined me in the project. Through her father we had learned of a doctor who prescribed birth control pills to unmarried women without asking too many questions. We had also found a pharmacist who was willing to cooperate – which meant, in 1968 in a small town, actually handing over the pills without keeping a record of names and other personal details. Two other friends had provided harder-to-come-by and far riskier information: the names of a couple of abortionists who were relatively reliable. So in effect what we had created was an underground network of information and support services for campus women who had nowhere else to go.

I myself used the services. I went to see the physician, had birth control pills prescribed, and used them. I took the pills for a year. But during that year, I had a lot of problems with them. After only a couple of months, the only time I felt well was the week I'd be off the pills. Later, much later, I learned that these pills had been very high on estrogen and very wrong for me. As far as I know, all the women who saw this physician had had the same pills prescribed to them.

I believe it was the summer after my sophomore year that I went to visit my parents in Argentina, where they were living at the time. During my three-month stay there, the nausea, dizziness and depression I had begun to identify with my use of the pills began to get worse and worse. My mother noticed that I was taking birth control pills. She didn't ask me any questions about that nor did she harass me in any way. But she did offer some words of caution: 'You have to be careful with these pills, Mirtha. Nobody knows yet what long-range effects they have on women's bodies.' She was the first person to make any comments to me about the possibility that not all might be okay with birth control pills.

I returned from my trip to my home in Boston, where I

was now attending school. Soon afterwards, I discovered that I had infectious hepatitis. Since my parents's neighbours in Argentina had also contracted it, it was assumed that I had gotten sick when I was there. Somehow though, I felt that the birth control pills had contributed to my illness. But of course I wasn't sure. I didn't have any information about what birth control pills could do to one's liver. The doctor I saw immediately took me off the pills and told me that I could not use them again; he did not give me any explanation, however, despite my insistence.

As soon as it was medically safe to do so, I became sexually active again. I didn't want to get pregnant, so I went to a community health clinic – probably one of the first in the city of Borton to provide 'hassle-free' birth control services. There, I encountered the IUD for the first time. The Dalkon Shield. I had to have it inserted twice before it 'stayed,' and the insertions were very traumatic. The first was so excruciatingly painful that I was hardly able to make it to a phone to call my boyfriend and ask him to pick me up. I was sure I would not be able to get home on my own. The second was not much better, but I decided to put up with it because I couldn't take birth control pills and didn't want to take any chances. At the time, diaphragms were not being discussed much, I guess. Their use was not offered to me as an alternative to the pill or the IUD. In fact the diaphragm did not even come up in conversation during any of my visits to this clinic.

I used the Dalkon Shield for about two years, during which I got married and moved to Chicago where my parents were now residing. In Chicago, with the IUD still in place, I got pregnant. I didn't know I was pregnant when I started to have blurred vision, to see double, to swell up (I could hardly put on my shoes). I felt continuously nauseous and generally awful. At the point that I realized that I had missed two periods, I said to myself: 'It's unlikely, but I better check to see if I'm pregnant.' I had no idea about what was wrong with me otherwise, and I was *scared*.

I went to the health center at the University of Illinois, Chicago Circle, where I was a student. I requested a pregnancy test which turned out to be positive. Needless to say, I was not pleased, but my displeasure turned into mild panic when the lab technician who did the test told me I absolutely and immediately had to see a doctor. Ironically, it was he, and not the doctor, who gave me the information about the first legal abortion clinic in Milwaukee. What I got from the doctor, as I remember, was that indeed there were serious complications that had to be attended to right away (apparently I had toxemia – so early in the pregnancy!). Yet all he did was give me an appointment for two or three weeks later and send me home.

I decided to take no chances and have an abortion. I didn't have any money, so that was a problem. Fortunately, there was a feminist group on campus which was lending money to women who needed it just for that purpose. I borrowed the $200, took a Greyhound bus to Milwaukee early one Saturday morning, and had the abortion.

The experience itself was unproblematic. Everything went well. The whole procedure (suction method) was clearly explained to me, and I had the opportunity to discuss my situation, including my various options, before signing any papers, committing myself to the abortion, or paying any money. Plus, the clinic setting couldn't have been better – clean, modern, colorful and cheerful. And the staff was warm and friendly. As I recall, most of the health workers there were women, though this was not a feminist clinic.

Though I personally experienced no difficulties, I met other women at the clinic who had a very hard time. In particular, I remember a Guatemalan woman who was living in the US illegally. She was cleaning houses and taking care of children in order to support her family back home. This woman went through the same procedure I did and received the same care and attention. Nevertheless, she was very traumatized by her abortion. She cried nearly non-stop throughout the five or six hours we were there. In between sobs she told me over and over how much she had wanted to have the child. Her boyfriend had paid for the abortion, but apparently she would have preferred that he ask her to marry him and help her raise the child (he was North American). Being a single mother seemed to be completely out of the question for her. . . .

Since this woman and I both lived in the Chicago area,

we were able to keep in touch afterwards and discuss our 'post-abortion' progress. We both faithfully took the anti-biotics that had been prescribed to us at the clinic; I had no trouble, but she ended up having a serious infection for quite a long time. And, while I felt no regrets, she remained un-consoled about having had the abortion. If I was not aware of the fact when I went in to have the abortion, I quickly realized that there was a great deal more to this kind of experience than the public discussion on the topic would have led one to believe.

At the time, my relationship with my husband was very poor. He was a very violent man and I was trying to get out of my marriage. Two months after the abortion I got pregnant again. This time, I felt I really wanted to have the child. I started reading absolutely anything and everything I could find on childbirth. I realized that I knew very little about it and somehow nine months did not seem like a hell of a long time to learn everything I thought I needed to learn. I think perhaps I was a little too obsessive about the whole thing.

Virtually the only concrete information I had about childbirth was that my mother had lost her first child in connection with very poor medical attention during delivery. She had almost died herself. She had not been the one to tell me about this experience, but I had heard about it anyway. I wanted to have the 'best pregnancy and childbirth possible,' so I began to read whatever kind of material I could get my hands on – from books for the general public to medical textbooks on childbirth and gynecology.

During that period, I was coordinator of a predominantly Latino, family health clinic in the Near North Side of Chicago. It was a pilot community project that had been set up as a result of local pressure during the height of the community health movement in the early 1970s. Also, I was getting a degree in medical anthropology and had developed close ties with faculty and other students who were very much involved in doing advocacy work in community health. So, in effect, my job and school contexts provided access to information and resources which I hoped would ease my pregnancy and childbirth experience.

I was very nervous about my pregnancy, especially

because I wanted to divorce my husband and also because questions about my sexual identity continued to be a problem for me. But, I was very excited as well; I was not having the kinds of problems I had had during the first pregnancy, and I was feeling very much like 'mother earth.' My parents were getting ready to leave the country again, this time to go to work in Brazil. I was not very happy about the prospect of giving birth without having at least my mother with me, but as long as they were in town, I knew I could count on them for the emotional support I needed. I had many, many acquaintances in the city, but I felt then, as I had felt since I immigrated to this country, that I was very much alone.

I started to bleed during the third month. One of the nurses at the hospital where I worked told me that sometimes that meant that I could have a miscarriage. Somewhat alarmed, I decided to see one of the hospital out-patient clinic physicians. He wanted to give me a shot of Depo-Provera. I asked him to explain to me what that was, what it would do for me and/or to me. He got furious at me, screaming in his little examining room 'If you want to know so much, why don't you go to medical school. I can't afford to waste my time teaching my patients medicine. Don't you trust me?' I told him: 'Frankly, I don't. I've had enough trouble already. I need to know what it is I'm taking. . . .' He insisted that I choose to have or not to have the shot right on the spot and on the basis of his unexplained recommendation only, so I chose not to. Afterwards I did a little investigating and found out that Depo-Provera was often prescribed to women who started to bleed during pregnancy, though it had not been definitely established that it prevented miscarriages.

I continued to spot, so I made an appointment to see another doctor. Before I was able to see him, however, I began to bleed more heavily. I called him and he decided to prescribe another form of synthetic progesterone (pills). He never examined me. He just called a pharmacy and presto! All I needed to do was to pick up the pills. This man and I had never met; he didn't have my medical history. If anything else was wrong with me neither of us knew about it nor about the possible effects that these pills could have on me. I was rather hesitant to take the pills, but at that point I was feeling desperate; I did not want to lose the child. I took the pills, but the bleeding wouldn't stop.

One early evening, I went shopping with my husband. Suddenly I began to bleed so heavily that I came very close to fainting. It was just awful, everything seemed to be going around and around in circles and I felt extremely weak. But I was so proud that I couldn't imagine allowing myself to pass out in public, in the middle of a crowd. It took every bit of energy I had, but I managed to hold on to myself until we got home.

By then I was passing huge blood clots as well as bleeding 'fresh' blood. I feared that I was going to hemorrhage and die. My husband, instead of helping, started to accuse me of being overly dramatic. I thought, 'Here I am, laying on a couch barely able to move, and this man is shouting at me!' I finally decided that I couldn't count on him for my life, so I practically dragged myself to the kitchen 'phone and called the doctor who had prescribed the pills. He was nowhere to be found. I was convinced that he *didn't want* to be found. Luckily I was able to get a hold of my parents who contacted their doctor. He arranged for me to go to a hospital that was relatively close to the house.

In the middle of all these proceedings I figured that it might be important to have a blood clot or two for the lab to analyze, so I took a couple of samples and wrapped them up in tin foil. Once I knew that the situation was more or less under control and that I was doing all I could to help myself, I was able to relax. My husband, however, continued to be hysterical and utterly abusive: 'Imagine, collecting blood clots. You're crazy, you're completely crazy.' I was ever so grateful that my parents were still in town.

Even before we arrived at the hospital I knew what to expect: a long wait, questions to answer, and papers to fill out before anyone would see me. I thought 'no way.' Just as I was being told to sit down and wait for my turn, I staged a theatrical performance. I pretended I was about to faint. It worked! A wheelchair was immediately brought to me and I was taken care of right away. As it turned out, if I had *not* been taken care of when I was, I may have lost my life. The doctor who saw me later told me and my husband that I had come 'very close' to hemorrhaging. I had been bleeding heavily for hours.

I was told that I had not lost the fetus. But, for the first time in my life, I had to stay overnight in a hospital. I was put in a room with a woman who had ovarian cysts. This woman had been in the hospital for several days and had not yet seen the same doctor twice. She was very much in pain and, while I was there, the pain apparently got so bad that she couldn't stop screaming. And no one paid attention to her. It was unbelievable! Finally, after a couple of hours of calling for a doctor, the poor woman was prepared for emergency surgery and taken away. It was really devastating for me to be witness to such cruel treatment, and I swore that I was going to get out of that place as soon as possible and, if I could help it, never set foot in a hospital as a patient again.

Earlier that evening, the doctor had told me that if I did not stop bleeding altogether, I would have to have a D and C (dilation and curettage) in the morning. But there was no way on earth that I was going to have a D and C, I was sure of that. I absolutely did not want to undergo any treatment that resembled surgery. I did not want any instrumental interference with my body, any tampering with my reproductive organs. I realized at that point, that my abortion had been interference enough for me. . . .

I said to myself 'You are going to stop bleeding. You are going to be just fine and ready to leave the hospital in the morning.' I was determined to be all right, and I was. Mind over matter, creative visualization, self-affirmation, whatever. It worked and I went home the next day. I thought I was still pregnant.

A week or two later, I discovered that I had milk in my breasts. I thought that this was not supposed to be happening, so I went back to see the doctor who had taken care of me at the hospital. He told me that I had had a spontaneous abortion (a miscarriage). I was devastated – angry at the doctor for having told me, back at the hospital, that everything was going to be fine, and at myself for having had that abortion a few months earlier. I was convinced that the abortion had been responsible for this miscarriage. I felt very alienated from my body, my body that had failed me. I felt confused, guilty and powerless.

I did not want to be the object of anyone's pity, so I did not show my disappointment, did not speak about my experience with anyone. I think that what was really going on was that *I* didn't want to confront what I was feeling. For the most part life continued as usual, but something did change. Suddenly I was unable to write. I had been writing fiction for quite some time, but after the miscarriage the creative flow immediately and mysteriously stopped. And it would be eight or nine years before I could do any creative writing again. To this day I haven't completely understood this experience.

I left my husband six or seven months after the miscarriage. Shortly thereafter I decided to give the IUD one more try. This time it was the Copper Seven (the Dalkon Shield had been taken off the market after several women had died in connection with its use). The Copper Seven was painful from the first day till the last, when I had to have it removed; it hurt continuously. While I was still using the Copper Seven, I found out more about the diaphragm. I was doing volunteer work at a women's self-help clinic and organizing in the area of women's health (particularly on the issue of sterilization abuse). I had the opportunity, for the first time in my life, to discuss in detail with other women issues that had concerned me since I started college.

At any rate, I started to use the diaphragm and was quite pleased with it. Less than two years after my divorce from my first husband, I remarried, but it was ultimately a matter of a relatively short period of time before I came out as a lesbian.

Being 'out' had a profound impact on practically all areas of my life. One thing I noticed immediately, though, was how *good* it felt not to have to worry about subjecting my body to contraceptives. No chemicals, no contraptions, no potential damage to my body in the name of . . . what? I realized that I had been very ambivalent about the use of contraceptives all along, that this issue had been a 'loaded' one for me. Not only because it had implied taking risks with my personal health and safety, but because I had associated this 'tampering' with a traditional heterosexual lifestyle (marriage and motherhood) that I had not consciously nor deliberately chosen for myself but that I had felt compelled to adopt. Against my deepest needs and best interests.

I felt very angry for myself and for those women who, like me, had had to struggle very hard to find their way to a lesbian lifestyle in a very heterosexist and racist world. But I also felt a great deal of empathy for heterosexual women, particularly Third World women, for whom reproductive abuses (not to mention all others) would continue to be a reality in their lives.

I stopped organizing in the area of women's health at some point during 1976. Nevertheless I have continued, to date, to organize around issues of women's sexuality and to participate in the feminist debate on sex and politics – particularly from the perspective of my being a Third World woman.[2]

Speaking as a Latina lesbian and Third World feminist, I would say that today's most pressing needs for Third World women working in the area of women's sexuality in the US are: (1) to establish *our own* private and public dialogues; (2) to determine *our own* political priorities and timetables and (3) to develop *our own* organizational strategies. So far, there has been little room in the women's movement (let alone anywhere else) for us to talk about our individual lives and thoughts, our shared experiences and concerns. And, *that* needs to happen before any theory of women's sexuality (ours, anyone's) can be considered 'valid.' Before any politically effective work can be carried out.

I can extrapolate that our cultural and class backgrounds and upbringing, our assimilation experiences, and the impact of racism, cultural imperialism, class discrimination, sexism and homophobia in this country play a role in shaping our sexual lives. But politics based on extrapolation can be at best ineffective and at worst destructive. I/we, want and need to *know*. Seventeen years of reading other people's stories, of studying other people's histories and theories, and of doing political work on the basis of that information, have taught me that there aren't too many folks out there knocking themselves out to learn about our lives, much less to help us change them for the better. So, all right, I accept the challenge: I'll help make our own sexual revolution.

## NOTES

1 The Third World Women's Archives is a project of the Third World Women's Educational Resources, Inc., a non-profit organization founded in 1981 by a group of Latina, Asian and Afro-American women. The Archives is dedicated to gathering any and all kinds of information about, by, and for Third World women in the US and abroad. Write to them for more information at: P.O. Box 159, Bush Terminal Station, Brooklyn, NY 11232.

2 See 'The complexity of desire: Conversations on sexuality and difference,' with Barbara T. Kerr. 1982. *Conditions*, 8; *Diary of a Conference on Sexuality*. 1982. (The Scholar and the Feminist. Towards a Politics of Sexuality Conference). Barnard College, NYC. April 24; *Compañeras: A Latina Lesbian Anthology*. Co-editor with Juanita Ramos, forthcoming; Third World Women's Archives bulletins – 'Up-coming events.'

## REFERENCES

Malinowski, B. 1953. *Sex and Repression in Savage Society*. Humanities Press. Atlantic Highlands, N.J.

Masters, W. and Johnson, V. 1966. *Human Sexual Response*. Little, Brown & Co., Boston, Mass.

# TEENAGE OPPRESSION AND REPRODUCTIVE RIGHTS

## Eleanor Trawick

This article, written by a teenager who is active in the reproductive rights movement, discusses some of the ways in which teenagers' sexuality and reproductive freedom are hindered by teenagers' position in society. Teenage oppression results in teenagers having very little freedom to choose goals and lifestyles free from sexist and heterosexist assumptions. Organizing teenagers in the reproductive rights movement would broaden the perspective of the movement and give support to teenagers to fight for their rights.

As a teenager who has worked on reproductive rights at my high school and now at college, I feel that in organizing and educating, teenagers it is essential to explain the full meaning of reproductive rights. Young people today are the victims of many of the governmental attempts to take away our reproductive freedom, yet while teenage women can often see the importance of individual issues – safe and legal abortion, for example – they many times do not recognize the importance of such nearly-related demands as *funding* for abortions, let alone the more distant ones – lesbian liberation, occupational choice and safety, etc. Work in our junior high and high schools (and in colleges too) is of tremendous importance in this period. But just as teenage sexuality and teenage organizing are vital to reproductive rights work, making connections between the many seemingly unrelated issues of reproductive rights is vital to our work with teenagers.

Reproductive rights means more than merely the choice 'to birth or not to birth.' We must have the freedom to choose our goals and lifestyles, free from sexist and heterosexist assumptions. We must have the freedom to question what has been set up as a norm, as what is 'right,' by society.

Teenagers, by our very position in society, are easily deprived of our right of choice — or simply never have it to begin with — and are the hardest hit when controls are imposed from above. Our problems are fourfold: social, moral, economic, and legal.

If society is to perpetuate itself as it is now, not just physically, by continued propagation and survival, but ideologically as well, it must instill in its young people the values that are held to be correct and that preserve the *status quo*. The sexist and capitalist society that we live in must preserve sexist and capitalist attitudes in its citizens. From birth to adulthood, children are taught the proper relationships between employers and employees, between individuals and the state, between men and women, and within the family. Continuity and stability are ensured — but at what price?

Young people are in a difficult position because many of the controls on us are argued to be justified on moral grounds. The innocence of youth must be protected at all costs, and young people must themselves be protected lest they become victims of the 'bad elements' (so called) in society. Yet how, we must ask, can they ever protect themselves if they are forced to remain naive and defenseless? Young people, it is also said, must not be taught about our own sexuality — and particularly should not know about 'deviant' sexual patterns — lest we become corrupted. Yet how, we must again ask, can anyone be virtuous if it is a virtue resulting from ignorance rather than conscious choice? By denying teenagers access to contraceptives and abortion, legislators are not promoting chastity, but only increasing the harmful effects of what they see as promiscuous behavior.

In this society, families are seen as economic units, not individuals. Those who are not seen as breadwinners have to struggle for any independence they may achieve, because they are seen as dependent parts of the family unit led by the salary earner. Minors, even more than women, are not seen as having any economic role, and hence they have no power. They are seen solely as wards of their parents or of the state.

And, finally, minors have few legal rights and almost no recourse to legal action. We are therefore an easy target for the New Right in its attacks on all women. Much of the legislation which has recently been proposed – or which has been on the books for many years – to limit women's reproductive freedom is aimed specifically at teenage women.

The so-called Teen Chastity Bill, a part of the more inclusive Family Protection Act, allocates as much as $30 million per year to promote teenage chastity and 'other family-centered approaches to the problems of adolescent promiscuity and pregnancy.' The name of the bill itself reveals the arrogant and abusive attitude toward teenage sexuality which characterizes not only the religious right, but much of mainstream society in the US. Money is provided for research into 'the negative consequences of abortion.' (Such 'research' as this, with the findings predetermined, is questionable, to say the least.) Under the terms of the bill, virtually no family planning centers would qualify for money; furthermore, all services that the Chastity Bill would provide would require parental notification and consent. It is interesting to note, as an aside, that the supposedly liberal Democrat, Senator Edward Kennedy, sponsors the Chastity Bill.

Another piece of legislation, dubbed the Squeal Rule, was recently stopped by a federal court injunction but is now being reintroduced. The Squeal Rule would limit teenagers' access to birth control by requiring parental notification. Such a rule would not only be a gross violation of young people's right to privacy, but would also be a major expense and burden on family planning centers. Interestingly enough, Education for Freedom of Choice Ohio (EFCO) surveyed a number of teenagers who were obtaining prescription birth control through centers and found that over half said their parents knew of their contraceptive use. Only 2 percent of those responding said that they would cease sexual activity if they could not obtain contraceptives without their parents' knowledge.

Although the Supreme Court decision in the spring of 1983 struck down many of the consent laws limiting teenage women's access to abortion, teenagers between the ages of eleven and fifteen may still need parental consent for an abortion in some places. In an ideal world, families function as close-knit support groups that young people may trust and feel secure in. Unfortunately, many families fall short of this ideal, and to assume such trust and security in all families is at best absurd, at worst quite dangerous to the young people involved.

While the legal position of teenagers jeopardizes our right to safe abortions and confidential, accessible birth control, it also puts us among the groups most victimized by compulsory sterilization. Young women, particularly if they are economically disadvantaged, of color, or do not speak English are considered too irresponsible to control their own bodies, and sterilization is seen as justified. Often a woman will go in for an abortion and be pressured into a sterilization operation – which too frequently is a hysterectomy rather than a tubal ligation. Depo-Provera, an injectable contraceptive (manufactured by Upjohn Company) not currently approved by the FDA for contraceptive use, is nevertheless given by some doctors to women who are seen as too irresponsible to use contraceptives on their own: it is effective for up to eight months, and takes control completely out of the woman's hands. Predictably, teenagers and young mothers are among the most common victims of Depo-Provera.

It is not enough that young people be free to obtain contraceptives and abortions, and not enough that we are free from compulsory sterilization. The concept of choice is invalid unless the choice is an *informed* one. Teenagers must know, to begin with, that we do have access to abortion and birth control, but we must also know the pros and cons of each option and know how to make use of each. The means of achieving this is through an adequate and accurate sex education program in schools. But this education must go beyond anatomy and pregnancy options to present various aspects of sexual choice. Virtually always, even in the best sex education courses, it is assumed that all the students are heterosexual; most of the time homosexuality is presented unfavorably, as a deviation or, at best, a sickness – or it is never mentioned.

The issue of gay liberation involves young people as it

relates to their sex education programs, but there is a second, perhaps more sinister, connection. In recent decades, at least, homosexuality has in large part been proscribed on the grounds that it is harmful to minors. The famous 'Save Our Children' campaign illustrates this focus, as does the law, in effect in many places, that elementary and secondary-school teachers cannot be gay. The theory behind the Save Our Children approach is, one supposes, that people who are 'unnatural' enough to prefer their own sex are unnatural enough, too, to molest small children. In practice, one group is being oppressed in the name and for the sake of a second group – a second group, ironically enough, which is also oppressed, although in different ways. Young people did not originate this demand for our 'protection,' and do not support it except in so far as they are inculcated with the prejudices of our parents and teachers. And the stunning absurdity in this whole line of reasoning is that there are plenty of *teenagers* who *are* lesbian and gay. Many gay adults, after all, were once gay teenagers, whether they were openly and admittedly gay or remained in the closet. The whole right-wing argument becomes ridiculously convoluted and contradictory if carried far enough.

The position of teenage lesbians and gay men is particularly difficult. Gay teenagers are much more vulnerable than gay adults, both legally and emotionally. Gay teenagers who come out to their parents risk being thrown out of the house or institutionalized. Often lacking any decent and accurate information about their sexual orientation, they may experience considerable difficulty and guilt coming out to themselves – let alone to others. When they and their peers are taught homophobia in the classroom, the difficulties are multiplied many times over. Recently we have seen the appearance of a number of works on this subject, books such as *One Teenager in Ten* (1983) and *Reflections of a Rock Lobster* (1981). But this can only be helpful in focussing attention on the problems of gay teenagers and emphasizing again the basic connection between various aspects of reproductive rights.

The struggle of gay teenagers is part and parcel of the struggle of gay people in general, but the oppression of young gay men and lesbians is also a part of the oppression of teenagers – part of the general process of suppressing an individual's sexual expression and her or his choices regarding important questions – questions as vague as which life-style is preferable, or as specific as whether or not to carry a pregnancy to term. Like the fight for abortion rights and for available, accessible birth control, gay rights and gay liberation for teenagers are an important part of fighting the rigid controls of our sexist and homophobic society. The goal of the reproductive rights movement is to free all people from the notion that sexuality must be kept within 'correct' bounds – bounds, that is, which are acceptable to legislators and to a vocal part of the population. To give women a choice and allow us to control our own bodies is to free us from the narrow concept of sex as reproduction, where sexuality is reduced to an assembly-line function of turning out babies. Abortion, contraception, and homosexuality are seen as somehow 'wrong' in such a society, because they divorce sexuality from reproduction.

When, as reproductive rights activists, we go into high schools and into youth groups, we can certainly go in knowing that what we say has relevance to teenagers. Many of the major attacks on the availability of abortion and birth control have been concentrated on teenagers. Teenagers, particularly those who are economically disadvantaged, are among the primary victims of sterilization abuse and birth control means such as Depo-Provera. And teenagers, more than adults, are the victims of heterosexism and homophobia. Surely if reproductive rights is an issue of concern to anyone it is of concern to young people.

There *are* teenagers out there who see and understand the problems. We can attract them, help solidify their feelings of outrage, and help them make the connections between the various aspects of reproductive rights. In turn, incorporating the perspectives and experiences of teenagers into the reproductive rights movement will help us build a more effective movement. A movement that will challenge the separation that our society foists on people because of sex, class, race, body characteristics and age.

# REFERENCES

Fricke, Aaron. 1981. *Reflections of a Rock Lobster*. Alyson, Boston, Mass.

Heron, Ann, ed. 1983. *One Teenager in Ten*. Alyson, Boston, Mass.

# REFUSING TO TAKE WOMEN SERIOUSLY: 'SIDE EFFECTS' AND THE POLITICS OF CONTRACEPTION

## Scarlet Pollock

Women who complain of symptoms which may be linked to their contraceptive method are rarely taken seriously by their doctors. Symptoms are dismissed while women are presumed to have 'other reasons' for complaining. Side effects are treated as having less to do with contraceptives than with the fact of being a woman. Headaches, depression, low sex drive and vaginal discharge are portrayed as 'natural' for females — even when the women who experience them insist they are not. It is too late to recognise side effects as serious only when they begin to threaten a woman's health and, perhaps, her life.

Heterosexual intercourse, by common and legal definition, is the penetration of a man's penis in a woman's vagina culminating in his ejaculation. It is the form of sexual activity likely to result in conception, and for the most part, it is taken to be what sex is. Yet, most women do not want to get pregnant most of the times they have sex with men.

Sexual excitement and pleasure is geared towards what turns men on since, according to 'normal' heterosexual intercourse, male orgasm but not female orgasm is, by definition, sex. The woman's sexual feeling, whether pleasant or unpleasant, is irrelevant for 'sex' to happen. Her enjoyment is an optional extra dependent upon her partner's sensitivity and willingness. The consequences of such heterosexual intercourse, however, are distributed quite differently: it is women who run the risk of pregnancy, childbearing and childbirth, and it is women whose lives will be most affected by having children.

Contraceptive research and the distribution of

contraceptive methods are based upon this male-centred version of sex. Of central concern is how to prevent pregnancy and thus control the birth rate. It is *not* to question why it is women who bear the consequences of 'normal' sex; nor is it to ask what is so sacred about this male-oriented form of sexuality. The goal of government, pharmaceutical and medical organisations is to develop and distribute contraceptives which are most likely to prevent pregnancy while least likely to interfere with men's enjoyment of heterosexual intercourse.

Side effects, health risks and long-term effects of using contraceptives have been minor considerations in the development of birth control. Women's demands to control their own fertility have been in direct opposition to the policy of maintaining the stability of patriarchal family life. Medical 'knowledge' is based upon assumptions of male control over sexuality and family life. This is the political context in which women have had to manoeuvre between sex and pregnancy, contraceptive reliability and other effects.

The purposes and assumptions underlying the development of contraceptive technology cannot be separated from women's experiences with the use of contraception. Definite notions about the proper place for women, the characteristics of 'real' womanhood, the desired quality and quantity of the population, the morality of abortion, the varying suitability of different types of birth control to women of different ethnicity/nationality/economic class – all these are tied into the information we receive about contraceptives and how available they are to us.

Deciding which contraceptive method to use – and whether to use any at all – at any particular time involves women in transactions with their sexual partner and, depending on which method is chosen, with one or more doctors. The position of women in these negotiations is a defensive one. Social subordination of women places women's concerns about contraception amidst a body of ideas and practices which assert men's privileges and interests over and above those of women. Men's sexual arousal and enjoyment is portrayed to be vitally important while women's contraceptive side effects and health risks are undermined and said to be not very serious. Taken-for-granted notions about contraception, as taken-for-granted ideas about sex, are much more comfortable to live with for men than they are for women.

## FINDING A 'SUITABLE' CONTRACEPTIVE METHOD

I recently talked with fifty women in England about their experiences of contraception. All were attending full-time, postgraduate courses at university; their cultural backgrounds were varied, most were white and their families of origin were largely middle-class. They ranged in age from 23 to 38 years, and in experience with contraception from six months to fifteen years. Only three of the women had children, and a fourth woman was pregnant. Despite this range of differences amongst the women, their experiences of sexuality, contraception and family planning services were remarkably similar.

The general lack of information received before they actually began to have sexual relations was emphasised by almost all of the women. Lessons of morality, animal reproductive cycles, and/or guidance for marriage and motherhood had seemed to have deliberately neglected any practical advice about sex and birth control. The protectiveness of knowledgeable, experienced males proved to be more of an image than a reality when it came to taking contraceptive precautions. The knowledge women gained was through trial and (mostly) error.

To start with women used the method which seemed easiest and was generally considered 'the thing to use'. It was not until things went wrong that women began to question why they used that particular contraceptive method and wonder whether there was anything else that might be more suitable. What went wrong might include worry or experience of pregnancy; their partner's dissatisfaction with disruptions of his sexual enjoyment; or symptoms which women felt to be related to the contraceptive they used.

In spite of the technological developments of the

twentieth century there is today no contraceptive method which provides 100 percent reliability and has neither adverse effects upon health nor interferes with 'normal' heterosexual intercourse. Choices are therefore made in the context of limited information about less than perfect contraceptives. Finding a 'suitable' method means finding one alternative which is better – but still not ideal – in the particular woman's situation, than others.

Finding this relatively more suitable method depends upon being able to try out different methods. For the women I spoke with, however, this usually meant taking more risks of becoming pregnant than they wanted to take. The uncertainty of being able to have an abortion, the social pressures against doing so, and the concern for the personal stress this might involve left most women in the position of needing 100 percent reliability from their contraceptive method. They therefore felt greatly constrained in experimenting with different contraceptives.

Because sex is geared to intercourse and male enjoyment, contraceptives which affect 'the sex act' least – at the peril of women's health and comfort – are those predominantly chosen. It seems to me that under these circumstances, the least we could expect would be a close and careful scrutiny of women's reactions while using the pill, the coil and injectable contraceptives. Yet, in the experience of the women I spoke with, this does not happen. Negotiating symptoms, their relation to contraception and what should be done about them was complicated by the refusal of doctors to take women seriously.

## SIDE EFFECTS

Few women received from their doctors any information about side effects and health risks. Some were given advice about which contraceptive method to use; others were simply prescribed a particular brand of the pill or fitted with a specific sort of coil. Health risks were dismissed as negligible while side effects were demeaned as unimportant. The link between symptoms, possible side effects and the early indication of damage to women's health was rarely made. Women were discouraged from experimenting with contraception by their doctors, and advised to be content with what they had. Especially in view of the reliability of the pill and the coil, women were told that they were or ought to be 'happy on it' and that 'it would be silly to change' unless serious side effects were recognised.

Here lies the catch. Whether or not the symptoms women experience are interpreted as side effects; whether or not they are seen as serious; and who has the power to decide if they are and what should be done about them – determine the extent to which women are able to be flexible and to find the most suitable contraceptive method for them. As long as symptoms are not recognised to be possible side effects nor regarded as serious, there appears to be no problem – except for the woman. In her doctor's eyes, she is 'happy' or should be.

Women's symptoms are commonly dismissed by doctors who show little interest in women's problems with contraception. Yet women do not have the luxury of being able to dismiss their doctors so easily. Medical control over the availability of birth control makes women acutely aware of the significance of their doctor's attitudes. Women are forced to be concerned about their doctor's opinions about contraception, abortion, sexuality and proper womanhood in order to obtain or change their contraceptives to those distributed by medics.

When medics cast suspicion upon the reliability of the statements made by patients, they protect their own views from challenge or change. Their legitimacy as the proper decision-makers in contraceptive or other health matters is reinforced. This form of legitimization is frequently used by dominant social groups to safeguard their position. The medical prerogative to reference an individual's physical or mental state as unhealthy is a powerful means of bringing that person's rationality or reliability into doubt. Whether people are portrayed as weakened, diseased, over-anxious, sickly, hysterical, pathological or neurotic, the result is the same – they appear to be incapable and unreliable.

These adjectives are applied most often to women. And

they are applied regardless of any individual woman's state of health or illness. Medicine as a profession has played a central role in defining women to be intellectually incapable, lacking in physical stamina, periodically polluting, sexually dangerous and emotionally unfit solely on the grounds of being female and not male (Oakley, 1976; Duffin, 1978; Ehrenreich and English, 1979; Scully, 1980; Elston, 1981). It was not surprising that the women I talked to had encountered all of these attitudes over several years of using contraception. Medical dominance, accentuated by male dominant perceptions of women, resulted in frequent conflicts between women and their doctors. Convincing her doctor that she is a rational and responsible human being, and not 'another neurotic female', is not always an easy task for a woman.

## IS IT RELATED?

'Come back if you have any problems' was the extent of the advice most women received when first prescribed the pill or fitted with the coil. The first problem they had was trying to work out what sort of problem was likely to be considered a problem associated with the contraceptive. When symptoms occurred which women thought might be related, and these were reported to their doctors, more often than not women found their complaints were dismissed or invalidated. Yet the advice remained the same:

> I've complained before of what I thought might be side effects of the pill and they very much pooh-poohed it, saying: 'You're getting neurotic about it, hearing a lot of stories, whereas in fact it doesn't do this.' Every time I go to the family planning clinic they say: 'Oh it's nothing, it's nothing.' When I told them I'd been on it (the pill) for six years and wanted to know whether I should take a break off it, they said: 'Well, it's a mild one so it doesn't particularly matter. As soon as you have any side effects, then it's time to start thinking about coming off it.'

How could the woman in this example find such advice reassuring when she had over several years been reporting symptoms which included cramps, migraine, depression, loss of sex drive and vaginal thrush (yeast)? How was it even possible for her to follow the advice she was given? As each time she asked about a symptom she thought might be a side effect, it was dismissed as nothing or treated in isolation, she was unable to work out whether her symptoms indicated that it was time to start thinking about coming off it.

Only three out of the fifty women had never used either the pill or the coil. Of the rest, 85 per cent had had symptoms which they considered were likely to be side effects of their birth control method. It should be pointed out that women did not connect symptoms with their contraceptive method until they continued over a length of time or became severe. That is, they were unlikely to relate the two until they felt they had substantial evidence.

Medical studies often imply that women do not make such judgments carefully and dismiss the possible side effects women report as the result of the greater likelihood of women to report symptoms when using contraceptives. This is referred to as 'over-reporting' and is said to provide for a 'biased' view of the symptoms associated with contraceptive use. A notable example in Britain is the Royal College of General Practitioners' survey of medical reports on 46,000 women over eight years of use with oral contraceptives. This study suggests that because women know they are using the pill, they will be more concerned about themselves, have a better doctor-patient relationship and greater opportunity to report symptoms to their doctors than other women. Therefore they may report symptoms which they would otherwise not report. The 1974 Report provides an interesting survey of medical research of the effects of oral contraceptive use as well as the interim results of its own study. Throughout, evidence of adverse side effects are undermined by references to over-reporting leading to bias and, repeatedly, the conclusion is drawn that the evidence is not 'convincing'. The report winds up its discussion by pointing to the substantial reporting of adverse symptoms of a 'vague and subjective' nature: these include migraine and headache, vaginal discharge, depression, chicken pox and other virus infections (a positive correlation with the pill, thought to result from lowered immunity), and loss of libido. An amazing feat is then accomplished. The report suggests that we accept that the evidence of these symptoms is 'largely, if not entirely, due to bias' and thereby dismiss them. It is only once we have done so that we are not completely astounded by the unlikely conclusion to the evidence presented. The estimated risk of using the pill, says the report, 'is one that a properly informed woman would be happy to take' (pp. 84–5).

If it is assumed that women are likely to over-report their symptoms, then evidence of contraceptive side effects is not recognised. The low-risk-few-side-effects viewpoint is confirmed by a self-fulfilling prophecy. As women are thought to have 'other reasons' for complaining of symptoms, it appears as if it is the women themselves who are to blame for complaining.

Doctors of the women I spoke with seemed to have very definite opinions about the side effects and risks involved in using contraceptives – so definite that what the women said about their reactions often made very little difference. In some cases women were left wondering whether they hadn't really imagined it all; neither their symptoms nor their questions appeared to make any impression upon their doctor:

> It was as if I was imagining them. It was really absurd. You'd think they would touch you or act as if you were complaining of something. . . . It's almost as if they can't hear you. They go on with the same sentence that they've been saying. And you say something new that you think really ought to change things and they somehow manage to evade it as if you hadn't said it. They somehow manage to sidetrack you so that you forget that you've asked it, and you only remember later.

The experience of having their symptoms and questions invalidated was combined with the general atmosphere of medics being too busy and having more important things to do than turn their attention to women who were complaining of nothing. So, women grew less inclined to discuss their symptoms with doctors. Over time, many doubts were raised in the women's minds about the general level of medical expertise. Indeed, cynicism increased with experience of consulting doctors.

Medical control over distribution of many birth control measures meant that women had to continue to negotiate with their doctors even if they would rather not. Learning how to negotiate included assessing which symptoms their doctors were likely to consider as possible side effects. One criterion emerged as particularly significant: could the symptom be measured independently by the doctor? That is, if the medic did not have to rely upon the woman's word for evidence but was able to use measures such as bacterial cultures, weight scales or blood pressure levels, it seemed more likely that it would be recognised as a side effect. Less tangible symptoms, including mood changes, headaches, reduced sex drive, cramps, and other pains and discomforts, were less likely to be said by doctors to be related to the contraceptive method. Instead, being female and/or being unfeminine were implied to be the source of the women's symptoms.

In practice, 'other reasons' for symptoms were associated by doctors with patriarchal ideas about the 'normal' characteristics of females or 'abnormal' and unladylike behaviour. Women inferred from their doctor's approach that it was nothing unusual for women to experience, or think they experienced, untoward symptoms. Vaginal discharge and discomfort, for example, were treated as natural despite the insistence of the women involved that this was not so:

> If you approach a doctor it's got to be with a very specific angle which they're prepared to discuss up to a point. When my vagina was very sore and irritated it took a lot for me to go to the doctor. When it proved not to be an infection they thought it wasn't a problem. If it's not an infection, you're all right and if you're uncomfortable, well that's too bad.

> I've tried to talk to them but you never seem to get anything but put-off replies like: 'Females always have a certain amount of infection in their vaginas.'

It was women's 'normal' genital state and, also, their mental state which doctors seemed to regard as unhealthy. Mood changes and high emotional levels, for instance, were more likely to be regarded as side effects of being female than of contraceptive technology:

> His attitude was just: 'Don't be so silly.' He said it (loss of sex drive) was purely emotional. I knew that it wasn't but he wasn't interested in that.

> I went along for some Valium or something (for depression) and said that I was taking the pill. I got the Valium but no discussion about the pill. He just gave me the pills and that was that.

Women's denial or challenge of their doctor's view were easily discounted on the same basis as their symptoms – that women are typically over-anxious and mentally unsettled.

Unladylike, or unfeminine, behaviour offered medics a second reason to discount a woman's symptoms. Sexual 'promiscuity' was commonly pointed to as the cause of symptoms which could be viewed as no more than a woman's 'just deserts':

> He was implying that if I had sexual relationships with more than one person, then I couldn't help but pick up thrush (yeast) and vaginal infection – just assuming that because I wasn't married I did that.

Remarks such as this were frequently made during vaginal examinations, making it extremely difficult for women to object and defend themselves:

> They put you in the most unladylike position they can, you can imagine, for the ordinary internals. They put you in this big seat, you know, with your legs apart, sort of naked from the waist down. It's a position in which you're totally powerless to do anything. And even if you can sort of get at people verbally, which I'm not very good at, it doesn't seem to carry much weight in that position.

Pre-marital or extra-marital sexual relations, having more than one sexual relationship, having had an abortion, or even 'delaying' pregnancy once married were examples of what was taken to be unfeminine behaviour and reasons for ill health. Stepping outside of a woman's proper place in subordinating her sexuality and fertility to one man in marriage would, it seemed to be assumed, quite rightly make her sick.

This patriarchal mistrust and contempt for women provides the basis of medical assessment of individual women's symptoms. The potential to correct this image of women is destroyed by the continuous dismissal of what women have to say about the experience of using contraceptives. Patriarchal medical 'knowledge' inhibits the perception of possible side effects of contraceptives.

This is a very serious problem for women. It can and frequently does result in the failure to quickly assess and deal with symptoms which may indicate or develop into serious health problems. It forces women to live with unnecessary discomfort and pain. The invalidation of our experience precludes the possibility of finding further evidence about side effects, their relation to health risks and the effects of using contraceptives over many years. The acknowledged ignorance about long-term effects of contraceptives such as the pill, the coil, and Depo-Provera; the high proportion of women world-wide who use them; and the length of time over which women have and will continue to use them make it urgent that this problem be confronted.

## IS IT SERIOUS?

Who decides what is serious and for whom? How are women to decide whether symptoms are serious enough to warrant changing contraceptive methods? When does a symptom indicate a risk to the woman's health rather than simply a discomfort to put up with? Questions such as these are continually part of women's experiences and dilemmas of contraception. Medical ignorance of these issues is not helped by the dismissal of the questions as unimportant; by the dismissal of women as unimportant; by the dismissal of contraception as a social issue – except when it comes to sharing medical powers over birth control; nor by the dismissal as insignificant health risks which do not appear to be fatal.

The women I talked with had a great deal of difficulty trying to find out from their doctors whether their symptoms were something to be concerned about, and what should be done about them. Medical assumptions about contraceptive technology as low-risk-few-side-effects overrode what women reported as their experience. Hence, women found it hard to have a decent conversation with their doctors about what was happening to them:

> I began to have a strong reaction to alcohol (1–2 glasses of wine; never occurred when off the pill). As soon as I had a drink I would have such a headache I could hardly see. But the doctor just laughed and said: 'That's probably the drink.' He just told me not to worry.

> He just gave me this speech on how 'Going on the pill is no more dangerous than going on a holiday for two weeks on the Norfolk Broads.' He didn't give me any advice about what type of pill would be best, just: 'We'll put you on this.' When I went back because I was having trouble, he just automatically said: 'Oh take this; have this instead' and didn't even discuss it with me. The next time I started having trouble I swapped over to the woman doctor because I felt that he was an idiot and didn't appreciate what was happening.

As in the experience of this second woman, female doctors were found to be relatively better than their male colleagues at taking women and their symptoms seriously. Women spoke of their female doctors as being more supportive, listening more carefully, showing greater understanding and being more competent. This allowed for a more detailed exploration of problems and solutions with women doctors. However, the medical privilege of having the final say in which contraceptives and treatments were to be made available to women, kept women patients dependent upon their female as well as their male doctors.

Women found that their doctors did not consider their symptoms, even where they were recognised to be side effects as serious because they did not seem to present life-threatening hazards. Thus for the majority of women little attention was paid to their symptoms:

> They seem to think that if something isn't really, really serious – if it isn't going to kill you – then it isn't an important side effect, when it is! Somehow they maintain such a distance and say: 'Oh, yes, well, you do get a certain amount of side effects when you're on the pill. Just keep on it and if it's still there in another few months. . . .' I just thought: 'Well God Almighty there I am having to sleep with my legs on top of a pillow they're so sore when they're lying flat– there's something wrong.'

This disregard for women's pain and discomfort was sometimes compounded by moralistic or punitive sexual attitudes:

> So I went to the doctor and the first thing she said was: 'Are you on the pill?' and I said 'Yes.' 'Oh, well, that's why then. If you go on the pill you expect to get these things. I'm not going to treat you. There's nothing wrong with you.'

The relationship between symptoms which were seen as 'merely' side effects and those which indicate life-threatening illnesses was rarely discussed. Side effects and health risks seemed to be regarded in medical 'knowledge' as two entirely separate issues. Side effects were taken to be common but insignificant while health risks were significant but uncommon. The potential for discovering the relation between them was thus completely missed.

What women are prepared to accept defines a contraceptive method's 'acceptability' in family planning research. This emphasis upon acceptability factors has less to do with the side effects and health risks of using contraceptives than it has with women's willingness to use them. For example, the problem with the pill in recent years is not defined by evidence of changes in women's health, but by the fact that women have increasingly come to see its associated symptoms as a risk to health. Family planning services either 'reassure' women about the risks of the pill or encourage them to use another method which women have not – as yet – come to see as unacceptable. Such an approach directs research efforts to find methods of contraception over which women have little control. The IUD and Depo-Provera have been heralded for the 'advantage' that women have little control over them once inserted or injected (Roberts, 1979; Rakusen, 1981).

It is obviously too late to recognise symptoms as serious only when they begin to threaten a woman's health and perhaps her life. As so many women are affected by the contraceptives available in adverse ways, we need a much clearer understanding of side effects and their relation to women's health. The only way to obtain more information is to take women seriously, to take our symptoms seriously, and to share and accumulate this evidence. When symptoms can be recognised as having a possible relation to contraception, women are in a better position to weigh up whether or not this is something to be concerned about. Changes can be noted, discussed and assessed regularly. The experience of other women is essential in judging our own symptoms. Too many women have suffered side effects and damage to their health as a result of women's symptoms not being taken seriously. We must learn from this experience before almost an entire generation of women pay the consequences in terms of our health.

# REFERENCES

Beral, Valerie. 1976. 'Cardiovascular disease, mortality trends and oral contraceptive use in young women'. *Lancet*, 13 November: 1047–51.

Duffin, Lorna. 1978. 'The conspicuous consumptive: woman as an invalid' in S. Delamont and L. Duffin, eds. *The Nineteenth-Century Woman*. Croom Helm, London.

Ehrenreich, Barbara and Deirdre English. 1979. *For Her Own Good: 150 Years of the Experts' Advice to Women*. Pluto, London.

Elston, Mary Ann. 1981. 'Medicine as "old husbands' tales": the impact of feminism' in D. Spender, ed. *Men's Studies Modified*. Pergamon, Oxford.

Oakley, Ann. 1976. 'Wisewoman and medicine man: changes in the management of childbirth' in J. Mitchell and A. Oakley, eds. *The Rights and Wrongs of Women*. Penguin, Harmondsworth.

Rakusen, Jill. 1974. 'The pill report: information or progaganda?' *Spare Rib*, 32: 6–8.

Rakusen, Jill. 1978. 'The pill . . . as bad as we thought'. *Spare Rib*, 67: 44–5.

Rakusen, Jill. 1981. 'Depo–Provera: the extent of the problem. A case study in the politics of birth control' in H. Roberts, ed. *Women, Health and Reproduction*. Routledge & Kegan Paul, London.

Roberts, Helen. 1979. 'Women, social class and IUD use'. *Women's Studies International Quarterly*, vol. 2, no. 1: 49–56.

Royal College of General Practitioners. 1974. *Oral Contraceptives and Health*. Pitman Medical. London.

Scully, Diane. 1980. *Men Who Control Women's Health: The Miseducation of Obstetrician-Gynecologists*. Houghton-Mifflin, Boston.

Seaman, Barbara and Gideon Seaman. 1977. *Women and the Crisis in Sex Hormones*. Rawson, New York.

Walsh, Vivien. 1980. 'Contraception and the growth of a technology' in Brighton Women and Science Group, eds. *Alice Through the Microscope: The Power of Science Over Women's Lives*. Virago, London.

# WOMEN AS TARGETS IN INDIA'S FAMILY PLANNING POLICY

Vimal Balasubrahmanyan

India's Family Planning (FP) programme is zooming in on women. Possible adverse effects on women's health are being disregarded. The IUD campaign of the 1960s was a disaster because of the poor back-up health services. The vasectomy drive of the 1970s dislodged the government of the day. The current Indian government's plan to establish widespread Pill distribution, the impending introduction of injectable contraceptives and the hormonal implant are ominous signs of the government's iron will to achieve population control on the backs of women. Not enough facilities exist for safe abortion or adequate obstetric care and it is poor women who suffer most. The current FP policy has an inbuilt potential for abuse, especially when applied to an uninformed and illiterate population.

India was the first developing country to adopt in 1951–2 a national policy of population control through a family planning (FP) programme. If one looks at the pattern of the programme from the early years, when the rhythm method and the condom were advocated, to the present time when the introduction of both the injectable and the hormonal implant are imminent, a very distinct picture emerges. Over the years in India's FP programme women have become targets, objects and victims. The population controllers have been intent on drastic curbing of the birth rate at any cost, and the fulfilment of FP 'quotas'. The latest FP target for 1983–4 announced by the health ministry is: fifty-nine *lakh*[1] sterilisations, twenty-five *lakh* IUD insertions, seventy-nine *lakh* 'conventional' contraceptive users, and eleven *lakh* oral Pill users. In practice there has been insufficient attention (though lip service is paid to such concepts) to improvement in the quality of women's lives or to change in the man-woman relationship wherein reproduction has been a major instrument of women's oppression.

In the 1960s an intensive programme of IUD insertions was launched. It was a failure and women suffered. Initially 'successful' in the sense of recruiting 'acceptors', the IUD drive quickly showed a reverse trend. As the report of the Committee on the Status of Women (*Towards Equality*, 1975)[2] put it: 'Careless handling of IUD insertions by paramedical staff and inadequate follow-up treatment had caused a loss of popularity.' The Estimates Committee's Report (1971–2) to the Lok Sabha, quoting the health secretary, was even more forthright:

As regards the loop, it is correct that under pressure of our foreign advisers the programme was formulated and put into operation without thinking of the effects it would have on women. The result was that a large percentage of women suffered from harmful effects and the use of the loop went down subsequently. (Jain, 1975)

The 1969 evaluation report by the UN Advisory Mission remarked that the IUD drive had been adopted with 'insufficient preparation and undue optimism . . . little was known of the side effects and the public was taken by surprise by the common complaints of bleeding and backache.' (Jain, 1975)

The lessons of the IUD drive have not, however, been learnt. India is poised to launch social marketing (over-the-counter sale) and liberalised distribution of the Pill through village-level health workers (*Patriot*, July 13 1983) who are likely to be incapable of screening potential acceptors adequately. Meanwhile trials are going on with the injectable and the hormonal implant, both of which may be soon introduced, the targets once again being women. The basic requirement of a comprehensive health-care network, a precondition for the success and safety of any hormonal contraceptive drive, remains unfulfilled.

The 1970s saw the launching of an intensive sterilisation drive with emphasis on vasectomy. It is now well-known that the aggressive and coercive methods employed to achieve targets resulted in political disaster for Mrs Indira Gandhi's Congress Party at the 1977 general election. Ever since 1977 the emphasis in FP has put increasing pressures on women. Feminists in India feel that this policy shift is based on the belief that women, whatever be the FP onslaughts on them, will not express their displeasure through the ballot box. The IUD disaster lost no votes for the ruling party while the vasectomy compulsions did result in decisive votes *against* the Congress government.

Today the government's emphasis on laparoscopic sterilisation, the Pill, the IUD and soon perhaps the injectable and the implant are proof of the overwhelming concentration on women in the FP programme, regardless of the potential abuses inherent in this approach and the resultant adverse impact on the health of women.

Studies conducted by the government in the 1960s and 1970s had shown that the Pill is not acceptable in the Indian illiteracy-cum-poverty milieu. The discontinuation rate because of side-effects is high. (Jain, 1975) There is a definite danger of irregular Pill users becoming pregnant and a consequent risk of foetal abnormalities. The lessons of liberalised Pill distribution and consequent disaster can be learnt from umpteen studies in neighbouring Bangladesh.[3] Further, it is possible that pressures on health personnel to achieve targets and fulfil quotas will over-ride all health considerations. Doctors as well as feminists in India have urged the health minister to desist from launching the proposed Pill programme which is poised to take off soon.[4]

In January 1983 the deputy director-general of the Indian Council of Medical Research (ICMR), Dr G. P. Saxena, told the press (*Patriot*, Jan. 27, 1983) that an injectable contraceptive had been 'successfully' tested on 2,600 women and that no 'serious' side effects had been observed. In March the minister of state for health, Mrs Mohsina Kidwai, told parliament that a decision regarding the injectable would be taken soon. (*Patriot*, March 23, 1983) Meanwhile Dr Saxena has announced that trials are going on with the implant.

Soon after news about the injectable became known, the Centre for Education and Documentation (Bombay) published, in March 1983, an eighteen-page booklet, *Injectables:*

*Immaculate Contraception?* which detailed the abuses inherent in a mass programme with the injectable. On the basis of news from other Asian and African countries as well as reports on the misuse of the injectable on blacks and browns in the UK, health groups in India have expressed concern over the directions being taken in Indian FP policy. The CED researchers have described the controversies surrounding the safety of Depo-Provera in an effort to educate the public. They have pointed out that very little is known about the safety and long-term effects of the particular injectable used in Indian trials, Net-En (norethisterone enanthate) supplied by the West German firm Schering. When the CED approached the Institute for Research in Reproduction (one of the ICMR units) in Bombay, they were told that no information on the injectable could be released.

An editorial in the March 1983 issue of the *Medico Friend Circle Bulletin* (the MFC is a forum for socially conscious doctors) warned that steroidal contraceptives are being pushed through with a frightening urgency. We in India feel that the strategy of the government and the medical establishment will be to launch the injectable without much pre-publicity (hence the tight-lipped response to requests for information on side effects) before too many questions are asked or objections raised. By avoiding use of the controversial Depo-Provera, objections could be circumvented by arguing that the new injectable drug is blameless. However, as the CED points out, whether the injectable used is DP or Net-En, what is of concern is the possible use of the injectable on a mass scale, with all the abuses inherent in such a programme, as evidence from other countries has amply demonstrated.

It is true that arguments in favour of the injectable have been voiced by some feminists. In an interview with *Spare Rib* (March 1982), Dr Hari John logically spelled out the reasons for her pro-injectable stand. But, as others have argued, the injectable in the hands of a concerned, sympathetic person like Hari is quite different from the injectable in the hands of target-oriented, quota-filling, syringe-happy health personnel, especially when they are operating in the most backward and illiterate regions. Whatever its short-term benefits for oppressed women in a patriarchal structure, the long-term abuses and the lessons from other countries make most feminists and health activists in this country oppose the very introduction of the injectable, be it DP or anything else. And as the CED booklet points out, arguments in favour of the injectable (as the only contraceptive that women can use without the knowledge of husbands) only serve to strengthen the sexist status quo.

Another point raised by those concerned over India's FP priorities is: why is there no research and emphasis on male contraception and barrier methods? Today the cap and the diaphragm are practically non-existent in India. (*Medico Friend Circle Bulletin*, 1983) It is doubtful if doctors here would even know how to fit a woman with one of these devices, assuming a woman could get hold of one. Recently it was announced that a vaginal contraceptive sponge would soon be on sale in the UK and USA (*People*, 1983) and that at one dollar each the sponge would be beyond the reach of Third World women. The question is: if the Pill and the injectable can be subsidised for mass use why shouldn't a safe and non-controversial sponge be subsidised to reach the same masses?

Whenever population controllers speak enthusiastically of the Pill and the injectable they keep saying that the health risks of these are far outweighed by the risks of repeated pregnancies. It is true that the health of Indian women is affected by repeated pregnancies. But the direct causes are malnutrition and inadequate ante-natal and obstetric care and hardly anything is being done to remedy these conditions. Even though the FP programme is supposed to be integrated into maternal and child health schemes, in reality the emphasis has always been predominantly on FP and the aspect of maternal health is largely neglected.

There are several other dimensions to the FP programme's impact on women. The organisation of 'camps' for sterilisation and IUD insertions has resulted in careless insertions of IUDs with no follow-up care and reports of septic conditions and even deaths following sterilisations. Recently, the health minister warned that laparoscopic operations should *not* be done in camps so as to avoid complications which may result in the method itself falling into disrepute. (*Hindu*, April 24, 1983) But the camps continue because that is the only way in which targets can be achieved.

An auxiliary nurse midwife working in a rural area has written revealingly in *Manushi* (January–February 1983) of the pressures on women like her from senior medical officers: 'These days the government is laying stress on family planning. Every month the SMO scolds us saying that our family planning work seems to be nil . . . . he is interested in family planning because it affects his post and promotion.'

In 1981 the Feminist Resource Centre of Bombay organised a workshop on Women, Health and Reproduction. Many pertinent points were raised by feminists and doctors who participated in the workshop. It was pointed out that in spite of the large sums of money spent on FP, and in spite of the programme affecting so many women, the women's movement in India has yet to take serious note of the directions of the government's FP programme. The fact is that issues like dowry deaths, rape, employment opportunities, etc. have so much greater immediacy, that the feminist movement as a whole has yet to turn its attention to FP policy in a big way. However, there is today, especially because of the emerging health activist movement against harmful drugs and harmful health policies, a wider awareness of the issues involved in FP policy and its impact on women.

The 1981 conference in Bombay focussed on poor follow-up after IUD camps, hormonal contraceptive research on Indian women, inadequate access to safe abortion, and the general trends visible in India's FP programme. It was stressed that the majority of women have no access to menstrual regulation and safe cheap abortion, even though the Medical Termination of Pregnancy Act of 1971 has made abortion legal. The government's anti-natal propaganda has made it possible for urban abortion clinics to advertise their services in a big way through hoardings and press advertisements. And yet easy abortion today is available only to those who can afford the services of the private clinics. The Committee on the Status of Women (1975) had noted:

Several medical practitioners are reluctant to perform this operation because of ethical considerations, long recording procedures and paper work, and lack of proper medical facilities especially in rural areas. We were informed that some hospitals insist on sterilisation or the husband's consent before performing abortions. . . . imposition of such conditions will only drive women to unqualified persons and defeat the main purpose of the Act. (i.e. the MTP Act)

Concern was expressed at the Bombay conference over the widespread testing of hormonal contraceptives by the country's prestigious medical research institutes. Very little information is available regarding identity of the women who are being experimented upon, except that they must inevitably belong to the poorest and most deprived sections. The concept of informed consent for participating in clinical trials is practically ignored in medical research programmes. If there is any token consent it is certain that not enough information is given to make it genuinely informed consent as it is understood in the West.* Elitist medical researchers generally argue that informed consent as a concept is not feasible when the subjects are illiterate and that in any case all medical experimentation is only being done for the good of the people at large.[5] (Balasubrahmanyan, 1983) Civil liberties activists in India are yet to wake up to the attack on human rights inherent in the prevailing unethical medical research programmes. Meanwhile, since contraceptive research has high priority, women continue to be unwitting guinea pigs.

News items in Indian newspapers periodically refer to this or that new contraceptive drug being tried out and developed by the medical research institutes. In April 1983, for example, it was announced that the ICMR would start a joint project with Swedish Nobel Laureate, Dr Sune Bergstrom, for developing contraceptives based on prostaglandins. (*Patriot*, April 19, 1983) The project, it was reported, was soon to enter the clinical trial phase. By the end of 1983 neither women's groups nor human rights activists had asked any questions about the project, who the subjects are, how were they approached, whether they are aware that they are being experimented upon.

* Editors' note: However, informed consent is frequently lacking in Western medical practice.

This article on Indian FP priorities has so far dwelt on contraception. There are some other aspects too in the context of women's health and their reproductive role. Last year, after intensive campaigning by health and women's groups, the combination estrogen-progesterone hormone drug, widely misused for pregnancy testing, was banned by the government.[6] (*Lancet*, 1982) Although the West has long been aware of the risks of foetal defects caused by the drug when used for pregnancy testing, many doctors in India are still ignorant of these findings and the drug has been misused not only for pregnancy testing, but also has been often prescribed to cause abortions, though it is *not* an abortifacient. However, drug companies, including the multinationals, Organon and Ciba-Geigy, have obtained a stay order on the ban by claiming that the drug is needed for treating other gynaecological disorders. (*Economic Times*, 1983) At the time of writing the matter is still in court. Although it is a prescription drug it can be easily bought over the counter and it continues to be misused by the ill-informed. Some brands carry warnings in microscopic print, but many brands carry no warning at all. Many doctors too are unconvinced about foetal risk and continue to prescribe it for pregnancy testing. Last December it was reported (*Patriot*, Dec. 28, 1983) that in a survey of outpatients coming for abortion at an Ajmer hospital, 75 per cent had already consumed the drug on the advice of private practitioners. There is no data on the number who consume the drug and do not seek abortion, whose babies have been exposed to the drug. The Ajmer survey was done several months after the ban was announced and after there had been a fair amount of media exposure regarding foetal risks.

Today in India urban maternity and abortion clinics do thriving business but good obstetric care and safe abortion are beyond the reach of the poor. There is big money in abortion and although amniocentesis for the purpose of sex selection has been banned officially, there are enough loopholes to allow its continued misuse for selective abortion of female foetuses. Many gynaecologists have expressed the view that there is nothing reprehensible in selective abortion of female foetuses because: (a) it is a method of 'balancing' the family and is therefore a legitimate FP tool; (b) if abortion is morally permissible selective abortion is equally so; (c) after all, the women themselves desperately want it.

Again, there is big money in hysterectomy, which women see as a final solution to the inconvenience of menstruation and the fear of uterine cancer. According to a report in *Manushi* (No. 12, 1982), hysterectomy has become the 'mainstay of some nursing homes' and one estimate refers to 1,500 hysterectomies performed every month in one district of Andhra Pradesh alone. No systematic study has yet been done to gauge the extent of prevalence of unnecessary hysterectomies, unnecessary caesarian sections, drug-induced labour to suit the convenience of the attending doctors, etc., although periodic reports on all these do appear in the press. There are also continued reports of baby food multinationals like Nestlé persisting in maintaining links with doctors, health personnel and mothers in maternity clinics, and continuing to distribute free samples of baby food.

This report would be incomplete without a mention of infertility and the desperation it causes among most Indian women. The FP programme being emphatically anti-natal, there is no priority within it to help the childless though expensive expert gynaecological advice is within the reach of those who can afford it. Mahmood Mamdani in his classic, *The Myth of Population Control* (1972), evaluates the Khanna Study in Punjab, the first major birth control field study in India. He shows how the population controllers failed from the start to understand the perceptions and needs of their human targets, men and women. One quote from a woman in one of the villages covered by the study is relevant in the context of this article: 'It's strange that they gave free medicine to stop women from bearing children but had nothing to help those who could not bear children. That's where medicine could have been of use to us.' In another book, *Poverty and Population Control* (Bonderstam and Bergstrom, 1980), a similar example is given, reflecting the unfulfilled need for help to overcome infertility. In a chapter on FP in a Tamil village there is a reference to a Swedish nurse and former volunteer in a health programme. She became famous in the village for her ability to help women overcome

infertility and, during her time, people were coming from
far-off villages to be treated by her.

Today the government's FP programme is not only concentrating on women and on methods that are expected to
achieve quick results, but there is a distinct tilt towards the
introduction of disincentives for those who have more than
two babies. Primarily such disincentives attack women's
rights. In June 1983, the Justice G. D. Khosla Committee on
behalf of the Family Planning Foundation of India recommended denial of maternity leave and increase in hospital
charges for women who have a third or subsequent child.
(*Patriot*, June 10, 1983) Other disincentives proposed by the
committee include low priority in admission to educational
institutions for the 'surplus' children as well as low priority
in housing, bank loans, etc. for such families.

Whether or not these heinous suggestions are accepted
by the government, they are a clear indication of the climate
of opinion among the population control establishment of the
country and the fact that such an attitude is conducive to the
introduction of anti-women policies.

At the moment, however, the dominant focus is on incentives – prizes in cash and kind – for those who accept sterilisation or the IUD. During special 'family planning weeks' the
additional gifts sometimes announced are TV sets and
pressure cookers for women, over and above the usual cash
incentive. The fact remains that large numbers opt for
sterilisation because they desperately need the cash. Last
year, when laparoscopy camps were started and higher
incentives were offered to volunteers, there was such a
scramble for the operation in a Madras camp, that the
organisers ran out of funds. (*Hindu*, Feb. 15, 1982)

To sum up, women in India definitely need access to safe
and inexpensive contraception as well as safe and inexpensive abortion. They also need emancipation from poverty,
unequal male-female relationships, job opportunities and
economic independence, as well as transformation of the
socio-cultural structure which is patriarchal and oppressive
to women. Access to birth control has not progressed hand-in-
hand with fulfilment of these other needs. The result is that
within the FP programme women have been mere objects and

while they have sometimes received what they want and need, often they have not had access to methods they would choose if they had a free choice and an informed choice. Further, the lessons of the past and the lessons from other developing countries with comparable socio-cultural conditions have not been taken into account by FP policy makers. The result is that India is poised to repeat the FP mistakes which have already been experienced within the country and in other countries of the Third World. These are avoidable mistakes. And the tragedy is that the mistakes will be made and the lessons learnt all over again in India, *mainly at the cost of Indian women.*

## NOTES

1 *Lakh* is an Indian unit of measurement. One *lakh* means 100,000 (of anything).
2 The Committee on the Status of Women in India was appointed to prepare a report which was released on the eve of the International Year of Women. This report, *Towards Equality* (1975), resulted in fresh emphasis on women's issues and an important women's studies programme was initiated by the Indian Council of Social Science Research.
3 Loes Keysers (1982) describes in detail the disasters of Pill promotion in Bangladesh, which included the dumping of high-dose pills, a massive drop-out rate because of side effects, and a 'pill-induced population explosion' caused by pushing the Pill to breastfeeding women. When the latter's milk decreased they abandoned the Pill and thus also lost the contraceptive protection they would have had from uninterrupted lactation. Prolonged breastfeeding is an important reason for natural birth-spacing and has worked well in traditional societies.
4 In March 1983 the Hyderabad branch of the Indian Women Scientists Association wrote to the health minister explaining the dangers of the proposed Pill drive and urged him not to launch such a programme.
5 Recent months have seen a few press reports on medical experimentation without informed consent but the exposures have failed to move either the government or the medical authorities.
6 The campaign against the hormone pregnancy test was the first of its kind in India; health groups, feminists and journalists joined together and compelled the health ministry to respond.

## REFERENCES

Balasubrahmanyan, Vimal. 1983. 'Blind Spot in Medical Ethics.'
   *Mainstream*, March 13.
Bonderstam, Lars, and Staffan Bergstrom, eds. 1980. *Poverty and
   Population Control*. Academic Press, London.
Centre for Education and Documentation. 1983. *Injectables:
   Immaculate Contraception?*, Counterfact no. 3. CED Health Cell
   Feature. March. Bombay.
*Economic Times* (Calcutta edition). 1983. January 14.
Feminist Resource Centre. 1981. Report of The Workshop on
   Women, Health and Reproduction. Bombay.
*Hindu*. 1982, February 15; 1983, April 24. Newspaper published
   from Madras.
Indian Council of Social Science Research (on behalf of the
   Committee on the Status of Women). 1975. *Towards Equality*.
   New Delhi.
Jain, S.P. 1975. *A Status Study on Population Research in India*, vol.
   II, *Demography*. Family Planning Foundation. New Delhi.
Keysers, Loes. 1982. *Does Family Planning Liberate Women?*
   Institute of Social Studies, The Hague.
Keysers, Loes. 1982. 'Does Family Planning Liberate Women? (a
   summary).' *Insisterhood*. Journal of the Institute of Social
   Studies, The Hague.
*Lancet*. 1982. Round the World column. August 28.
*Mainstream* is a current affairs weekly from New Delhi.
Mamdani, Mahmood. 1972. *The Myth of Population Control*.
   Monthly Review Press, New York and London.
*Manushi*. 1983. Jan–Feb.; and 1982. issue no 12. Bimonthly feminist
   journal published from New Delhi.
*Medico Friend Circle Bulletin*. 1983. Editorial. March. Monthly
   published from Puna.
*Patriot*. 1983. January 27, March 23, April 9, June 10, July 13, July
   18, December 28. Newspaper published from New Delhi.
*People*. 1983. vol. 10, no. 3.
*Spare Rib*. 1982. March. Interview with Dr Hari John.

# CALLING THE SHOTS? THE INTERNATIONAL POLITICS OF DEPO-PROVERA

Phillida Bunkle

Despite serious questions of safety, the three-monthly contraceptive injection Depo-Provera has the fastest growing sales of any contraceptive worldwide. New Zealand is a small, apparently insignificant part of that global market. This paper examines the way the manufacturer of this drug has been able to use New Zealand women to produce 'safety' data that are favourable to Depo and its own interests. Pharmaceutical companies not only manufacture drugs, they also manufacture most of the information about them. This article shows how the process by which medical data is produced, endorsed and validated systematically excludes the experience of women. It examines the way the economic power of a multinational corporation has been used in New Zealand to produce medical data that favour its own interests. Depo-Provera provides an example of how the 'objectivity' of medical data is polluted by the interests of the corporations who pay for and control its production.

Depo-Provera, the three-monthly contraceptive injection, is a case study in the dilemmas posed to women by the development of the new reproductive technology. On the one hand Depo's easy administration and contraceptive efficacy makes contraception potentially convenient for millions of under-privileged women; on the other hand these very features make it a powerful tool for the control of women.

Depo is exclusively manufactured by the multinational Upjohn Corporation. Upjohn not only manufactures the drug – it also manufactures most of the information about it. Responding 'rationally' to the economic system, naturally they promote knowledge favourable to their product.

Depo, or medroxyprogesterone acetate, is a progestogen, that is, an artificially created drug which has some properties similar to naturally occurring sex hormones called progesterones. Upjohn started testing Depo as a contraceptive in the early 1960s.

In 1967 Upjohn applied to the United States Food and Drug Administration (FDA) for a licence to sell Depo as a contraceptive (*The Depo-Provera Debate*, 1978). In the following year Upjohn began the seven-year dog and ten-year monkey studies required by FDA.

The dog trials showed dose-related increases in both benign breast nodules and breast cancer. As a result of initial findings in dogs, the oral form of the drug, called Provest, and four other progestogen contraceptive preparations were withdrawn in 1970. Controversy has surrounded the use of the injectable long-acting Depo form ever since.

In 1974 FDA responded to the licensing application by allowing marketing with very stringent restrictions (ibid.: 223–7). Even with these conditions final permission was stayed on request from a Congressional Committee. The debate continued with a series of Congressional Hearings. In 1978 FDA finally rejected the application to market Depo as a contraceptive in the United States. In an extraordinary move Upjohn appealed against the decision. A Public Board of Enquiry heard this appeal in early 1983 (*Science*, 1982; *Time*, 1983). As of September 1983 the results of this and a similar appeal in the UK are not known.

The FDA ban meant effectively that Depo could not be manufactured in the USA. New Zealand, which had approved it for use in 1968, imports its supplies from an Upjohn subsidiary in Belgium. Not only was the company denied the lucrative US market, but, more importantly, because State Department policy prevented USAID (the main channel for American overseas aid) from supplying drugs banned in the US, Upjohn could not manufacture there for the huge Third World market (*Export of Hazardous Products*, 1980; Shaikh and Reich, 1981). Until President Reagan changed this policy in 1981 this was the primary cause of the company's concern. The ban not only inhibited willingness to buy by making the product look suspect, it cut off the large market that AID funds would make available.

Various population agencies were led, by their perception of the overriding need to make contraception available to all women, to evade this restriction (Ehrenreich, Dowie and Minkin, 1979; Sarra, 1982). It is alleged, for instance, that AID funds passed to International Planned Parenthood Federation (IPPF), whose headquarters are in London. IPPF purchased Depo for worldwide supply to national family planning associations. In this way family planning associations (FPA) became major sources of Depo, although many of their well-intentioned medical workers are not aware of this background. When the propriety of laundering funds was questioned, IPPF defended their action by convening an international committee of medical experts especially to consider Depo. Some committee members had worked with FPA supplying Depo in their various countries. Their report was highly reassuring, as were the expert evaluations provided by other interested parties, the World Health Organisation and AID (*Bulletin of the World Health Organization*, 1982; *IPPF Medical Bulletin*, 1980; 1982; AID, *Report to USAID of the Ad Hoc Consultative Panel*, 1978). Sometimes FPA doctors who prescribe Depo in New Zealand appear to have only information from these reports and package inserts supplied by the company.

## WHO USES DEPO-PROVERA?

The market potential of Depo was enormous. With half the world's population as potential users and manufacturing costs low, the market for contraceptive drugs is particularly large and profitable. In the West market saturation for contraceptive pharmaceuticals was reached with the pill by the late 1960s. Thereafter development of new products slowed. Market expansion depended on developing methods of administering contraceptives that would reach new populations. Here the interests of the drug companies and population controllers coincided. Unlike other expensive drugs, contraceptives are ones which Third World governments and international agencies are willing to spend money on. Although long-acting injectable drugs were ideal, the US ban meant that Upjohn had to work hard to develop the market potential. Between 1971–4 Upjohn spent over $4 million in bribes to foreign governments and family planning officials to encourage the use of the drug (*Export of Hazardous Products*, 1980: 184–7). Upjohn's persistence in challenging FDA decisions kept the safety issue 'open' and kept the debate focussed on the distant issue of cancer rather than more immediate adverse effects, until Depo was firmly established as brand leader.

Sales increased throughout the 1970s, reaching 7 million doses per year in 1978 and 8 million by 1983 (*Population Reports*, 1983. K-21). Of the countries with the highest rates of use, Jamaica, Thailand, New Zealand, Mexico and Sri Lanka, only New Zealand is not a third world country (ibid.). In most rich countries, for example, in the USA, Australia and Great Britain, Depo is banned or heavily restricted (Rakusen, 1981). In these countries there is, however, significant use in sections of the population which most resemble Third World stereotypes. Depo is, for example, reportedly used extensively on West Indian and Asian women in Britain and Aboriginals in Australia (*Cultural Survival*, 1981; Floreman, 1981: 17; Lucas and Ware, 1981; Savage, 1983; Thomas, 1982; *The Times*, 1981).

In New Zealand it is used disproportionately on Polynesian women. One statistically reliable survey of family practice found that

> Maori and Non-Maori women had similar overall
> contraception consultation rates, but there was a striking
> difference between races in the type of contraception used.
> Maori women were much more likely to get the Depo
> Provera injection. (Gimore, 1983: 8)

In this study Depo was prescribed to Maori women more often than any other form of contraception.

Company sales figures suggest that between 80,000 to 100,000 injections are sold in New Zealand each year. Dr Charlotte Paul of the University of Otago Medical School has estimated from surveys of contraceptive use that approximately 15 per cent of Pakeha (paleface) and 25 per cent of Maori women have used it at some time (Paul, 1981). A disturbing proportion of us, especially Maoris, will be at risk from any long-term effects Depo many turn out to have.

## DEBATE OVER THE SAFETY OF DEPO-PROVERA

Upjohn's assertion that Depo 'is probably the safest hormonal contraceptive drug available' is based on their claim that after fifteen years' use and millions of prescriptions there is a 'low reported incidence of side effects' (Upjohn Corporation, 1980: 314). The company has a vested interest in not looking for such evidence. But the absence of information does not establish the safety of a drug.

Upjohn claims that Depo is one of the most studied drugs available. None of these studies, however, conclusively answers vital safety questions. This is apparent even from an exhaustive evaluation of the medical evidence that is very favourable to Depo by Ian Fraser, Australia's foremost advocate of Depo and consultant to WHO and FPA (Fraser and Weisberg, 1981).

The example of this review shows why the medical evidence does not answer women's questions. Fraser's review was published as part of the *Medical Journal of Australia*. Printing costs were, however, paid by Upjohn. Having paid for production, Upjohn distributes this 'reputable' medical opinion as part of their promotional literature. Corporate production of 'academic' knowledge is not usually so blatant. Political science journals do not carry party manifestos even as supplements. The medical literature is generally reassuring about Depo, not because the drug is safe, but because of the way medical knowledge is constructed and disseminated.

The claim made by medical literature that Depo is safe cannot in fact be scientifically evaluated because the evidence available is either (i) the result of experiments performed or funded by the Corporation and constructed to give them favourable results, (ii) is 'proprietary information', or (iii) has never been systematically examined at all. To illustrate this I shall examine each of the safety issues using these three categories.

## (i) The corporate construction of knowledge
*Cancer*

Three cancer sites are involved, the breast, cervix and uterus. There are questions about the carcinogenicity of oestrogen pills and IUDs, especially copper IUDs, but if Depo were licensed it would be the first contraceptive drug accepted by FDA which is known to have caused cancer in test animals.

Controversy has centred on the applicability of the findings of cancer in the dog and monkey studies to women. Upjohn argued, and the population control agencies echoed, that the dog study is not significant because in Upjohn's view the beagles used in the dog studies were uniquely susceptible to breast cancers. Critics reply that while these results do not prove that Depo causes breast cancer in humans it must nevertheless be treated as presumptive evidence. Since animal tests have proved predictive for other known carcinogens, at the very least they shift the onus of proof of safety onto the manufacturer (Epstein, 1977).

When the results of the monkey study became available they added fuel to the controversy. At the end of the ten years, two of the high dose animals had endometrial cancers, and it was later revealed that three had had breast lumps. The debate on the validity of species-to-species extrapolation was promptly repeated for the monkeys. There has been little independent study of a possible cancer link in women. The evidence on breast cancer is described as 'sparse' (Fraser and Weisberg, 1981: 11). Upjohn rebuts the possibility that Depo causes uterine cancer by citing a 'study' done by Malcolm Potts in Thailand (McDaniel and Potts, 1979). In 1978 Potts, former medical director of IPPF, joined the International Fertility Research Program (IFRP), an organisation funded by USAID with lesser contributions from IPPF, Upjohn and others. IFRP has led the campaign for Depo. Potts went to Thailand for one month and with Edward McDaniel, the main distributor of Depo in Northern Thailand, he was able to trace nine of the sixty women who had been admitted to the region's hospital with uterine cancer (Minkin, 1981). He ascertained that none of the nine had had Depo. The inadequacies of the 'study' are obvious, indeed laughable, yet it has been cited repeatedly as 'evidence' that Depo does not cause cancer in women.

Very recently, Dr Potts, Dr Shelton from AID and others have published evidence from 5,000 black American Depo users showing no increase in breast, uterine or ovarian cancers (Liang, 1983). Unfortunately, short exposure, a limited follow-up period and wide 'confidence limits' prevent the study from being anything other than inconclusive.

In the meantime, however, concern had arisen over a possible relation in humans between Depo and cervical cancer, which is a much greater cause of concern than relatively rare uterine cancer. This is the shakiest, but in some ways most suggestive, human evidence on the carcinogenicity of Depo.

The human trials required from Upjohn were reported with no controls, little information of concurrent drug usage and zero follow-up. In 1974 an FDA analyst giving testimony to a Congressional Sub-Committee showed, however, that if the Third National Cancer Survey was used as a control to the Upjohn supplied data then it appeared that women on Depo had rates of cervical cancer in situ much greater than expected (Johnson, 1976).

FDA rejected the validity of using the National Cancer Survey as a control because the Upjohn group had been subject to more intense diagnostic scrutiny. Feminists were dissatisfied with FDA's dismissal of such suggestive evidence. They found two similarly screened groups to use as controls for the Upjohn data. Both suggested elevated rates of cervical cancer in Depo users (Corea, 1980).

Upjohn now needed evidence to refute the suspicion. The New Zealand Contraception and Health Study was the response. The 'primary objective' of the study 'is to examine the relative association between contraceptive practices and the development of dysplasia, carcinoma in situ, or invasive carcinoma of the cervix' (*Protocol*, 1982: 2). The study has a most prestigious executive committee, including the senior obstetrics/gynaecology professors from both New Zealand medical schools. The chairperson of the executive, Professor

Liggins, from the National Women's Hospital, vehemently maintains that the study is independent and was initiated by him (*Close Up*, 1983). This is disputed by some scientists who were first consulted by Upjohn personnel. The fragmentary documentary history made public at a recent Statistical Association conference would seem to support the view that the early stages were initiated and designed by Upjohn (Renner, 1983a). The company seems less concerned than academics to maintain the appearance of independence from the study; their 'media package' says 'Upjohn is currently conducting long range studies in New Zealand' (Upjohn Interview, 1982). There appears to be no other study to which they might be referring.

New Zealand is convenient for an investigation of a possible link between Depo and cervical cancer. New Zealand has a higher rate of use than any other country with a social and ethnic composition similar to the United States and a comparable standard of health care. An internal Upjohn memo notes the public health care system as an advantage, presumably because it will relieve the company from having to pay for any medical treatment incurred by subjects (Weisblat, 1977). The minister of health, dedicated to the 'free market' of ideas, eschews any regulation of privately funded research, even on human subjects. More significantly, welfare state legislation precludes the possibility of suing a doctor or drug company for damages. Regulatory freedom and legal immunity must be extremely attractive to a company which is a party to multi-million dollar suits for damages from American women who feel they have been injured by DES or Depo.

The New Zealand Contraception and Health Study is a prospective observational study following three groups of 2,500 subjects using Depo, IUDs, or combined pills for five years. A PAP smear is taken at each annual examination and a questionnaire completed by the doctor. Completed questionnaires are forwarded to the study office located in a partitioned section of the Upjohn warehouse in Auckland, which is leased by the Executive Committee from Upjohn, with Upjohn funds. 'Sealed patient questionnaires are not opened in New Zealand' (*Protocol*, 1982: 13) but are sent direct to

Upjohn headquarters in Kalamazoo, Michigan, where data are stored on the company computer (ibid.: 21). Data will be analysed by company scientists under the director of an Upjohn 'project manager' (ibid.). There is no undertaking to publish all or any results.

Professor Liggins maintains that this constitutes complete independence from the Upjohn Corporation (*Close Up*, 1983). There has been some discussion internal to the medical profession about why the pathology for the study is not being handled in New Zealand, where the capacity to process PAP smears is well developed. Similarly the Protocol says that 'All data processing and analysis will be performed in Kalamazoo' (*Protocol*, 1982: 21). Some biostatisticians have asked why the statistical analysis has not been designed and carried out in New Zealand. The Report of the Survey Appraisals Committee of the New Zealand Statistical Association, which is critical of the study, draws attention to the fact that there will be no independent access to data to facilitate 'peer review' (Deely, 1983).

The design of the study will crucially affect its results. Papers by a statistical consultant at recent Statistical Association and Epidemiological conferences show that the duration and sample size are too small to allow the study the statistical power to discriminate even large increases in cervical dysplasia or cancer (Renner, 1983a; 1983b; 1983c). Study design will therefore ensure reassuring results, justified or not. Only one medical doctor in New Zealand has publicly voiced concern about the study (*Close Up*, 1983). Next day he was verbally assailed by the head of National Women's Hospital and told that his professional standing was in jeopardy. These remarks were later withdrawn but the collective silence of the medical profession is perhaps not surprising. It is unlikely that aspiring obstetricians and gynaecologists will risk their career prospects by publicly criticising senior professors of both medical schools, on an issue of little personal concern to themselves.

The most outspoken medical advocate of Depo in New Zealand is John Hutton, formerly junior colleague of Professor Liggins, and recently promoted to the chair of obstetrics and gynaecology at Wellington Clinical School. At his aptly entitled inaugural lecture, 'Depo-Provera: Are the critics justified?' (Hutton, 1981; 1983), Professor Hutton defended Upjohn paying for a study in which they have a vested interest, on the grounds that 80 per cent of all medical research worldwide is funded by drug companies. Upjohn funding for this study was, he said, comparable to the annual budget of the Medical Research Council, the government source of medical research funds in New Zealand. Of course, such funds are important to those whose careers and prestige depend upon attracting them. By lending their names to research funded by drug companies, academics notch up the publication titles essential to career success. The more they do this, the more successful and powerful they will become, and the more able to attract funds (Mangold, 1983).

Upjohn money may also have influenced liberal doctors, many of whom work for FPA. Through affiliation with IPPF, FPA became the single largest supplier of Depo in New Zealand. FPA is chronically poorly funded. The company pay them $25 plus a consultation fee for each woman recruited into the study.

Upjohn have spent a great deal of money on the New Zealand Contraceptive and Health Study. It is unlikely that their funds will be wasted.

## (ii) Corporate control of knowledge

Cancer is not, however, the only safety issue with Depo-Provera. In 1979 Stephen Minkin published a critical review of the evidence on Depo in which he claimed that company reports of the animal studies spoke of cancers but did not reveal other very important adverse effects, in particular that many dogs actually died of uterine disease (Minkin, 1979). Minkin's work has been widely discredited, especially for lax citation (Hutton, 1980). Some of these criticisms are justified, but nevertheless the central charge that important evidence of side effects was not released remains unrefuted (Corea, 1980). Since the company 'owns' the evidence it is not available for scrutiny and the charge cannot be evaluated. The safety debate has focussed on cancer with little investigation on other health risks to women.

Depo has been promoted worldwide as the ideal

contraceptive for lactating mothers. This is a critical issue for Third World women. In New Zealand this is when it is likely to be prescribed for white, middle-class women. Apart from one study on rats, there is no evidence about the effect on neo-nates of Depo, absorbed from breast milk (Satayasthit et al., 1976). That Depo should have been promoted for this purpose before its effects on infants was established is another example of unwillingness to look for evidence that might injure prime markets.

## Teratogenic effects

The concern arises because of the known teratogenic effects of progestogens (Shapiro, 1978). Exposure during gestation is different and more significant but is nevertheless reasonable grounds for caution in exposing breast-fed neo-nates. As with cancer the evidence is a pattern of suggestive animal studies, backed by fragmentary human evidence.

In animal studies progestogens given in utero cause masculinisation of female foetuses. There is some slight but disturbing corroborative evidence from children who have been treated with Depo during gestation. Girl babies exposed to large doses of Depo in utero have been found to have 'clitoral hypertrophy'. 'Clitoral hypertrophy is an increase in the size of the clitoris in relationship to the size of the baby.' (*The Depo-Provera Debate*, 1978: 75–80). The doctors who gave this evidence to a Congressional Committee, however, testified that they found no evidence of birth defects. Clitoral enlargement 'becomes less obvious as the girl grows up' (ibid.) so that although it was a defect apparent at birth it was not a 'birth defect'.

Upjohn have used this remarkable logic to discredit critics concerned about a possible link between Depo and growth abnormalities (*Export of Hazardous Products*, 1980: 332). Now-you-see-it-now-you-don't definitions enable them to evade disturbing evidence and at the same time discredit opposition.

A recent evaluation in the prestigious *Journal of the American Medical Association* turns the lack of research on this issue into an argument for wider use to facilitate further experimentation (Rosenfield et al., 1983: 2925).

Upjohn recognises that more evidence is needed. In their submission to the FDA Board of Enquiry Upjohn say: 'follow-up of children exposed in utero is one aspect of the prospective observational study being conducted in New Zealand'. (Upjohn Corporation, 1982: 5)

The study *Protocol*, however, has no mention of such children. The *Protocol* simply provides no evidence for the existence of this aspect of the study (*Protocol*, 1982: 5, 10). This is similar to the 'six years of clinical trials' that the Upjohn consumer information pamphlet claims have taken place in New Zealand, but of which there is no trace (*Close Up*, 1983).

### (iii)  The invisibility of women's experience in medical research

If advocates of Depo discount animal evidence because it is animal, they also discount women's experience with the drug because it is 'subjective'.

When women report to their doctors effects of the drug unrelated to its contraceptive efficacy it does not appear to raise doubts about the drug, but, rather, reinforces the stereotype of women as 'complaining' or 'over-anxious'. Effects may be attributed to women's nature rather than recognised as drug-related. Many women have been told that the problems they report are 'most unusual'. The implication is that the problems are 'in' the women rather than 'in' the drug.

Women's experience has not been heard at all in the Depo debate. The definition of medical knowledge excludes the personal and invalidates our testimony. I have been part of a New Zealand feminist health group evaluating the medical evidence and asserting the primacy of women's experience in the debate. By gathering together many women's accounts of how they were prescribed Depo and their experience using it we have been able to reassure many women that they are not alone or unusual in experiencing adverse effects. For many women it has been a huge relief to feel it is not something 'wrong' with them.

In trying to gather information about the use of Depo in New Zealand, our group has been hampered not only by our lack of resources but also by the belief that we are paranoid or neurotic. Not being scientists or doctors, we are made to feel that we have no 'right' to such information. Our health and our bodies are none of our business. The chief O & G (obstetrician/gynecologist) of New Zealand described the letters that come to National Women's Hospital on 'forced sterilization and Depo-Provera' as 'not usually true, grossly distorted or psychotic' (Bonham, 1980). Feminist research is seen as the exaggeration of distorted minds having problems with 'authority'. This may seem like rather primitive abuse of psychiatric labels but it is effective in discrediting our individual and collective experience.

Some of the women who shared their experience with us found Depo helpful and experienced few side effects; others experienced side effects but considered them worthwhile for effective contraception; others experienced very severe effects. Because it is important that negative experiences be made visible I draw on them here.

### Bleeding

The medical literature recognises that bleeding 'disturbances' are the most common side effect of Depo. What is unacknowledged is how disabling these 'disturbances' can be.

> *Ruth:* Within 24 hours of the injection I started bleeding. I flooded for 14 weeks. In that time I lost 3 stone (42 lbs). I couldn't go out. Sometimes I could only crawl around.

Upjohn does now admit that 1–2 per cent of women will have heavy bleeding on Depo. Bleeding is difficult to quantify. It has therefore been consistently minimised. Few studies investigate it. One study which does do so speaks of bleeding 'episodes' of eleven–thirty days a month (Nash, 1975; Toppozada, 1978). But how heavy, for how many months? Bleeding is perceived as a problem because it is the main reason of 'discontinuance'. The significance of side effects are measured by the effect on 'acceptance ratios'. This orientation is reflected in a World Health Organization study which set out to test how 'legitimate' women's reasons were for discontinuing Depo. They found that stopping Depo was

positively correlated with bleeding 'episodes' of eighty days
or more (WHO, 1978)!

There is no recognition in the medical literature of the
meaning to otherwise healthy women of these 'disturbances',
or of the utter debility they can cause. One 'expert' said 'one
woman a week was admitted to National Women's Hospital
with uncontrollable bleeding from Depo Provera' (Taylor,
1980). The issue is not just how many incapacitated women
this adds up to, but that it trivialises women's, sometimes
devastating, experience.

*Christine:* Christine is a maths teacher. She is married to a
senior lecturer (assistant professor) of accountancy. She
was given Depo in the maternity hospital after the birth of
her second child. She believed it was administered
routinely to all her doctor's patients and did not feel she
had a choice. It seemed to make all her post-natal
symptoms worse. She felt debilitated by the following
eighteen months spotting and bleeding which was
accompanied by sharp stabbing pains in the uterus. But it
was feeling afraid to go out of the house because she had to
be near a toilet that contributed most to her depression.
She was prescribed psycho-active drugs but the
gynaecologist offered no treatment for the bleeding.

When we talk openly of women's experiences and what
they mean we are said to be 'sensationalising' the issue. The
fact that they are often accompanied by acute distress and
depression is used to discredit the testimony. We are accused
of 'frightening' women but their months of fear are ignored.

There seems to be a discrepancy between what women
experience and the evidence in the medical literature. The
New Zealand Contraception and Health Study provides an
example of how this discrepancy can come about. The study
devises useful measures of bleeding 'disturbances'. The
'exclusion criteria', however, exclude subjects who stop their
method of contraception within ninety days (*Protocol*, 1982:
7). Ninety days is only relevant to Depo. It means that women
who only have one shot will be dropped from the study.
Although heavy bleeding sometimes occurs when the drug is
withdrawn, usually the worst bleeding occurs immediately

after the first shot. The most severe bleeding will therefore be excluded by the study and will not be measured at all.

Such knowledge is constructed to discount women's actual experience. 'Objective facts' like these are used to show how feminists exaggerate.

Science is projected as 'pure', that is, independent of the interests that produce it. The authority of science obscures the political process in the construction of scientific knowledge. The 'facts', however, directly reflect the structures that create them.

The process by which facts are validated is very important in defining what is 'known'. Only events recorded in medical literature are recognised, yet such documentation is quite haphazard. The experience of our group suggests significant underreporting of serious effects. Fraser's review of the medical literature found 'one case of anaphylactic shock has been reported' and 'There does not appear to be a single well substantiated case' of permanent infertility 'in the literature' (Fraser and Weisberg, 1981: 8). Our group knows of four women who have had life-threatening anaphylactic reactions. Two followed the first and two followed the second injection. The ninety-day 'exclusion criterion' will predictably result in under-representation of anaphylaxis in the New Zealand Contraception and Health Study, which will contribute to 'knowledge' about the rarity of such events.

*Infertility*

Similarly, we know of four women, two of 'proven fertility' who, having been regular before, have not had a period since taking Depo.

*Gail* had previously had a child. 'I took Depo 8 years ago and my cycle has never returned to normal. I have never had a period since then unless I took the pill.' Gail was later able to conceive with the help of fertility drugs.

*Jane* had previously had a child. 'I had two shots of Depo 7 years ago. I have not had a period since.' Jane has recently had some treatment with fertility drugs. She hopes they will make her fertile again as she felt that being made infertile was one reason why her relationship broke up.

The absence of 'objective' evidence of permanent infertility is used to show that continuing concern about Depo is irrational. Four women may not be many, but for them being unusual is no comfort.

The long delay in the return of fertility can cause havoc in women's lives. It is hard to plan your life when you are waiting in limbo to conceive, or worrying that you may be either pregnant or sterile.

The manufacturers do admit that there is a lengthy delay in the return of fertility. Two studies are quoted which show that, two years after stopping Depo injections, conception rates are comparable to the pill and higher than the IUD (Pardthaisong, 1980; Gardner and Mischell, 1970). The medical literature shows that, eighteen months after discontinuance, 85 per cent of women are menstruating again (*Population Reports*, 1983). The 15 per cent who are not disappear from the literature. Reversibility is of vital concern to women, yet it is given little attention in the research. Women's needs do not determine scientific priorities.

## Depression and permanent weight gain

No attempt at all is made to gather information on some 'side effects', no matter how important they are to women. Medical research tends to equate 'real' with 'quantifiable'. 'Real' means you can add it up. Everything else is psychosomatic or subjective. Evidence that does not fit into the objective quantifiable mode, such as depression, cannot be measured and is readily dismissed. There is an assumption that only clearly physical effects can be caused by a drug. It is a short step to seeing the person who reports such 'unreal' effects as unreal or unstable too.

Many women have told us how depressed they seemed to become while taking Depo. Most women recognised that it was difficult to tell whether Depo was a 'cause' of their depressed mood, although some said that they had never felt depressed before taking it. Quite a few women had treatment for depression while taking Depo. Depo is frequently given to women who are experiencing difficulties. It is routinely given to many mental hospital patients. No-one knows how much it may contribute to keeping them in this state.

Women who are given Depo post-natally may have weight gain, sexual turn-off and depression anyway, but Depo isn't going to help the situation. These women may have to struggle harder to climb out of their condition. The medical literature shows that the average weight gain is 5–10 lbs (*Population Reports*, 1983: K-27). Quite a lot of women are, however, really distressed by very large weight gains which they find hard to reverse. The literature shows gains of up to 45 lbs in a year. For some women this was associated with a sense of helplessness that contributed to depression.

## Sexual turn-off

The effect of Depo about which most women complained to us was that of being sexually turned off. Depo is used in two American clinics to chemically castrate male sex-offenders (Barry and Ciccone, 1975), but it is used on millions of women without any consideration of its effects on their sex lives. In the medical literature on Depo, the only discussion of this as a problem I have found was from a Chilean doctor who said that they gave up using six-monthly injections of a double dose because 'it caused a rather marked regression of the internal genitals that was accompanied frequently by poor libido and lack of orgasm, a matter that meant some conflict with the husband' (Zanartu, 1978). What it meant for the women themselves is not considered. It simply isn't important that women experience sexual pleasure. Is contraception for women, but sex for men? Only sexist science sees the chemical castration of women as a technical advance.

Two women who shared their experiences with us said they thought Depo was a good contraceptive but also said that they lost interest in sex. Some women are so concerned about pregnancy that they find being turned off an acceptable price to pay for secure contraception. That some of us do not feel free not to have sex we do not enjoy is probably a comment on how closely sex is associated with our dependence on men, rather than our pleasure. It is a telling measure of our powerlessness in a sexist society.

I have been told repeatedly that being turned off cannot be investigated at all because it would rely on what women say. It would mean believing that women actually know whether they are turned on or not. Such a belief cannot be incorporated into science. 'Hard' science has 'objective' evidence that women do not know the difference between an orgasm and a shiny floor.

## Who calls the shots?

Depo is not unique. It is one example of the creation of authoritative knowledge in our society (Spender, 1981: 1–9). Technological knowledge is both a function and a source of power. Women must insist upon becoming informed participants in public debate over technology. But it is hard. We have been told we are incapable of this type of understanding. Not only do we have to convince ourselves that we can crack the medical code but be confident enough to offer a basic criticism of the distortions of male-defined science (Elston, 1981; Overfield, 1981).

Committed to an empirical, value-free mode, medics find it hard to perceive the basic contamination of the 'objectivity' of their data by the processes and structures within which it is defined and constructed (Fee, 1982; Whitbeck, 1982). From the industry's point of view the health care system exists only to market its products. The integration of the medical profession and corporate enterprise is obvious in marketing but is actually cemented in the production of medical data itself.

Contraception is an example of the technology created by the structures of capitalist patriarchy. The 'knowledge' on which it is based reflects these interests. It is not 'value-free' but generated to serve the interests that create it. Many doctors pass on the fruits of this knowledge in good faith because they do not see their own place in the structure that perpetuates such 'truths'. They then find themselves unable to treat the problems it creates.

The overwhelming reason most women who spoke to us use Depo is that they cannot solve the contraception problem. Many had run the gauntlet of contraceptive methods. All the other methods demand that we face the conflict over and over again, every day. Here at last is a method that promises we will not have to face the problem for a few weeks. No wonder it sounds attractive. For some it worked, but for some it was a false promise. For most of those of us who need birth control there is no answer to the problem.

The technology is the end product of the system that produced it. That system has nothing at all to do with women's needs. No wonder our needs are not met by it. Depo-Provera gives the illusion that women can control their reproductive destiny. Our need for that control is exploited. Our desire for that control is used against us. We are made to pay an enormous price for our reproductive 'power'.

## REFERENCES

Agency for International Development. 1978. *Report to USAID of the Ad Hoc Consultative Panel on Depot Medroxyprogesterone Acetate.* AID. New York.

Barry, D. and J. Ciccone. 1975. 'Use of Depo-Provera in the treatment of aggressive sexual offenders: Preliminary report of three cases.' *Bulletin of the American Academy of Psychiatry and the Law*, 3 (179).

Bonham, Professor. 1980. Family Planning Course for Counsellors and Nursing Staff. Auckland. 22 September.

*Bulletin of the World Health Organization* (WHO). 1982, vol. 60, no. 2, pp. 199–210.

*Close Up.* 1983. TVNZ. 13 April. Producer Chris Mitson.

Continho, Elsimai. 1978. 'Statement of Dr. Elsimai Continho, Professor of Obstetrics and Gynaecology, Federal University of Baluci, Brazil.' *The Depo-Provera Debate*: 75–80.

Corea, Gena. 1980. 'The Depo-Provera Weapon.' In Holmes, Helen B., ed. *Birth Control and Controlling Birth: Women Centered Perspectives.* Humana Press, New Jersey: 107–16.

*Cultural Survival*, 1981. 5(4): 6.

Deely, J. J. Convenor, Survey Appraisals Committee of New Zealand Statistical Association. 'The New Zealand Contraception and Health Study: the Appraisal of the Protocol.' *New Zealand Statistician*, vol. 18, no. 2, Dec. 1983, pp. 6–11.

*The Depo-Provera Debate: Hearings Before the Select Committee on Population, United States House of Representatives.* 1978. Ninety-fifth Congress, Second Session, August 8, 9, 10. Chairman Scheuer.

Ehrenreich, Barbara, Mark Dowie and Stephen Minkin. 1979. 'The Charge: Gynocide, the Accused: The U.S. Government.' *Mother Jones*, November.

Elston, Mary Ann. 1981. 'Medicine as "Old Husband's Tales": The Impact of Feminism.' In Spender, Dale, ed. *Men's Studies*

*Modified: The Impact of Feminism on the Academic Disciplines.*
Pergamon, Oxford: 189–211.

Epstein, Samuel. 1977. 'Cancer and the Environment.' *Bulletin of the Atomic Scientists*, 24, 25, 29.

*Export of Hazardous Products: Hearings before a Sub Committee on International Economic Policy and Trade of the Committee of Foreign Affairs, United States House of Representatives*, 1980. Ninety Sixth Congress, Second Session, June 5, 12 and Sept. 9.

Fee, Elizabeth. 1982. 'A Feminist Critique of Scientific Objectivity.' *Science for the People*, July/August: 5–33.

Floreman, Ylra. 1981. *Lyckopillret. Reportage, Falun, Sweden.*

Fraser, Ian and Edith Weisberg. 1981. 'A Comprehensive Review of Injectable Contraception with Special Emphasis on Depot Medroxyprogesterone Acetate.' *Medical Journal of Australia*, 1 (1). Supplement 1: 1–20.

Gardner, J. and D. Mischell. 1970. 'Analysis of bleeding patterns and resumption of fertility following discontinuation of a long acting injectable contraceptive.' *Fertility and Sterility*, 21 (4): 286–91.

Gimore, Lyn and Judith Madarasz. 1983. 'Women's Involvement in Primary Health Care.' *A Report on the Women's Health Network National Conference.* New Zealand Women's Health Network. Tauranga.

Holmes, Helen B., ed. 1980. *Birth Control and Controlling Birth: Women Centered Perspectives.* Humana Press, New Jersey.

Hutton, John. 1980. 'Depo-Provera, A Critical Analysis of the Published References.' Typescript. Postgraduate School of Obstetrics and Gynaecology. National Women's Hospital, Auckland.

Hutton, John. 1981. DMPA and the Press in New Zealand in McDaniel, Edwin, ed., *Second Asian Regional Workshop on Injectable Contraceptives, Chiang Mai, Thailand.* World Neighbours, Oklahoma.

Hutton, John. 1983. 'Depo-Provera: Are the Critics Justified?' Inaugural address to the Wellington Clinical School. Wellington. Aug. 3.

*IPPF Medical Bulletin.* 1980. 14 (6).

*IPPF Medical Bulletin.* 1982. 16 (6).

Johnson, Anita. 1976. 'Depo-Provera – A contraceptive for poor women.' *Public Citizen.* Washington DC Health Research Group.

Liang, Arthur et al. 1983. 'Risk of Breast, Uterine Corpus, and Ovarian Cancer in Women Receiving Medroxyprogesterone Injections.' *Journal of the American Medical Association*, 249 (21): 2902–12.

Lucas, David and Helen Ware. 1981. 'Fertility and Family Planning in the South Pacific.' *Studies in Family Planning*, 12 (8/9): 303–15.

McDaniel, Edwin, ed. 1981. *Second Asian Regional Workshop on Injectable Contraceptives, Chiang Mai, Thailand.* World Neighbours, Oklahoma.

McDaniel, Edwin and Malcolm Potts. 1979. 'International forum update: depot medroxyprogesterone acetate and endometrial carcinoma.' *International Journal of Gynaecology and Obstetrics,* 17 (3): 297–9.

Mangold, Tom. 1983. 'Relationships between Doctors and Salesmen are Lurching Out of Control.' *Listener,* London. Jan. 2.

Minkin, Stephen. 1979. *Depo-Provera, A Critical Analysis.* Institute for Food and Development Policy, San Francisco.

Minkin, Stephen. 1981. 'Nine Thai Women had cancer . . . None of them took Depo-Provera: Therefore Depo-Provera is Safe . . . This is Science?' *Mother Jones,* November: 34–50.

Nash, H. 1975. 'Depo-Provera: A Review.' *Contraception,* 2 (4): 377–94.

Overfield, Kathy. 1981. 'Dirty Fingers, Grime and Slag Heaps: Purity and the Scientific Ethic.' In Spender, Dale, ed. *Men's Studies Modified: The Impact of Feminism on the Academic Disciplines.* Pergamon, Oxford.

Pardthaisong, T. et al. 1980. 'Return of fertility after discontinuation of depot medroxyprogesterone acetate and intra-uterine devices in Northern Thailand.' *Lancet,* 1 (8167): 509–12.

Paul, Charlotte. 1981. Unpublished paper, Department of Preventative and Social Medicine, Medical School, Otago University, Dunedin.

*Population Reports.* 1983. 'Injectables and Implants.' May. Series K no. 2. N.B. This publication is 'supported by' USAID.

Potts, Malcolm. 1978. 'Statement by Dr Malcolm Potts, Executive Director, International Fertility Research Programme.' *The Depo-Provera Debate:* 15–18.

*Protocol, New Zealand Contraception and Health Study.* 1982. Auckland.

Rakusen, Jill. 1981. 'Depo-Provera: the extent of the problem – a case study in the politics of birth control.' In Roberts, Helen, ed. *Women, Health and Reproduction.* Routledge & Kegan Paul, London.

Renner, Ross. 1983a. *Depo-Provera: A Study in Weak Design.* A paper delivered on 29 June 1983 at the 34th Annual Conference of the New Zealand Statistical Association.

Renner, Ross. 1983b. *Scientific Objectivity and Social Responsibility: A Critique of the Protocol of the New Zealand Contraception and Health Study.* A paper presented to ANZSERCH Annual Conference, 25–7 May, at the Clinical School, Wellington.

Renner, Ross. 1983c. 'Depo-Provera: the New Zealand Contraceptive and Health Study.' *New Zealand Statistician*, vol. 18, no. 2, Dec. 1983, pp. 20–33.

Roberts, Helen, ed. 1981. *Women, Health and Reproduction*. Routledge & Kegan Paul, London.

Rosenfield, Allan et al. 1983. 'The Food and Drug Administration and Medroxyprogesterone Acetate: What are the Issues?' *Journal of the American Medical Association*, 249 (21): 2925.

Sarra, Janis. 1982. 'The Case Against Depo-Provera.' *Healthsharing*. Fall: 20–3.

Satayasthit, N. et al. 1976. 'The effect of medroxyprogesterone acetate, administered to the lactating rat, on the subsequent growth, maturation and reproductive function of the litter.' *Journal of Reproduction and Fertility*, 46 (2): 411–12.

Savage, Wendy. 1983. 'Taking Liberties with Women: Abortion, Sterilization, and Contraception.' *New Zealand Women's Health Network Newsletter*, April, 1 (36).

*Science*. 1982. 'Depo-Provera Debate Revs Up at FDA.' July 30, 217: 424–8.

Shaikh, Rashid and Michael Reich. 1981. 'Haphazard Policy on Hazardous Exports.' *Lancet*, October 3: 740–2.

Shapiro, Samuel. 1978. 'Evidence Concerning Possible Teratogenic Effects of Exogenous Female Hormones and Statement of Dr. Samuel Shapiro, Drug Epidemiology Unit, Boston University Medical Center.' *The Depo-Provera Debate:* 87–91.

Spender, Dale, ed. 1981. *Men's Studies Modified: The Impact of Feminism on the Academic Disciplines*. Pergamon, Oxford.

Stimpson, Catharine and Ethel Spector Person, eds. 1980. *Women: Sex and Sexuality*. Chicago University Press, Chicago.

Taylor, John. 1980. Statement at Family Planning Course for Counsellors and Nurses, Auckland. September 18.

Thomas, Helen. 1982. 'Girls Injected with Contraceptive U.S. has banned.' *National Times*, October 31.

*Time*. 1983. 212 (4): 49.

*The Times*. 1981. 'Aborigines given birth control banned in U.S.' March 23.

Toppozada, Mokhtav. 1978. 'Effects of Depo-Provera on Menstruation.' *The Depo-Provera Debate*: 438–77.

Upjohn Corporation. 1980. Commentary on Depo-Provera, submitted by the Upjohn Corporation. Appendix 8. *The Export of Hazardous Products*.

Upjohn Corporation. 1982. *Depo-Provera for Contraception: Information for the Public Board of Inquiry for Depo-Provera: Response to the Board's Questions*, June 25: 5.

Upjohn Interview. 1982. *Controversy Continues to Cloud Facts about Depo-Provera*. Upjohn Interview is a trade mark of the Upjohn Company.

Weisblat, D. 1977. *Memo to D. Weisblat, From N. Mohberg, J. Assenzo, and P. Schwallie, Subject: Review of Depo-Provera Study Proposed.* November 1: 1–7.

Whitbeck, Caroline. 1982. 'Women and Medicine: An Introduction.' *Journal of Medicine and Philosophy* 7 (2): 119–32.

World Health Organization. 1978. 'Multinational Comparative Evaluation of Two Long-Acting Injectable Contraceptive Steroids: Norethisterone Enanthate and Medroxyprogesterone Acetate.' *The Depo-Provera Debate*: 662–85.

Zanartu, J. 1978. *The Depo-Provera Debate*: 79.

# SUBTLE FORMS OF STERILIZATION ABUSE: A REPRODUCTIVE RIGHTS ANALYSIS

Adele Clarke

Sterilization abuse is often thought to mean forced sterilization against a person's will. But, as reproductive rights activist Adele Clarke points out, sterilization abuse can take on subtle guises when the social conditions of people's lives constrain our capacity to exercise genuine reproductive autonomy. Currently, the subtle forms of sterilization abuse are becoming increasingly prevalent. In this paper, Adele Clarke points out ten of the most common forms of subtle sterilization abuse, and makes recommendations for political changes that would affirm the reproductive choices of all people.

In 1977, women workers in the lead pigment department of an American Cyanamid plant in West Virginia were given the 'choice' of being sterilized or moving to lower-paying jobs. Laws against sterilization abuse did not protect these women — after all, they were 'free' to remain fertile! All that would involve was leaving their current jobs — at $225 per week plus overtime — and transfering to jobs as janitors — at $175 per week maximum. Five of these women 'chose' to be sterilized. Several have regretted their decisions (Mereson, 1982: Stellman and Henifin, 1982).

Sterilization is today the most common method of birth control worldwide, and its use is rising (Kessel and Mumford, 1982; Stepan et al., 1981). There are several means of sterilization available and all should be considered *permanent* (e.g. see NWHN (National Women's Health Network), 1981). As in the situation above, however, not all sterilizations are genuinely desired by those who are sterilized.

*Sterilization abuse*, the coerced or unconsenting

sterilization of women and men, occurs in both blatant and subtle forms. *Blatant* abuse includes forced sterilization against a person's will, sterilization without telling the person they will be sterilized, and (in the US) sterilization without the patient's informed consent to the procedure.

*Subtle* sterilization abuses include situations in which a woman or man *legally consents* to sterilization, but the *social conditions* in which they do so are abusive – the conditions of their lives constrain their capacity to exercise genuine reproductive choice and autonomy. While blatant abuses continue to occur in the US (though seemingly less frequently), subtle abuses appear to be much more common today.

This paper presents a reproductive rights analysis of subtle sterilization abuse. I begin with an examination of the reproductive rights perspective. Ten basic types of subtle sterilization abuse are then delineated and discussed. I conclude with some recommendations for policies and activities to enhance women's and men's exercise of their reproductive rights and reduce subtle sterilization abuse.

In the feminist tradition, the ideas presented here grew collectively.[1] I have worked for several years with the sterilization group of the Committee to Defend Reproductive Rights, a San Francisco-based feminist women's consumer activist organization.[2] I have also taught a variety of courses on women's health over the past decade. In all our discussions of reproductive rights, there has been a characteristic tension between the personal and the political. How can we relate our personal reproductive experiences to larger social policy issues? It is through our joint attempts to address such contradictions that we have come to understand subtle sterilization abuse and what genuine reproductive freedom might be.

## REPRODUCTIVE RIGHTS PERSPECTIVES

The central argument of reproductive rights is that reproductive issues must be viewed in their specific social, historical and institutional contexts. Further, reproduction is a *fundamental human right*: neither the state nor the actions of others should deny any person autonomy over their reproductive processes.[3]

Reproductive freedom is prerequisite for any kind of liberation for women. The right to decide whether and when to bear a child is fundamental to a woman's control of her own body, her sexuality, her life choices. Involuntary motherhood precludes self-determination. This is why abortion, the final line of defense against an unwanted pregnancy, is the bottom-line requirement of the reproductive rights movement.[4,5]

Reproductive freedom, as Petchesky (1980: 665) has ably noted, is irreducibly social and individual at the same time because reproduction itself 'operates at the core of social life, as well as within and upon women's bodies.' Reproductive rights work, then, must address issues such as sterilization abuse at *both* social and individual levels of action to enhance women's and men's reproductive autonomy.

In sharp contrast, several opponents of reproductive rights – population controllers, corporate privilege advocates and medical professionals exercising their own authority over patients' reproductive decisions – all subscribe to what I call *market analyses* of people. Such analyses measure human worth by an 'economic test of fitness' in terms of an individual's assumed capacity for self-support or potential for becoming a burden to the state (Carver, 1929; Kittrie, 1971).[6,7,8] These three perspectives also assume a *commodification of children*, who are viewed as luxury items in the marketplace of individual or familial consumption (cf. Rothman here). Children become something to be afforded – in terms of money, time and energy. Both quantity (numbers) and quality (the anticipated health and well-being) of children are evaluated in commodified forms.

While such a commodity orientation currently appears predominantly in more industrialized nations, it may be spreading to less developed areas as people have fewer children (Folbre, 1983). This is due in part to the awesome level of investment in international family planning made by the population control establishment (Population Information Program, 1983a). Because of its permanence, sterilization is especially favored among population controllers, and extensive surgical training for physicians from less developed countries is provided by the US Agency for International Development (Wagman, 1977). Thus, while this article primarily addresses sterilization abuse in the US, the problem is certainly international in scope.

## FROM BLATANT TO SUBTLE STERILIZATION ABUSE

Patterned *blatant* sterilization abuse began in the US in the late nineteenth century (Bajema, 1976; Haller, 1963). It continued quite actively under the authority of state eugenics (better people through better breeding) laws until about 1960, focused on the unconsenting and/or coerced sterilizations of the (usually incarcerated) mentally retarded, physically disabled and mentally ill, often immigrants (Fox, 1978; Robitscher, 1973).

During the 1950s and 1960s in the South, a new form of blatant sterilization abuse emerged: numerous cases of Black women and girls sterilized without their knowledge and/or consent came to the attention of civil rights workers. There were also several fresh state proposals for compulsory sterilization (mostly for illegitimacy). Both of these issues were taken up by the national press in 1964, when the Student Nonviolent Coordinating Committee also published a pamphlet 'Genocide in Mississippi' on these and similar issues (Paul, 1968). Sterilizations became so common in the South that they are known as 'Mississippi appendectomies' (Rodriguez-Trias, 1982: 150).

Blatant sterilization abuse became a core focus of the reproductive rights movement in the early 1970s as the result of several especially horrifying cases, including the Relf sisters (two young Black girls sterilized without their knowledge in Alabama), Norma Jean Seren (a Native American woman sterilized without her knowledge for 'socioeconomic reasons' in Pennsylvania), the patterned sterilization abuse of Native American women by the US Indian Health Service, and the series of abuses in Los Angeles of Mexican American women known as the Madrigal case (Ad

Hoc Women's Studies Committee, 1978; National Lawyers' Guild, 1979; NWHN, 1981; Women Against Sterilization Abuse, 1977). Extensive abuses were also reported in Puerto Rico and of Puerto Rican women on the mainland US (e.g. Rodriguez-Trias, 1982).

In response to these cases, reported extensively by the media, reproductive rights and civil rights activists organized and pushed for the enactment of *regulations* to protect women and men against such abuses through more rigorous required informed consent procedures for the surgeries. Today in the US, federal regulations cover all federally-funded (Medicaid) sterilizations. Additionally, New York City and the state of California both have similar regulations which cover 'private pay' (third party/insurance and personal pay) patients.

Reproductive rights activists gradually began to understand that blatant abuses are really the tip of a much larger iceberg of sterilization abuse. Most abuse is likely to be *subtle and privatized*, taking place in physicians' offices, hospitals and even at home where women and men 'choose' sterilization as a means of contraception under constraining circumstances with inadequate and erroneous information about it and its consequences.

## FORMS OF SUBTLE STERILIZATION ABUSE

Ten major situations in which the majority of subtle sterilization abuses occur have been identified by reproductive rights activists.

### 1 Lack of abortion options

Despite extensive efforts by the anti-abortion /'Right to Life' movement (English, 1981; Merton, 1981), abortion remains *legal* in the US. In many areas, however, that movement has succeeded in impairing women's *access* to abortion.[9] Also, providing high quality, accessible abortion services has not been given adequate social policy priority in this country. In some whole states and many rural counties there are no abortion facilities or providers (NARAL, 1980). Moreover, since the 1977 Hyde Amendment, federal

Medicaid coverage of almost all poor women's abortions has ceased.[10, 11]

But what does access to abortion mean in terms of an individual's 'choice' of contraception? Some data are available. In Illinois, newspapers reported that 'the poor are turning to sterilization as the ultimate means of birth control as a result of restrictions on government-funded abortions'; in that state in 1980, when Medicaid abortions were no longer easily available, the number of sterilizations rose to 6,219 compared to 3,625 in 1979 (UPI, 1981: A10). Crucially, when the federal government reimburses states for abortions, only 50 per cent of the actual costs of the abortion are covered. In sharp contrast, 90 per cent of sterilization costs are reimbursed, making sterilization more immediately cost-effective for the state.

Obviously, reproductive rights or even individual choice are meaningless when abortion and other birth control access is limited. Abortion is our last line of defense against an unwanted pregnancy; if it is unavailable, *all* our contraceptive options *except* sterilization are much less attractive.

## 2  Unnecessary hysterectomy

Hysterectomy is the most common major surgery in the US; if present rates continue, 50 per cent of all women in the US will have had this surgery by the time they are sixty-five years old (Scully, 1980: 141). Since 1975, hysterectomy has ceased to be recommended as appropriate for solely contraceptive purposes (ibid.).[12]

The potential for subtle sterilization abuse through medically unnecessary hysterectomy is tremendous. Too many physicians are paternalistic, classist, racist and/or sexist and assume they should be the ultimate arbiters of women's fertility, especially that of poor women and women of color. This is a classic example of professionals exercising their autonomy over and against that of patients. For example, the highest rates of hysterectomy and tubal ligation in the US are in the South (Center for Disease Control, 1980; 1981), likely in part to reflect racism in reproductive care.

Some physicians have urged 'hysterectomy especially for

those who usually fail to comply with medical and contra-ceptive management' (Roach et al., 1972). This is a common euphemism for poor women, women of color, and women for whom English is a second language who are often derogated as incompetent in the medical literature on sterilization (Arnold, 1978: 15).

Scully (1980), Fisher (1982, 1983) and West (1983) have studied doctor/patient interaction around hysterectomy decisions; all noted patterns of actual abuse and coercion. They found that poorer and minority women were especially likely to be hustled by physicians into pro-hysterectomy decisions.

Last, it has historically been common medical practice to hysterectomize mentally retarded girls and women to prevent childbearing (Bass, 1967) and to eliminate men-struation which is claimed to be 'unhygienic' (see Finger, in this volume). Recent reports indicate that this practice con-tinues, especially in states where there are no regulations prohibiting the sterilization/hysterectomy of institution-alized people or requiring informed consent of the individual (e.g. Donovan, 1976; Macklin and Gaylin, 1981; Petchesky, 1979).

## 3 Economic constraints upon reproductive choice

There are two basic issues here. First, some workplaces abusively require women to be sterile or sterilized in order to qualify for employment. (To my knowledge, there have been no such requirements for men.) The classic case is the American Cyanamid Company's requirement described earlier. Stellman and Henifin (1982) have documented many similar cases in other industries. Routine gender-based employment discrimination simply manifests itself in new guise when employers attempt to claim corporate privilege in policies stating 'no fertile women need apply.'

The potential for damage to male fertility, likely to be at greater risk from industrial hazards (Castleman, 1980; Cooke and Dworkin, 1981), is routinely ignored in employ-ment policies. But, seven male Dow Chemical Company workers recently won $5 million in damages for on-the-job pesticide-induced sterility (Sward, 1983).

Second, economic constraints are also manifest in our personal lives in high unemployment, deindustrialization and profound economic and social insecurity. Despite the absence of so-called 'medically effective' methods of contraception (the Pill, IUD, sterilization), birth rates dropped drastically during the Great Depression of the 1930s (Gordon, 1976; Petchesky, 1981). Over the past few years, how many women and men have 'chosen' sterilization because they 'can't afford' a child, another child or the costs of hospital delivery (which often must be paid in advance by those lacking medical insurance)? How many might be able to 'afford' the child but not the childcare necessary for them to continue working?

A recent news story (Joyce, 1983) documents couples giving babies up for adoption, often for several thousand dollars. One father commented, 'We're having trouble providing for the kids we have now. By giving the child up, it gives us a chance to get on our feet,' Such 'selling' of babies as 'adoption' has even been advocated as an alternative to abortion by anti-abortion spokeswoman Phyllis Schlafley.[13,14] Economic constraints upon reproductive choice are at the heart of the commodification of children.

## 4 Lack of knowledge of the permanence of sterilization

Many people do not fully understand that the surgery of sterilization is in almost all instances permanent and irreversible.[15,16,17,18] In one study, some 39 percent of all the women interviewed did not know sterilization was permanent; among Black women – 45 percent, Hispanics – 59 per cent, and whites – 24 per cent. (Carlson and Vickers, 1982: 35). Of the previously sterilized women surveyed, 40 per cent thought they could become pregnant again (ibid.: 22).

Why is there such lack of information and so much misinformation about sterilization? It is likely a variety of factors come into play, including:

media highlighting of medical success stories – such as reversals of sterilizations – with inadequate coverage of the difficulties, costs, and medical risks involved (e.g. Hamilton, 1982);

'puritanical' attitudes on the part of providers or patients which can limit the amount and quality of information given and/or received;

providers assuming knowledge and understanding without adequately checking with patients; and, conversely, patients indicating that they do understand something when they do not;

provision of information in language that is too technical – or not technical enough: for example, a 'tied' tube implies that it could be 'untied' while, in fact, tubes are rarely actually tied, and can only very rarely be untied;

provision of information in a language that is foreign to the patient;

inadequate emphasis in sterilization counseling upon its permanence.

Overall, the lack of knowledge of permanence of sterilization trivializes the meaning and value of women's and men's reproductive capacities. This certainly serves the interests of population control perspectives. Further, when providers do not provide full and complete information to patients, they enhance their own control over the patient at the patients' expense. This has the flavor of the exercise of patriarchal professional authority – whether it is over women or men. There is too long a tradition of 'doctor knows best,' especially in terms of women's health (Ehrenreich and English, 1978; Ruzek, 1978).

## 5 Lack of knowledge or access to other means of contraception

If sterilization is the only available contraceptive option, there is no choice. Lack of *knowledge* of and real access to alternative methods and their risks and benefits leads to subtle sterilization abuse. Carlson and Vickers's (1982) study of over 600 New York City women found no significant differences by race, income, religion or education with respect to the number of methods *heard of*. However, significant differences were found in *usage*: wealthier, better educated women had used more methods than poorer women; Black and Hispanic women had used fewer methods than white women and discussed fewer methods with their providers (ibid.: 20–2).

In New York City, health workers have improved required sterilization counseling procedures so that patients are more likely to give genuine and fully informed consent. An important aspect is providing information on contraceptive alternatives to sterilization. In one municipal (largely Medicaid) hospital, 35 per cent of the women counseled for sterilization in this way did not return for the procedure; in another private pay hospital, 50 percent of the women counseled did not return (Barron and Richardson, 1978; Shapiro-Steinberg and Neamatalla, 1979). These ambitious sterilization counseling programs may provide many woman with needed birth control information which then preempts their desire for sterilization for contraception.

The regulations requiring counseling toward informed consent advocated by reproductive rights groups have long been opposed in principle and in the courts by professional groups (e.g. the American Medical Association and its affiliates), by population control and related organizations (e.g. the Association for Voluntary Sterilization) and by some advocates of individual choice perspectives (discussed below).

## 6 Simultaneous sterilization and childbirth or abortion

Historically, blatant sterilization abuse often occurred in conjunction with childbirth, as in the Madrigal case (CARASA, 1979), and in conjunction with abortion, as 'package deals' in which women were offered 'free' abortions unavailable elsewhere if they allowed simultaneous sterilization (National Lawyers' Guild, 1979). As one doctor said, 'Unless we get those tubes tied before they go home (from abortion or childbirth), some of them will change their minds by the time they come back to the clinic' (Rodriguez-Trias, 1982: 152). In both instances, women were unnecessarily pushed to consider sterilization in situations of urgency and emotional stress.

Because of such abuses, reproductive rights advocates pushed to include in the regulations both a prohibition against obtaining consent during childbirth or abortion and a 'waiting period' between the time of *consent* to sterilization and the actual surgery. US federal regulations require a thirty-day wait. Research has supported such a waiting period in terms of reduction of subsequent regret (see section 10 below).

The one-month waiting period, while still engendering some regret, seems to be the best compromise between fair access to sterilization and prevention of regret. Thus pregnant women could decide during their pregnancies – but *not* on the delivery table – and women who had decided to be sterilized and then discovered an unwanted pregnancy could have simultaneous surgeries if desired.[19,20,21]

The issue of a waiting period essentially pits regulatory *protection of all women* against *individual convenience and preference*. It particularly demonstrates the differences between reproductive rights and individual choice supporters who have historically opposed regulations which constrained full freedom of choice. For example, in 1977, the Californian chapter of the National Organization of Women (NOW) testified against having any 'private pay' sterilization regulations in that state because they would constrain ease of access to sterilization.

NOW has historically reflected the opinions of middle-class women (Fee, 1975). Such women had themselves been victims of yet another kind of sterilization abuse – they were denied access to sterilization as a means of contraception unless and until they fulfilled the '120 rule.' This was an unofficial rule of thumb of the American College of Obstetricians and Gynecologists until about 1970, under which a woman's age multiplied by the number of children she had must equal 120 or more for her to obtain a sterilization for contraception (National Lawyers' Guild, 1979: 25). Obviously, the 120 rule is a classic example of 'doctor knows best' paternalism in action, this time against the reproductive autonomy of middle-class women.

The protection of women through regulations is complex and often difficult to formulate while respecting the diverse needs and desires of *all* women. Reproductive rights activists advocate giving primary consideration to the protection of the most vulnerable – the poor, the disabled, and people of color – who have historically suffered the most abuses.

**7 Iatrogenic (medically-caused) sterility or infertility**

Sterility (inability to conceive) or infertility (difficulty in conceiving) caused by medical treatment or its lack is epidemic. The National Center for Health Statistics' estimates for the US find only 56 percent of married women of childbearing age fertile; 18 percent sterilized for contraception, 10 percent for other reasons, and 16 percent unable to conceive for unknown reasons (United Press, 1983: 2). (These figures do not account for infertility among non-married women – heterosexual and lesbian – who might be desirous of bearing children.) In this study, possible causes of growing infertility rates include:

increased rates of *socially transmitted diseases* (STDs), such as gonorrhea and syphilis, infections which can cause a build up of scar tissue leading to infertility, especially if inadequately or un-treated;

the 600 percent increase in women using *IUDs* which increase risk of Pelvic Inflammatory Disease (PID), another infection leading to the build up of scar tissue and possible infertility (ibid.; Population Information Program, 1983b).

Other possible sources include:

inappropriate overuse of *cone biopsies and hysterectomies* for the medical diagnosis and treatment of cervical dysplasia (Clarke and Reaves, 1982);

use of *Depo-Provera*, an injectable contraceptive, which has a wide range of severe side effects for many women, often including sterility (Hatcher et al., 1982; Rakusen, 1981);

*inadequate treatment* of STDs and PID for several reasons:

1 cutbacks in Medicaid and limited providers for Medicaid patients (Gonski, 1983);

2 physicians attempting to protect husbands from their wives' awareness of outside sexual activity resulting in infection and therefore inadequately treating the wives (Corea, 1977);

3 physicians' traditional dismissal of many female patients' complaints as psychosomatic rather than functional (Ruzek, 1978).

Certainly 'doctor knows best' professional autonomy is being exercised here. Population control perspectives are also manifest in two ways. First, physicians exercise less caution to protect the reproductive capacities of women whose fertility they do not see as valuable or worthy of protection (e.g. see Scully, 1980). Second, the push for population control has historically directed contraceptive research toward high technology methods that are physician-controlled rather than woman-controlled (Blake, 1983; Holmes et al., 1980; Norsigian, 1979; Roberts, 1981). Such methods include the IUD and Depo-Provera, both extensively implicated in infertility (e.g. Rakusen, 1981).[22] Researchers (including physicians, endocrinologists, physiologists, etc.) are likely to support this 'high tech' direction considerably as it provides ongoing, even endless, career opportunities for research, publication and employment. It would be difficult, as Ruzek has noted, to build a medical or research career on the diaphragm or the new contraceptive sponge.[23] Thus contraceptive research has valued stopping *conception* more than enhancing *control over reproduction*, especially control in women's hands.

## 8 Disproportionate sterilization of welfare women

Reproductive rights activists long suspected that women on welfare were more likely to be sterilized than their non-welfare counterparts. For example, 97 percent of physicians in one study favored the sterilization of welfare mothers who had borne 'illegitimate' children (Silver, 1972). Recent research in the US (Shapiro et al., 1982: 20), using data on over 18,000 women from the US Survey of Family Growth, found that women on welfare with three or more children were, in fact, 67 percent more likely to be sterilized than non-welfare women with the same numbers of children. The researchers concluded, 'something occurs in the process of delivering publicly-assisted family planning health care that channels services in the direction of more permanent services,' such as sterilizations, which are 'immediately cost effective' (ibid.: 21).

A parallel situation exists among Native Americans, who generally receive care from the welfare-like US Indian

Health Services (IHS). Blatant sterilization abuses were found in the IHS in 1976, including inadequate record-keeping, lack of counseling for informed consent, and thirty-six clear violations in 3001 cases (including several sterilizations of women under twenty-one years old) (Women Against Sterilization Abuse, 1977: 2–3). Lee Brightman, President of United Native Americans, estimates that of the US Native population of about 800,000, as many as 42 percent of the women of childbearing age and 10 percent of the men have been sterilized (*Akwesasne Notes*, 1977a, 1977b; Jones, 1979: 29).

The disproportionate sterilization rates among welfare and IHS women reflect, I believe, a patterned institutional discrimination on the basis of population control of poor people and people of color, that is, class, race and welfare related.[24,25]

## 9 Ideologies of 'appropriate' family size and structure

We do not know the ultimate nature or extent of the influence of ideologies of small families as 'ideal' upon decisions to contracept or become sterilized. Further, we do not know how ideologies of 'proper' family structure affect reproductive decisions – for example, a view of the youngish heterosexual couple as the only appropriate unit for childbearing. Chico's research (forthcoming) on people seeking sex preselection revealed an ideology of the 'complete family' composed of a mother and father and at least one child of each sex. It seems likely that this ideology is widely shared.[26]

Different racial and ethnic groups hold varying ideologies regarding favored family size, structure, what is known as 'legitimacy' and what is called 'the family' (e.g. see Davis, 1981; Mora and del Castillo, 1980; Stack, 1974). It is around the issue of 'proper' family size that population control groups (such as Zero Population Growth) have been most influential. In sharp contrast, reproductive rights groups have questioned this small nuclear family as the 'ideal' for all, especially as it ignores cultural as well as health differences.

Both reproductive rights and individual choice perspectives emphasize the autonomy of women in determining the number and timing of children they choose to bear. Especially challenging to us as feminists is how to simultaneously support women who genuinely choose to have children and even many children, while also supporting women who genuinely choose to have none. This issue of supporting a diversity of childbearing options must be extended to supporting a diversity of appropriate family structures as well.

## 10 Lack of counseling to prevent regret of sterilization

In a recent review of the literature on post-surgical regret, Chico (forthcoming) notes that worldwide estimates of the number of sterilizations during the 1980s are as high as 180 million procedures. Even if regret *rates* are relatively low, say 5 per cent, by 1990 there would be in absolute numbers *9 million* more women in the world who regretted their sterility. Moreover, estimates of *actual* rates of regret range from 1.5 percent to 43 percent (ibid.). This is, then, a problem of considerable magnitude.

Some proportion, perhaps even the majority of post-surgical regret, could be prevented through counseling focused on factors associated with such regret. Such factors include *age* at the time of surgery as younger women are more likely to regret (Carlson and Vickers, 1982; cf. Chico, forthcoming). Many people regret their sterilizations upon *remarriage* after the surgery, due to the desire to 'start a new family' (see Chico, forthcoming). Other factors, discussed earlier, are *poor contraceptive information* both on the permanence of sterilization and on alternative birth control, *shorter length of waiting period* between the decision to be sterilized and the actual surgery, and *sterilization simultaneous with childbirth or abortion*. Since Black and Hispanic women and poor women have reported higher rates of regret (Carlson and Vickers, 1982), counseling to prevent regret should especially address their reproductive needs and goals.

These factors associated with regret demonstrate the intensely *social* nature of the decision to become sterilized for contraceptive reasons.

# CONCLUSIONS

While contraceptive technologies have enhanced *control* over reproduction, economic and social *supports* for childbearing and rearing have become issues at the core of highly controversial policy debates around reproduction. The technologies of reproductive control do *not* intrinsically or necessarily bring about a social world which supports genuine reproductive freedom.

Understanding both increasing rates of contraceptive sterilization and its blatant and subtle abuse requires careful analysis. It should be clear that in each specific situation described, participants may or may not be conscious of the perspectives influencing their decision-making. One goal of the reproductive rights agenda is, in fact, to help women and men to become more fully aware of reproductive issues and related medical information.

Specific activities to enhance women's and men's exercise of their reproductive rights and to reduce blatant and subtle sterilization abuse do emerge from this analysis. They include, but are far from limited to:

encouraging second and even third opinions regarding hysterectomies of women of childbearing age, with rigorous informed consent procedures and printed information (in various languages) regarding alternative treatments (as has just been required regarding breast surgeries in California);

working toward legal, accessible, safe and affordable abortion services in the community;

working against sterility as a job requirement or preference for *either* sex, against genetic screening for employment and for safe workplaces for all;

working toward the separation of sterilization from both abortion and childbirth;

enhancing women's and men's knowledge of all forms of contraception;

pushing for more contraceptive research on methods which can be controlled by the user, including more low technology contraceptive options for both women and men;

implementation of 'private pay' sterilization regulations in
the currently unprotected forty-nine states;

improved monitoring and enforcement of the existing
federal, state and city sterilization regulations;

educational outreach toward broader understanding of the
permanence of sterilization;

countering population control/overpopulation
perspectives with those of reproductive rights, including
enhanced legitimacy of families of various sizes and
structures;

fighting for improved perinatal care and nutrition,
especially for poor women and women of color, to reduce
infant and maternal mortality and morbidity;

targeted support to welfare women and men and welfare
rights organizations since this population appears most
vulnerable to both blatant and subtle abuses;

particular outreach to providers of medical care to promote
their protection of fertility in all areas of treatment, and to
pressure them to improve reproductive counseling,
especially around sterilization, toward the prevention of
regret.

Because of its permanence, contraceptive sterilization high-
lights problems which pervade reproductive health care. The
concept of subtle sterilization abuse helps to extend our
understanding of the interrelation of reproductive issues.
This fundamental interrelation of social, medical, personal
and political issues is at the core of the reproductive rights
perspective. It must continue to inform us in our struggle
toward reproductive freedom for all.

## NOTES

1 I would like to express thanks to Sheryl Ruzek and Virginia
  Olesen of the Women's Health Program at UC, San Francisco for
  support of this research. Also the quality of the assistance of my
  writing group—Kathy Charmaz, Gail Hornstein, Marilyn Little,
  and S. Leigh Star—never ceases to amaze.
2 To Ruth Mahaney, Alice Wolfson, Sioban Harlow and Gail
  Kaufman, appreciation for initial direction and ongoing

comradeship. And to my sterilization group – Linda Okahara, Helen Wood, Valeria Purnell, Sandy Goldstein, Holly Finke and Anne Finger – this reflects all our work.

3 In *Skinner* v. *Oklahoma* in 1942, Supreme Court Justice Douglas said, 'The power to sterilize . . . may have subtle, far-reaching and devastating effects. In evil or reckless hands it can cause races or types which are inimical to the dominant group to wither and disappear.' (Kittrie, 1971: 297)

4 For information on the reproductive rights perspective, see e.g. CARASA, 1979; CDRR, 1983; Petchesky, 1980; R2N2, 1983.

5 To compare individual choice abortion views, see e.g. Fee, 1975; NARAL, 1980.

6 For recent actions by professionals' autonomy advocates, see e.g. Hubbard, 1982; Lynn, 1982; Fugh-Berman, 1983.

7 For the corporate privilege advocates, see Chavkin, 1979; Mereson, 1982; Stellman and Henifin, 1982.

8 For the population control perspective, see Bajema, 1976; Gordon, 1976; Haller, 1963; Jones, 1979; Kittrie, 1971; Maas, 1976; Michaelson, 1981; National Lawyers' Guild, 1979; Petchesky, 1979; 1981; Population Information Program, 1983a; Rakusen, 1981; Robitscher, 1973.

9 Various means have been used: picket lines at clinics, harassment of patients, firebombing, theft of equipment, kidnapping of physicians, and local ordinances aimed at limiting access (e.g. newsletters of NARAL and CDRR, 1976–present).

10 In 1980, it was state policy to pay for medically necessary abortions in Alaska, Colorado, District of Columbia, Hawaii, Maryland, Michigan, New York, North Carolina, Oregon and Washington.

11 Thirteen states were under state supreme court order to fund medically necessary abortions, including California, Connecticut, Georgia, Illinois, Louisiana, Minnesota, Missouri, New Jersey, Ohio, Pennsylvania, Virginia, West Virgina and Wisconsin (NARAL, 1980: 5).

12 Medicaid will not fund a hysterectomy for a poor woman *if* contraception is the primary or secondary reason for the surgery on the reimbursement form. Physicians, however, can put other reasons on the forms when contraception is the primary reason.

13 She did so on a radio program, *Spectrum*, broadcast by the CBS Radio Network on February 10, 1977.

14 For the anti-choice or 'right-to-life' perspective, see English, 1981; Leibman and Wuthnow, 1983; Merton, 1981.

15 While reversal of a sterilization is theoretically medically possible, there are numerous constraints. The tests for determining whether the reversal surgery is feasible usually

take several months, can be quite painful, and cost between $3000–6000.

16  Neither the tests nor the surgery are covered by Medicaid, nor are they covered by most medical insurance programs. Further, the best candidates for reversals are people who were sterilized within the past two years – often too brief a time to decide that reversal is desired.

17  The operation itself is a difficult microsurgery and can involve hours under anesthesia which increases the medical risks to the patient (Preciado-Partido, 1983).

18  Recently, instead of reversal, physicians have begun to recommend surgical removal of an egg from a woman's ovary followed by in vitro fertilization with sperm, and placement of the (hopefully) fertilized egg in the woman's uterus (Schmeck, 1983).

19  Some physicians argue for separating sterilization from both abortion and childbirth on medical grounds due to higher rates of thromboembolic complications (due to pregnancy, IUDs or the Pill) (Kimball et al., 1978; Hafetz, 1980).

20  Others cite increased risks of infection and hemorrhage (Hernandez et al., 1977) and reduced efficacy rates (Poma, 1980).

21  Post-surgical regret rates have also been found to be consistently higher for simultaneous surgeries (Cooper et al., 1981; Poma, 1980; Thompson and Templeton, 1978; Winston, 1977; Carlson and Vickers, 1982).

22  Recently, statisticians and physicians found that all intrauterine devices, not just the Dalkon Shield, cause severe infection, average rates above 25 percent. Substantial infertility follows (*Washington Post*, 1983: 22).

23  This analysis of research careers was made in a course offered by Sheryl Ruzek.

24  This pattern holds in terms of birth control as well: in one study, 43 percent of the women on welfare said their doctors had *not* told them of any risks associated with their birth control methods, compared to only 5 percent of the women not on welfare (Carlson and Vickers, 1982: 21–2).

25  Welfare women may thus be more vulnerable to iatrogenic sterility as well.

26  A fascinating dialogue on sex preselection is offered in Holmes et al., 1981; see also Hanmer, 1981.

# REFERENCES

Ad Hoc Women's Studies Committee Against Sterilization Abuse. 1978. *Workbook on Sterilization*. Available from

Women's Studies, Sarah Lawrence College, Bronxville, New York 10708.

*Akwesasne Notes*. 1977a. 'Sterilization Blasted: GAO Investigation Reveals Indians Used as Guinea Pigs.' January: 1.

*Akwesasne Notes*. 1977b. 'Killing Our Future: Sterilization and Experiments.' Early Spring: 1, 4–5.

Arnold, Charles B. 1978. 'Public Health Aspects of Contraceptive Sterilization.' In Newman, S. H. and Z. E. Klein, eds. *Behavioral-Social Aspects of Contraceptive Sterilization*. Lexington Press, Lexington, MA.

Bajema, Carl, ed. 1976. *Eugenics Then and Now*. Benchmark Papers in Genetics/5. Dowden, Hutchinson & Ross, Stroudsburg, PA.

Barron, Eugene and Jean A. Richardson. 1978. 'Counseling Women for Tubal Sterilization.' *Health and Social Work*, 3 (1): 49–58.

Bass, Medora. 1967. 'Attitudes of Parents of Retarded Children Toward Voluntary Sterilization.' *Eugenics Quarterly*, 14: 45–53.

Birke, Lynda I. with Sandy Best. 'Changing Minds: Women, Biology and the Menstrual Cycle.' In Hubbard, Ruth, Mary Sue Henifin, and Barbara Fried, eds. *Biological Woman – The Convenient Myth*. Schenkman, Cambridge, MA.

Blake, Constance. 1983. 'The Contraceptive Industry: Who Calls the Shots?' *Dollars and Cents*, January: 6–7.

Caress, Barbara. 1975. 'Sterilization: Women Fit to be Tied.' *Health/Pac Bulletin*, no. 62, January–February: 1–13.

Carlson, Jody and George Vickers. 1982. 'Voluntary Sterilization and Informed Consent: Are Guidelines Needed?' Manuscript available from UMCNews, 475 Riverside Dr., NY, NY 10115.

Carver, Thomas Nixon. 1929. 'The Economic Test of Fitness.' *Eugenics: A Journal of Race Betterment*, 2(7): 1–6.

Castleman, Michael. 1980. 'Sperm Crisis.' *Medical Self-Care*, Spring: 42.

Center for Disease Control. 1980. *Surgical Sterilization Surveillance: Hysterectomy in Women Aged 15–44, From 1970–1975*. September.

Center for Disease Control. 1981. *Surgical Sterilization Surveillance: Tubal Sterilization, 1976–1978*. March.

Chavkin, Wendy. 1979. 'Occupational Hazards to Reproduction: A Review Essay and Annotated Bibliography.' *Feminist Studies*, 5(2): 310–25.

Chico, Nan. 1983. 'The Elaboration of Improbable Possibilities: Unsuccessful Seekers of Sex Preselection Techniques.' Unpublished paper, Department of Social and Behavioral Sciences, UC, San Francisco.

Chico, Nan. Forthcoming. 'Sterilization Regrets: Who Seeks Reversals?' *Mobius* (early 1984).

Clarke, Adele and Martina Reaves. 1982. 'Cervical Dysplasia: The Ambiguous "Condition." ' *Second Opinion*, newsletter of the Coalition for the Medical Rights of Women, September: 1–2.

CARASA (Committee for Abortion Rights and Against Sterilization Abuse). 1979. *Women Under Attack: Abortion, Sterilization and Reproductive Freedom*. Available from CARASA, 17 Murray St., NY, NY 10007 ($2.50).

CARASA. 1982. *Sterilization: It's Not as Simple as Tying Your Tubes – Some Questions and Answers* ($1.00).

CDRR (Committee to Defend Reproductive Rights). 1983. 'Fighting for Private Pay Sterilization Regulations.' *CDRR NEWS*, March. Available from CDRR, 1638b Haight St., San Francisco, CA 94117.

Cooke, Cynthia W. and Susan Dworkin. 1981. 'It's Time to Take Male Infertility Seriously.' *Ms Magazine*, March: 37–8, 91.

Cooper, P. D. et al. 1981. 'Psychological and Physical Outcome After Elective Tubal Sterilization.' *Journal of Psychosomatic Research*, 25(5): 357–60.

Corea, Gena. 1977. *The Hidden Malpractice: How American Medicine Mistreats Women*. Jove, New York.

Davis, Angela. 1981. *Women, Race and Class*. Random House, New York.

DHEW (Department of Health Education and Welfare), Public Health Service. 1978. 'Sterilizations and Abortions: Federal Financial Participation.' *Federal Register*, 43 (217), Wednesday, November 8: 52146–75.

Donovan, Patricia. 1976. 'Sterilizing the Poor and Incompetent.' *The Hastings Center Report*, 6(5).

Ehrenreich, Barbara and Deirdre English. 1978. *For Her Own Good: 150 Years of the Experts' Advice to Women*. Anchor, New York.

English, Deirdre. 1981. 'The War Against Choice.' *Mother Jones Magazine*, February/March.

Fee, Elizabeth. 1975/1982. 'Women and Health Care: A Comparison of Theories.' In Fee, Elizabeth, ed. *Women and Health: The Politics of Sex in Medicine*. Baywood, Farmingdale, NY.

Fisher, Sue. 1982. 'The decision-making context: how doctor and patient communicate.' In DiPietro, Robert J., ed. *Linguistics and the Profession*. Abley, Norwood, NJ.

Fisher, Sue. 1983. 'Doctor talk/patient talk: how treatment decisions are negotiated in doctor/patient communication.' In Fisher, Sue and Alexandra Todd, eds. *The Social Organization of Doctor-Patient Communication*. Center for Applied Linguistics, Washington, DC.

Folbre, Nancy. 1983. 'Of Patriarchy Born: The Political Economy of Fertility-Decisons.' *Feminist Studies*, 9 (2): 261–84.

Fox, Richard W. 1978. *So Far Disordered in Mind: Insanity in California, 1870–1930*. UC Press, Berkeley.

Fugh-Berman, Adriane. 1983. 'Fetal Surgery: A Woman's Choice.' *Network News*. (NWHN) July/August: 13.

Gonski, Ann. 1983. Testimony for the Coalition for the Medical Rights of Women on R-2-82 (Proposed Changes in California 'Private Pay' Sterilization Regulations). Available upon request from CMRW, 1638b Haight St., San Francisco, CA 94117.

Gordon, Linda. 1976. *Woman's Body, Woman's Right: A Social History of Birth Control in America*. Penguin, New York.

Hafetz, G. 1980. *Human Reproduction*. Harper & Row, Hagerstown, MD.

Haller, Mark. 1963. *Eugenics: Hereditarian Attitudes in American Thought*. Rutgers University Press, New Brunswick, NJ.

Hamilton, Mildred. 1982. 'Overblock: A silicone plug that may mean sterilization without surgery.' *San Francisco Examiner and Chronicle*, December 12: 1–4.

Hanmer, Jalna. 1981. 'Sex Predetermination, Artificial Insemination and the Maintenance of Male-Dominated Culture.' In Roberts, Helen, ed. *Women, Health and Reproduction*. Routledge & Kegan Paul, London.

Hatcher, R. A. et al. 1982. *Contraceptive Technology, 1982–1983*. Irvington, New York.

Hernandez, Ingrid et al. 1977. 'Postabortal Laparoscopic Tubal Sterilization: Results in Comparison to Interval Procedures.' *Obstetrics and Gynecology*, 50 (3): 356–8.

Holmes, Helen B., Betty B. Hoskins, and Michael Gross, eds. 1980. *Birth Control and Controlling Birth: Women-Centered Perspectives*. Humana, Clifton, NJ.

Holmes, Helen B. et al. 1981. *The Custom-Made Child?: Women-Centered Perspectives*. Humana, Clifton, NJ.

Hubbard, Ruth. 1982. 'Some Legal and Policy Implications of Recent Advances in Prenatal Diagnosis and Fetal Therapy.' *Women's Rights Law Reporter*, 7(3): 201–28.

Hubbard, Ruth, Mary Sue Henifin, and Barbara Fried, eds. 1982. *Biological Woman – The Convenient Myth*. Schenkman, Cambridge, MA.

Jones, Paula. 1979. 'Three Million Dollar Suit Against Federal Government Underway.' *Akwesasne Notes*, Summer: 4.

Joyce, Fay S. 1983. 'Couples Who Give Away Their Babies.' *San Francisco Chronicle*, August 17: 34.

Kessel, E. and S. D. Mumford. 1982. 'Potential Demand for Voluntary Sterilization in the 1980s: The Compelling Need for a Nonsurgical Method.' *Fertility and Sterility*, 37(6): 725–33.

Kimball, Ann Marie et al. 1978. 'Deaths Caused by Pulmonary

Thromboembolism After Legally Induced Abortion.' *American Journal of Obstetrics and Gynecology*, vol. 132: 169–74.

Kittrie, Nicholas N. 1971. *The Right to be Different: Deviance and Enforced Therapy*. Johns Hopkins University Press, Baltimore.

Liebman, Robert C. and Robert Wuthnow. 1983. *The New Christian Right: Mobilization and Legitimization*. Aldine, Hawthorne, NY.

Lynn, Suzanne M. 1982. 'Technology and Reproductive Rights: How Advances in Technology Can Be Used to Limit Women's Reproductive Rights.' *Women's Rights Law Reporter*, 7(3): 223–7.

Maas, Bonnie. 1976. *Population Target: The Political Economy of Population Control in Latin America*. Charters, Ontario.

Macklin, Ruth and Willard Gaylin, eds. 1981. *Mental Retardation and Sterilization: A Problem of Competency and Paternalism*. Plenum, New York.

Mereson, Amy. 1982. 'The New "Fetal" Protectionism: Women workers are sterilized or lose their jobs.' *Civil Liberties*, July: 6–7.

Merton, Andrew H. 1981. *Enemies of Choice: The Right to Life Movement and Its Threat to Abortion*. Beacon, Boston.

Michaelson, Karen L., ed. 1981. *And the Poor Get Children: Radical Perspectives on Population Dynamics*. Monthly Review Press, New York.

Moore, Emily, ed. 1980. 'Women and Health in the United States, 1980.' *Public Health Reports Supplement*, September–October. US Public Health Service. Washington, DC.

Mora, Magdalena and Adelaida R. del Castillo, eds. 1980. *Mexican Women in the United States: Struggles Past and Present*. Occasional Paper no. 2, Chicano Studies Research Center Publications, UC, Los Angeles.

NARAL (National Abortion Rights Action League). 1980. Status of State Funding for Abortions.' *NARAL Newsletter*, 12(8): 5. Available from NARAL, 825 15th St NW, Washington, DC 20005.

National Lawyers' Guild, New York City Anti-Sexism Committee. 1979. *Reproductive Freedom: Speakers Handbook on Abortion Rights and Sterilization Abuse*. Available from NLG, 853 Broadway, 17th Floor, NY, NY 10003.

NWHN (National Women's Health Network). 1981. *Sterilization Abuse: What it is and how it can be controlled*. Available from NWHN, 224 7th St. SE, Washington, DC 20003.

NWHN. 1983. 'Dalkon Shield IUD: Device is Found Threat to Life.' *Network News*, July/August: 14.

Newman, S. H. and Z. E. Klein, eds. 1978. *Behavioral-Social Aspects of Contraceptive Sterilization*. Lexington Press, Lexington, MA.

Norsigian, Judy. 1979. 'Redirecting Contraceptive Research.' *Science for the People*, January/February: 27–30.

Paul, Julius. 1968. 'The Return of Punitive Sterilization Proposals: Current Attacks on Illegitimacy and the AFDC Program.' *Law and Society Review*, 3(1): 77–106.

Petchesky, Rosalind P. 1979. 'Reproduction, Ethics, and Public Policy: The Federal Sterilization Regulations.' *Hastings Center Report*, October, 9(5): 29–41.

Petchesky, Rosalind P. 1980. 'Reproductive Freedom: Beyond "A Woman's Right to Choose." ' *Signs*, 5(4): 661–85.

Petchesky, Rosalind P. 1981. ' "Reproductive Choice" in the Contemporary United States: A Social Analysis of Female Sterilization.' In Michaelson, Karen L., ed. *And the Poor Get Children: Radical Perspectives on Population Dynamics*. Monthly Review Press, New York.

Poma, Pedro. 1980. 'Why Women Seek Reversal of Sterilization.' *Journal of the National Medical Association*, 72(1): 41–8.

Population Information Program, Johns Hopkins University. 1983a. 'Sources of Population and Family Planning Assistance.' *Population Reports*, Series J(26), January–February.

Population Information Program, Johns Hopkins University. 1983b. 'Infertility and Sexually Transmitted Disease: A Public Health Challenge.' *Population Reports*, Series L(4), July.

Preciado-Partido, K., M.D. 1983. Personal communication.

Rakusen, Jill. 1981. 'Depo-Provera: the extent of the problem – A case study in the politics of birth control.' In Roberts, Helen, ed. *Women, Health and Reproduction*. Routledge & Kegan Paul, London.

R2N2 (Reproductive Rights National Network). 1983. *Newsletter*. Available from R2N2, 17 Murray St, NY, NY 10007.

Roach, C. J. et al. 1972. 'Vaginal Hysterectomy for Sterilization.' *American Journal of Obstetrics and Gynecology*, 114.

Roberts, Helen, ed. 1981. *Women, Health and Reproduction*. Routledge & Kegan Paul, London.

Robitscher, Jonas, ed. 1973. *Eugenic Sterilization*. Charles C. Thomas, Springfield, Il.

Rodriguez-Trias, Helen. 1982. 'Sterilization Abuse.' In Hubbard, Ruth, Mary Sue Henifin, and Barbara Fried, eds. *Biological Woman – The Convenient Myth*. Schenkman, Cambridge, MA.

Ruzek, Sheryl. 1978. *The Women's Health Movement: Feminist Alternatives to Medical Care*. Praeger, New York.

Schmeck, Harold M. 1983. 'New Help for Infertile Women.' *San Francisco Chronicle*, June 23: 25.

Scully, Diane. 1980. *Men Who Control Women's Health: The Miseducation of Obstetrician Gynecologists*. Houghton-Mifflin, New York.

Shapiro, Thomas, William Fisher and Augusto Diana. 1982. 'Family Planning and Female Sterilization.' Paper presented at the Annual Meetings of the American Sociological Association, San Francisco.

Shapiro-Steinberg, Lois and Georgianne Stiglitz Neamatalla. 1979. 'Counseling for Women Requesting Sterilization: A Comprehensive Program Designed to Insure Informed Consent.' *Social Work and Health Care*, 5(2): 151–63.

Silver, Morton A. 1972. 'Birth Control and the Private Physician.' *Family Planning Perspectives*, IV(2): 42–6.

Stack, Carol B. 1974. *All Our Kin: Strategies for Survival in a Black Community*. Harper & Row, New York.

Stellman, Jeanne M. and Mary Sue Henifin. 1982. 'No Fertile Women Need Apply: Employment Discrimination and Reproductive Hazards in the Workplace.' In Hubbard, Ruth, Mary Sue Henifin and Barbara Fried, eds. *Biological Woman – The Convenient Myth*. Schenkman, Cambridge, MA.

Stepan, J. et al. 1981. 'Legal Trends and Issues in Voluntary Sterilization', *Population Reports*, 6 (E): 73–102.

Sward, Susan. 1983. '$5 Million Verdict in Dow Pesticide Suit.' *San Francisco Chronicle*, April 15: 1, 4.

Thompson, P. and A. Templeton. 1978. 'Characteristics of Patients Requesting Reversal of Sterilization.' *British Journal of Obstetrics and Gynecology*, 85(3): 161–4.

United Press. 1983. 'Infertility Rate of U.S. Women Rises: Increase in Diseases Cited.' *San Francisco Chronicle*, February 10: 2.

UPI, 1981. 'With Lid On Abortions, Women in Illinois Turning to Sterilizations.' *San Francisco Chronicle*, October 4: A10.

Wagman, Paul. 1977. 'U.S. Goal: Sterilize Millions of World's Women.' *St. Louis Post-Dispatch*, April 22.

*Washington Post*. 1983. 'All IUDs Pose Threat, Report Says.' *San Francisco Chronicle*, August 12: 22.

West, Candace. 1983. 'Ask Me No Questions: An Analysis of Queries and Replies in Physician/Patient Dialogue.' In Fisher, Sue and Alexandra Todd, eds. *The Social Organization of Doctor/Patient Communication*. Center for Applied Linguistics, Washington, DC.

Winston, R. M. 1977. 'Why 103 Women asked for reversal of sterilization.' *British Medical Journal*, 2: 305–7.

Women Against Sterilization Abuse. 1977. 'Summary of General Accounting Office Report on the Permanent Sterilization of Native American Women.' Unpublished manuscript.

# ABORTION, A WOMAN'S MATTER: AN EXPLANATION OF WHO CONTROLS ABORTION AND HOW AND WHY THEY DO IT

## K. Kaufmann

Although there have been some gains in making abortion safe and accessible to women in many countries around the world, many of us still find abortion to be an experience of mixed and contradictory emotions: isolation and relief, pain and anger. A study of the legal and medical history of abortion reveals that we have many misconceptions and gaps in our knowledge of what abortion is and, more important, what it isn't. Throughout history, women have turned to abortion as a primary method of safe, effective birth control, a tool of reproductive choice. In patriarchal societies, however, it has too often become institutionalized as a weapon of men's reproductive control.

> 'It isn't a medical or a legal matter . . . it's a woman's matter.'
> Hazel Hunkins-Hallinan, twentieth-century feminist,[1] speaking about abortion in a 1982 interview with Dale Spender (Spender, 1983: 27)

## INTRODUCTION

When I think back to my abortions, I remember three things: the isolation, the pain and the relief.

From the time I realized I was pregnant — I always knew well before the test — it was like having a wall thrown up around me, closing me in and cutting me off from the people and things around me. I felt I had to hide my pregnancies and my plans for abortion, even from some of my closest friends and family members. I was afraid people would think that I

213

was a 'bad' woman; that I had either done something wrong or just been very foolish. I was a single woman; I had no 'steady boyfriend' or 'lover.' Both pregnancies were the result of short, casual sexual relationships and irresponsible attitudes, theirs and mine, toward birth control. Under the circumstances there was never the least thought of having a baby, either as a couple or a single parent. I received the result of the pregnancy test and made the appointment for the abortion with the same phone call. The waiting was the hardest: going to work, coming home; having to maintain an outward appearance of normality for coworkers, roommates and other acquaintances when I was constantly exhausted, sick and scared.

Both my abortions were first trimester, vacuum aspirations (suction) performed with local anesthetic by physicians at private, outpatient clinics. Counselors and friends do the best they can: hold onto my hands and smile, keep saying it's almost over; but they're not the one on the table. Doctor comes in – white, male, middle-aged and congenially brusque – some quick word or gesture of greeting. Everything goes fast except the pain. Local anesthetic doesn't numb a thing. Dilating rods in my cervix, and I'm screaming. Pump switches on, sucking sound, and I scream some more. Blood and a pad between my legs when it's over. Doctor pulls off the gloves. Another quick nod, and he's out the door; on to the next one.

In the recovery room there's ginger ale to sip, and Saltine crackers. In Boston in 1978, I ask to see my friend, but they won't let her in. In San Francisco in 1981, I have a friend with me the whole time and that makes it a little easier. Two days later, though, I get cramps in the middle of the night, so bad the pain wakes me. I start bleeding too. Next day I go to work but have to come home early: every time I try to stand up the pain wants to bend me over. I bleed for ten days.

But none of that matters when I walk out of the clinic with my stomach a little flatter than when I walked in. Nothing in the world matters except knowing I'm not pregnant. The wall's been lifted. I can breathe and laugh and be part again of people living. How can anything that feels this good be wrong?

Why then did both my abortions leave me bitter and angry in ways I could not, at that time, understand or explain to myself, let alone to other people? I did and still do define myself as a feminist. I believe absolutely in the fundamental right of all women to control our bodies. Why did I feel the need to hide my pregnancies and abortions? Why did the abortions hurt so much? I would become furious and defensive at the mere suggestion that I might or should feel guilty. Yet, for me there seemed to be a contradiction between everything I had ever read or thought about abortion and the lived experience, an enormous gap between the impassioned rhetoric of the political and moral arguments both for and against abortion, and the bloody reality of one scared woman screaming on a table.

I felt that somehow I, along with most of the women and men in our society, do not know what abortion really is about. There was, there had to be a larger vision, a more complex, a more essential meaning we have not been given.

For as long as women have been getting pregnant, we have been trying not to. A Chinese abortifacient (abortion-inducing) recipe, dating from the reign of the Emperor Shen Nung, 2737–2696 BC, appears in a medieval book of herbal remedies (Taussig, 1936). Aspasia of Miletus, the learned wife of the Athenian statesman Pericles, compiled a list of abortifacients and included instructions on how to prevent conception (ibid.). Forceps, dilators and curettes almost identical to modern instruments for dilation and curettage (D and C) have been found in the excavations of Pompeii and Herculaneum (ibid.). The word 'abortion' itself derives from the Latin *aboriri*, to fail to be born (ibid.).

Abortion is a universal phenomenon, occurring at all times, in all places and at all levels of human social development, from 'primitive' to 'civilized,' regardless of legal, religious or other cultural sanctions enacted against it (Devereux, 1955). It is the oldest, 100-percent effective and reliable method of birth control,[2] corresponding to women's real-life need to control our own bodies, specifically to define for ourselves and in our own terms our existence as physical, sexual beings and our ability to conceive and bear children.

For just as long as women have been trying to control our fertility, however, so have men. The great philosophers of ancient Greece, Aristotle and Plato, believed motherhood was women's duty to their husbands and the state, and should be controlled for the greatest benefit to both. In Plato's ideal republic of 5,400 citizens, abortion was seen as a tool of population control (Taussig, 1936). In the nineteenth century the campaign to outlaw abortion in the United States was built on a demographic panic over falling white, Protestant, American birthrates at a time of heavily Catholic immigration (Mohr, 1978). Population control has also been a primary concern of the Soviet Union, where abortion was first legalized in 1920 as a stopgap measure to keep birthrates low and free women for factory work during the economic collapse which followed the revolution. By 1936, with birthrates falling and long-term industrial development underway, women were called on to fulfill their duty to the state, to produce more socialist citizens, and abortion was decreed illegal (Knight). (Abortion was legalized again in the USSR in 1955.)

Throughout the course of Western patriarchal civilization, abortion has remained an historical constant. What has changed is the tolerance or intolerance of different societies, or more precisely the ruling classes of different societies, toward it, and at all times this can be directly related to economic and political expedients of population control.[3] The evolution of social attitudes toward sex and motherhood, of the medical technology and practice of birth control and, consequently, the individual woman's experience of abortion have been and for the most part continue to be determined by these patriarchal imperatives. In a patriarchal society, abortion is not a tool to enhance women's reproductive choice, it is a weapon to enforce men's reproductive control.

## HISTORY/ISOLATION

It's a peculiar thing about abortions: everyone has them, or at least knows someone who has, but no one ever really talks about them. Start talking about abortions and, more often than not, people start looking uncomfortable, or perhaps just very blank, and wait for you to pause for a breath so they can change the subject. Maybe that's why we know so little about them.

Dale Spender has theorized that men write history to suit themselves and to deny women a history of our own (Spender, 1982). As she puts it, women must 'reinvent the wheel' of feminism, and women's history with it, every fifty years (ibid.). Certainly our knowledge of the history of abortion fits this pattern.

Common knowledge about abortion does not stretch much beyond stories of the desperate back alleys, coat hangers and knitting needles of the 1930s–1960s, the nightmare world banished, hopefully forever, by legalization. Nor are we encouraged to think about abortion as an historical phenomenon, something women have been doing for centuries, or to question how and why it ever came to be illegal. Reconstructing the history of abortion is difficult, painstaking work. The few, so-called authoritative texts on abortion have been written mostly by male doctors, for other doctors. They are not widely known or available, and their coverage of the history of abortion is fragmentary, usually a few pages out of several hundred (Devereux, 1955; Potts et al., 1977; Taussig, 1936). Outside of these books, historical documentation on abortion before the nineteenth century appears to be almost nonexistent, and much of what can be found is indirect, hints and clues that must be read between the lines. (For a feminist approach to abortion in pre-industrial societies, see Gordon, 1976.)

A midwife's job description from ancient Greece, for example, lists as one qualification: 'She must not be greedy for money lest she give an abortive wickedly for payment' (Lefkowitz and Fant, 1982: 163), indicating, obviously, that women were obtaining abortifacients from midwives. Other historical records are more ambiguous and suggestive. 'You will be sorry to hear that your granddaughter has suffered a miscarriage,' a Roman citizen wrote to his wife's grandfather: 'Silly girl, through failure to recognize that she was pregnant, she neglected to take certain precautions and did

other things she should have avoided.' (Baldson, 1962: 195).
Is this an account of a spontaneous miscarriage or an
'accidental on purpose' abortion? Roman birthrates were low,
and, according to Juvenal, abortion was outlawed by
Septimus Severus in the second century AD (ibid.).

The picture of abortion assembled from such bits and
pieces seems very different from the scattered and sordid
images we have received through our patriarchal culture. A
tradition emerges of women's use of abortion to control and
define to some extent their roles as childbearers and rearers,
countered by the continuing and too often successful efforts of
patriarchal ruling classes to manipulate women's fertility to
serve and preserve their own economic and political interests.
This pattern can be clearly documented in the evolution of
abortion policies in the United States where ruling class
perceptions of the fall and rise of American birthrates have
been correlated with the criminalization of abortion, and all
birth control, in the nineteenth century and its legalization
in the twentieth (Gordon, 1976; Mohr, 1978).

Abortion was only illegal in the United States for about a
hundred years, from the 1880s to the Supreme Court decision
in the case of *Roe* vs. *Wade* in 1973. Prior to this time,
American women's right to abortion was protected under a
tenet of old English common law called the 'quickening
doctrine.' Quickening is the point about halfway, four-and-a-
half to five months, through gestation when a pregnant
woman first feels the fetus move within her. From medieval
times through the nineteenth century it was accepted as the
lower limit of fetal viability – independent movement =
independent life – both physical and legal. According to the
common law, a woman not yet 'quick with child' could terminate her pregnancy at any time and for any reason. The
Massachusetts Supreme Court confirmed this right in the
precedent-setting case of *Commonwealth* vs. *Bangs* in 1812,
and it continued to be upheld in courts and state laws around
the country until the 1860s (Mohr, 1978). Abortion before
quickening was viewed almost universally as safe, especially
in relation to the dangers of childbirth at the time. Doctors
and other health authorities included abortifacient recipes
and techniques in popular health manuals found in virtually

every American home. Newspapers regularly carried advertisements for a full range of abortifacient products and
services: from over-the-counter pills and powders to private
clinics, often run by midwives in cooperation with a friendly
boarding house (ibid.).[4]

Throughout the first half of the nineteenth century,
abortion became an increasingly common and significant
part of the lives of American women. Industrialization had
broken down the interdependent structure and function of
the rural or craft-centered family, and motherhood, representing the sexual division of labor, had become institutionalized as women's primary sexual and social role (Gordon,
1976). The 'maternal instinct' and women's 'duties,' sexual
and domestic, as wives and mothers were, according to the
dictates of repressive Victorian morality, the sole and
biologically ordained purpose of women's existence (ibid.).
Economically and sexually subject to the will of their
husbands and lacking any effective or reliable contraception,[5] women turned to abortion in an attempt to gain
some control over how many children they would have and
when they would have them.

Doctors recorded cases of 'respectable' married women
who spoke openly of past abortions and were equally frank
and determined in expressing their intent to terminate
future unwanted pregnancies (Mohr, 1978; Potts et al., 1977).
The philosophical distinctions over the origins of life had
little to do with abortion, wrote one woman to a feminist
journal of the time, and would not deter 'one out of ten, if it did
one out of one hundred . . . from the commission of the deed.'
(Mohr, 1978: 107) As late as 1888, an anonymous speaker
told the Medico-Legal Society that any attempt to outlaw
abortion was a farce 'due doubtless to the fact . . . that it was
against the common and universal sentiment of womankind.'
(ibid.: 109)

By the 1870s an estimated 20 percent of all pregnancies
in the US were ending in abortion (ibid.). Women of all
economic and social classes used abortion; however, the most
frequent users were white, American-born, Protestant
(WASP), married women of the middle and upper classes
(ibid.). Modern demographers have shown that after 1840 the

United States did experience a substantial decline in national birthrates, and the main factor in this decline was a sharp drop in the birthrates of American, as opposed to immigrant women (ibid.).

The fall in American birthrates was perceived by the ruling classes with fear and alarm. The higher fertility of immigrant women, particularly Catholic immigrant women, evoked visions of 'reverse Darwinism' ruining the nation as 'alien hordes' took power simply by outbreeding the white, Protestant Americans. 'Shall we allow our broad and fertile prairies to be settled only by the children of aliens?' demanded an 1867 report to the Ohio legislature, which blamed the crisis on abortion and American women's selfish desire to avoid 'the duties and responsibilities of married life.' (ibid.: 207–8) The threat abortion posed to the nuclear family was another area of ruling class concern. Both abortion and birth control opened the possibility of women's sexual autonomy, that is, a sexual identity separate from the patriarchal institutions of marriage and motherhood (reserved exclusively for men through the double standard) (Gordon, 1976). They were associated with the emergence, at about the same time, of the women's suffrage movement with its new and subversive ideas about women's roles in society, challenging the foundation of American industrialization: the sexual division of labor (Mohr, 1978).[6]

Between 1860 and 1880, the public image of abortion in the United States underwent a radical transformation: from a common, safe and legal method of birth control to a national crisis, a crime against the laws of God and man. Newspapers and medical journals began to regularly print sensational accounts of 'criminal' abortions and the 'quacks,' 'hacks' and 'doctoresses' who performed them. Citing recent advances in medical science, the American Medical Association declared that quickening had no significance as a stage in fetal development and launched a nationwide crusade against abortion. A new generation of home health manuals, mostly written by white, male doctors, focused on the physical dangers of abortion, specifically its damaging effects on women's fertility. In 1873, the US Congress enacted the notorious Comstock Act which outlawed the advertisement or publication of any information on abortion or birth control as 'obscene' and 'immoral.' At least forty other anti-abortion measures were passed by states and territories during this time (ibid.).

The campaign which led to this reversal of American laws and attitudes toward abortion had brought together three of the most influential and entrenched bastions of ruling-class power in the US: the law, the press and the American Medical Association (ibid.). Despite its high moral tone which focused on educating the public to the dangers and evils of 'criminal' abortion, the nineteenth-century anti-abortion campaign was essentially sex- and class-oriented. The success of the campaign reinforced women's sexual and social roles as mothers and specifically blocked American women's access to the information and technology of birth control (Gordon, 1976).

The disappearance and/or suppression of knowledge of the history of abortion has been one of the more subtle, but damaging results of criminalization. Isolated from its historic context of women's traditional birth control, abortion has become if not a single, then at least a contained issue. Many of the ideas and attitudes still widely held and believed about abortion and women's sexuality and role as childbearer in our society are rooted in nineteenth-century morality. The sexual division of labor has been modified to meet the needs of today's post-industrial economy, but it is certainly still in force. More and more women work double shifts in the home and office or feel themselves pressured into interrupting or sacrificing career plans for childbearing. The concept of abortion on demand is seen as a distinctly modern pheno-menon, a by-product of the sexual and feminist revolutions of the 1960s[7]; something other than and unrelated to birth control, which has become associated exclusively with con-traception. The separation of contraception and abortion has tended to perpetuate the Victorian double standard which still clings to abortion: 'good' women use contraception; 'bad' women have abortions.

The question remains whether the legalization of abortion is in reality a restoration of women's common law rights or a further attempt to regulate women's fertility. The division of human gestation into trimesters, the basis of the 1973 decision of the US Supreme Court in the case of *Roe* vs. *Wade*, is generally interpreted as a return to and reaffirmation of the quickening doctrine (Mohr, 1978). However, the Supreme Court decision also culminated a decade of increasing government concern about overpopulation and federal involvement and aid to birth control, following the post-World War II baby boom (ibid.). It has, in effect, legitimized the principle of patriarchal control over women's access to abortion.

## TECHNOLOGY/PAIN

Hippocrates, 'forefather' of modern medicine, denounced abortion and the use of abortifacient devices by women in ancient Greece. Not without compassion, however, the great physician was 'willing to permit and even to advise certain women as to a simple method of interrupting pregnancy . . . [although] he was opposed to putting agents for this purpose into the hands of the laity' because he had seen 'much of the injury to life and health produced by efforts to produce an abortion.' (Taussig, 1936: 33) Hippocrates' compassion and 'simple method' were demonstrated in his advice to a young, pregnant harp player upon whom, as the story goes, he took pity. He told her to jump in the air seven times, striking her heels against her hips. According to the legend, the young woman 'promptly aborted.' (ibid.)

In a modern variation of this story, the twentieth-century feminist, Hazel Hunkins-Hallinan, recalled doctors' advice to women seeking abortion in the 1920s:

> If you went to a doctor you really knew, and said you were pregnant but you didn't want to be, then as a favour he might give you some 'advice' and at the same time he'd disclaim any responsibility. He could know a *safe* way of carrying out an abortion, but because of the legal and medical entanglements you wouldn't get that. Instead, as a favour, you might get some very *unsafe* advice. Like 'go home and take aspros (which contained quinine) till your ears ring.' (Spender, 1983: 27)

Quinine was one of several commonly known, dangerous drugs used by women in nineteenth and twentieth centuries to induce their own abortions. Massive doses of the drug – 300 mg. every 1–2 hours, causing severe dizziness and ringing in the ears – were required to bring on an abortion. Some of the women who used quinine suffered permanent damage to their hearing (Potts et al., 1977).

An integral part of the historic battles over abortion, the struggle for control of the medical technology connected with it, has changed little in 2,500 years. The stories recounted above illustrate the ongoing hypocrisy of the male-dominated medical profession in its lack of concern for women's health in general and, more specifically, its obstruction of women's access to safe, effective choices in reproductive technology. The medical history of abortion presents an often bloody record of patriarchal manipulation of technology for economic and political purposes, and of the pain, permanent physical damage and deaths women have suffered in consequence.

The basic medical technology for safe, effective abortions has been known and available to medical practitioners since ancient Greece. The evidence of surgical instruments from Pompeii and Herculaneum clearly indicates that D and Cs were being performed, and additional archaeological findings of components for a simple vacuum pump suggest that the technology for vacuum aspiration may have existed even then (Potts et al., 1977). Certainly it had been fully developed by the middle of the nineteenth century, but was not widely known or used for almost a hundred years. Vacuum aspiration abortions began to be commonly performed in China and the Soviet Union in the late 1950s and early 1960s (ibid.). A woman gynecologist, identified only as D. Kerslake, introduced them to the English-speaking world in Britain in 1967 (ibid.). The historic dangers and abuses of abortion technology were not, as Linda Gordon has said of birth control in general, 'the result of lack of technology but of the suppression of technology' (Gordon, 1976: 46), and can be traced largely to patriarchal intervention in and/or control of women's health care.

It was not by chance that the chief instigators and agents

of the nineteenth-century anti-abortion campaign in the United States were American doctors. Throughout the first half of the nineteenth century, health care in the United States had become 'democratized.' America's 'regular' – university-trained and predominantly white, male – doctors had to compete for patients with a variety of alternative, 'irregular' practitioners, many of them midwives or other women healers who routinely performed abortions. The anti-abortion campaign launched by the AMA in 1859 was part of a much larger strategy to secure a professional and economic monopoly on medical technology and its practice in the US. While the AMA was lobbying for anti-abortion laws (in Vermont in 1867 the legislature voted in an anti-abortion law while doctors stood in the lobby, shouting their support), they were also pushing for strong medical licensing laws that would exclude the 'irregulars' from the health care market. In some states, such as Michigan in 1873, anti-abortion laws were passed in tandem with medical licensing laws. By the end of the century, midwives and other 'irregulars' had been barred from practice, and medical technology and its application were in the hands of the white, male doctors (Ehrenreich and English, 1973; Corea, 1977; Mohr, 1978).

The hypocrisy of the AMA's campaign against abortion was that it actually perpetuated the conditions it had – so the doctors said – set out to correct. Having blocked women's access to safe abortion, American doctors turned their backs on the dangers of the illegal abortion market which inevitably took its place. One of the most widely known and lethal abortifacients used by women in the late nineteenth and early twentieth centuries was a drug called savin, an extract of juniper berries also used to flavor gin. The abortifacient and toxic effects of savin have been recognized since ancient Greece, yet even at the height of its use as an illegal abortifacient, no systematic research or testing of the drug was undertaken. Or had been by 1977 when Malcolm Potts et al. wrote in their comprehensive study,

> *Abortion:*
> . . . the effect of savin in humans . . . has never been scientifically evaluated . . . no other therapeutic agent has

been so widely used, for so specific a therapeutic purpose
(i.e. abortion) and yet so little studied in animals and *never
once investigated in :nan – or woman.* (ibid: 172;
emphasis added)[8]

Abortion-related savin poisoning became so common at the
end of the nineteenth century that doctors were being
instructed to look for juniper needles in the stomachs of
female corpses whose deaths may have been caused by abortion (ibid.). By the 1930s, an estimated 8,000–10,000
American women per year were dying from illegal abortions,
while several times that number suffered permanent
physical damage (Taussig, 1936: 28).

Legalization has not essentially changed the abuse of
abortion technology by the male-dominated medical profession; in fact, it has actually strengthened its control. The
1973 *Roe* vs. *Wade* decision ensured doctors a professional as
well as cultural monopoly on abortion. Under the law only
doctors can perform abortions, and consequently we have
come to think of safe abortion as one performed by a licensed
physician. In fact, the vacuum aspiration method of early
abortion is a simple procedure and can be safely done by
well-trained laypeople. The illegal feminist abortion clinic
'Jane,' which operated in Chicago from 1969 to 1973, was run
entirely by women without any formal medical training. The
women learned how to do both first trimester vacuum and
second trimester saline abortions. In four years they performed thousands of safe abortions and had only one death, a
woman who came to the clinic with an incomplete, already
badly infected abortion (Bart, 1981).

The illegal clinics like 'Jane,' with their need for speed,
secrecy and anonymity, were the models for today's abortion
clinics, and many of the same procedures are used. The only
significant difference between then and now is that the
isolation and pain of abortion have become institutionalized,
often under doctors' control. In the South and Midwest of the
US, some clinics still call women by numbers or first name
only. Other clinics still do not allow a woman's husband,
boyfriend or other male or female friend to stay with her
through the abortion (Francke, 1978). The local anesthetics

used for vacuum aspiration abortions may do little to stop the pain both from the stretching of the cervix during dilation and from the severe cramping of the uterus when it is emptied. The local is a highly diluted anesthetic solution which is supposed to be injected at three points around the cervix and takes at least three minutes to reach full effect (Margolis and Goldsmith, 1973). Many doctors now performing vacuum aspiration abortions have no training in the procedure because it was illegal when they went to medical school (Bart, 1981). They may not wait for the anesthetic to take effect before beginning dilation. They may use a heavy metal speculum which can tear at the cervix, rather than a light plastic one, or they may use a larger dilating rod than is actually necessary (Francke, 1978).

Under these conditions, pain remains very much a part of women's experience of abortion, the 'natural,' i.e. deserved, result of an 'unnatural' act, and at present there appear to be few palatable alternatives. Barbiturates and pain killers, such as valium, and general anesthetics which can require an overnight hospital stay have been used with, at best, mixed results. A more exotic, but effective alternative is the gradual dilation of the cervix with laminaria tents, sticks of dried seaweed, a technique widely practiced in Japan but little known – though available – in the US. Inserted into the cervix twenty-four hours before the abortion, the seaweed absorbs moisture and expands, dilating the cervix slowly and painlessly. The tent is removed before the operation (Potts et al., 1977).

Often performed in hospitals rather than outpatient clinics, saline or other late abortions can be even more traumatic and punishing for women. In some hospitals, after the fetus is expelled it is left on the woman's bed until she also expels the afterbirth (Francke, 1978). One nurse who spent two months assisting in late abortion surgery recalled how hysterotomies, a kind of mini-Caesarian section, were performed:

The doctors would remove the fetus . . . and lay it on the table where it would squirm until it died. One Catholic doctor would call for sterile water everytime he performed

a hysterotomy and baptize [the fetus] then and there.
(ibid.: 52–3)

Some of the worst abuses of abortion technology have
occurred in Britain, where abortion has been legal since 1967
and is available to some women through the National Health
Service (NHS). In 1968, doctors sterilized an estimated 20
percent of all the women who had legal abortions in Britain,
including 20 percent of the married women who went
through the NHS (Potts et al., 1977). Administrative red tape
in the NHS can add one to two months to the time a woman
waits from her pregnancy test to the actual abortion.[9] For
many women this can mean the difference between being
able to have a vacuum abortion, being forced into a saline or
being refused entirely at the last minute because doctors
consider the pregnancy too advanced to terminate (Potts et
al., 1977; Williams and Hindell, 1972). In March 1983, four
abortion counselors quit their jobs at an NHS clinic in
Liverpool because, they said, doctors were not allowing them
to do their work, providing information and emotional
support to women coming to the clinic (*Off Our Backs*, June
1983: 10).

As long as doctors remain in control of abortion technology, such physical and psychological abuses seem likely to
persist. We may have made abortion safe and legal, but we
have yet to really bring it out of the back alley.

## EXPERIENCE/NO RELIEF

Three to five years ago, I worried about having babies I didn't
want, and I got mad. Mad because I felt throughout my
abortion experiences that I was being punished, being made
to pay in fear and pain and blood, when I hadn't done anything wrong. Today, committed to my work as a writer and a
feminist, I worry more about not being able to create for
myself the social and economic conditions that will enable me
to have the baby I do want, and, if anything, I get madder.
Madder because I know I haven't done anything wrong, but I
still feel like I'm being punished. The connection between

then and now is what Linda Gordon has called 'reproductive choice,' a term encompassing the many and complex social, sexual and economic issues which shape and determine women's experiences as childbearers and rearers in our society (Gordon, 1976).

In the course of researching this article, I have read the stories of many women who, like myself, have found abortion to be a contradictory experience, one which challenges in one way or another their beliefs about the conditions of their lives as women (Carter, 1982; Francke, 1978; Williams and Hindell, 1972; Woodhouse, 1980). Women who do not define themselves as feminists become aware of the connections between their personal situation of unwanted pregnancy and the social and economic environment in which they are confronting it. Teenage women, for example, discover the inherent unfairness of contraception: that it is the woman who takes the responsibility and the risks; that there is no completely safe, effective contraceptive that meets their physical and emotional needs (Woodhouse, 1980). On the other hand, women who do identify themselves as feminists often find that having an abortion is not as easy as they had expected. The conflict between their feminist ideals and their social realities, such as a decision to put career plans before childbearing, can touch off a storm of emotions: guilt or self-hatred; a deep sense of loss or sorrow (Carter, 1982; Francke, 1978). For these women, an experience which is supposed to affirm their right and power to choose, to define and use in their own terms their sexuality and creative energy, instead exposes how limited and illusory their choices really are.

In contemporary patriarchal cultures, 'safe and legal' abortion seems too often to become a panacea for lack of progress toward the social and economic conditions that would create true reproductive choices for women. It is worth questioning the significance of legalization in the United States, which has actually isolated abortion within the control of patriarchal institutions, when the more thoroughgoing changes in women's status envisioned under the Equal Rights Amendment remain beyond our power to achieve. Poor women are especially vulnerable in the present situation where, under the Hyde Amendment, safe abortion is a privilege reserved for women who can afford the $200-plus fees charged by most clinics. The potential for patriarchal abuse of abortion is currently being demonstrated in the USSR and the People's Republic of China, where implementation of legal abortion has had the effect of severely limiting women's reproductive choices. Legal abortion performed without any anesthetic in state-run clinics is Soviet women's primary method of birth control (Hansson and Liden, 1983). Under a rigid program of population control, Chinese women are reportedly being bullied by government cadres into having abortions (Mosher, 1983).

The history of abortion forms a continuous and irrefutable record of women's determination to make reproductive choices based on their own perceptions and definitions of their social, sexual and economic needs. Abortion and other forms of birth control were in all probability invented by women and passed from generation to generation as part of their traditional folklore and culture (Gordon, 1976). Anthropological studies have revealed women's abortion networks in hundreds of pre-industrial societies. In Africa, the women of the Riff tribes have special markets, kept secret from their men, where they sell abortifacients (Devereux, 1955). The illegal abortion clinics of the late 1960s, like 'Jane,' and, more recently, the use of menstrual extraction techniques by feminist groups in the US embody women's attempts to 'seize the means of reproduction,' to reclaim the technology of reproductive choice from patriarchal control (Bart, 1981; Potts et al., 1977; Rothman and Punnett, 1978).

The questions of who controls abortion and how and why they do it lead to larger, more challenging questions about women's reproductive choices in our society. Certainly, the legalization of abortion, in so far as it ensures open access to safe and timely termination of unwanted pregnancy for all women, does represent a positive choice. The criminalization of abortion in patriarchal societies has been and continues to be a real crime against women; its greatest outrage and injustice, that so many women have suffered and died unnecessarily. At the same time, the very existence of abortion brings into sharp focus the absence of sexual and social choices that correspond to the conditions of women's everyday lives. The problems go far beyond 'safe and legal' to fundamental questions about the structure of patriarchal economic and political systems. Control of the complex relations that define reproductive choice, such issues as the connections between women's work lives and sex lives, between contraception and childcare, between the economic value of women's work in the home and the cultural devaluation of childbearing and rearing, remain firmly in the patriarchal grip.

When the choices are not our own, what choice can women have?

## ACKNOWLEDGMENTS

To give credit where credit is due: I thank Renate Duelli Klein for her enthusiastic support and encouragement throughout the research and writing; Rita Arditti, Shelley Minden and Fay C. Budlong for their patient, persistent and very constructive criticism; and Sam Martin who sat in the Cafe Med in Berkeley and listened.

## NOTES

1  Hazel Hunkins-Hallinan (1890–1982) was born and raised in the western United States. She graduated from Vassar in 1913 with a degree in chemistry, but was unable to find a job because no laboratory would hire a woman chemist. In 1916, she joined the National Women's Party and soon after met and became friends with its leader, Alice Paul. During the fight for women's suffrage in the US, Hazel Hunkins-Hallinan was arrested and put in jail several times for picketing the White House. In 1920, she went to England where she lived and worked for women's equality for the rest of her life. Among her many friends were the pacifist Crystal Eastman and British feminists Vera Brittain and Dora Russell. She worked for birth control and legal abortion with Marie Stopes and, as a member and later president of the Six Point Group, a women's political discussion and action group, founded in 1921, for the passage of women's rights legislation such as the end to the marriage bar in the British Civil Service, the Sex Discrimination Act and the Equal Pay Act (Spender, 1983).

2 There is at this time only one other 100-percent effective and
  reliable method of birth control available to sexually active,
  heterosexual women: sterilization.

3 The presupposition of this article is that we live in a patriarchal
  society in which a system of economic and political oppression of
  women by men has existed throughout recorded history and
  remains institutionalized in all aspects of our culture. The well-
  quoted statistics compiled by the United Nations in 1980 support
  this view: women constitute half the world's population, perform
  nearly two-thirds of its work hours, receive one-tenth of the
  world's income and own less than one-hundredth of the world's
  property.

4 The legal basis of abortion, the quickening doctrine, also provided
  the practical basis of the wide availability of abortifacient
  products and services. Throughout the nineteenth century, in
  addition to establishing fetal viability, quickening was the only
  indisputable proof that a woman was pregnant. Before
  quickening, the symptoms of pregnancy could be construed as a
  late or 'blocked' period, and the treatment for this condition was,
  in effect, abortion. Relief for 'obstructed menses' or other 'female
  complaints' become the codewords used to identify abortifacient
  products and services. The subterfuge was, however, purely a
  matter of form: everyone – from the newspapers who carried the
  advertisements to the woman and man on the street – knew that
  what was being sold was abortion.

5 The diaphragm was not invented until 1880, and women's
  ovulation cycle, the basis of the rhythm method, was not
  accurately plotted until the 1920s.

6 The relation between abortion and the feminist movement in the
  nineteenth century was uneasy and paradoxical. While many of
  the women who had abortions did not identify themselves with the
  movement, the spread of feminist ideas throughout American
  society at this time seems likely to have influenced some in their
  decisions to limit the size of their families (Mohr, 1978). Caught
  between Victorian morality and their struggle to win the vote, the
  feminists appear to have been uncomfortable with sexual and
  reproductive issues and refrained from direct confrontation.
  Movement leaders, like Elizabeth Cady Stanton and Matilda
  Joslyn Gage, advanced the concept of 'voluntary motherhood,'
  arguing that abortion was the result of men's excessive sexual
  demands on women and sexual abstinence was the solution
  (Gordon, 1976). While voluntary motherhood emphasized the
  principle of women's right to choose, it did not challenge either the
  sexual division of labor or the Victorian double standard (ibid.).
  Ironically and to their own disadvantage, the feminists
  ultimately supported the anti-abortion campaign.

7 As Dale Spender has amply documented in *Women Of Ideas And What Men Have Done To Them: From Aphra Behn to Adrienne Rich* (1982), the contemporary women's movement is not an isolated phenomenon or even the 'second wave' following the women's suffrage movement of the early twentieth century. Feminism is a continuous historical tradition, expressing women's opposition and resistance to patriarchy, which stretches back at least 300 years and probably much further.

8 The last statement is not entirely true. Ely Van de Warker, a nineteenth-century American physician, did test savin on himself and recorded the results:

> A violent pain in the abdomen, vomiting and powerful cathartic action, with tenesmus (ineffective, painful straining to empty bowels or bladder), strangury (painful discharge of urine), heat and burning in the stomach and rectum and anal region; intoxication, flushed face and severe headache. (Potts et al., 1977: 171)

9 British abortion procedures are significantly more complex and bureaucratic than in the US. In order to have a legal abortion, two gynecologists must certify that the woman needs the operation for reasons of physical or psychological health. To qualify for certification, a woman must first have her pregnancy confirmed by her regular doctor or GP who must then refer her to a gynecological consultant. Every appointment, from pregnancy test to abortion, must be made separately, and especially under the NHS, there can be two- to three-week waiting periods between appointments.

## REFERENCES

Baldson, J. P. V. D. 1962. *Roman Women: Their History And Habits*. Bodley Head, London

Bart, Pauline. 1981. 'Seizing The Means Of Reproduction: An Illegal Feminist Abortion Clinic – How And Why It Worked.' In Roberts, Helen, ed. *Women, Health And Reproduction*. Routledge & Kegan Paul, London and Boston: 109–28.

Carter, Diana L. 1982. *Getting Beyond An Abortion*. Pamphlet published by author.

Corea, Gena. 1977. *The Hidden Malpractice: How American Medicine Treats Women As Patients And Professionals*. Morrow, New York.

Devereux, George. 1955. *A Study Of Abortion In Primitive Societies*. Thomas Yoseloff, London.

Ehrenreich, Barbara and Deirdre English. 1973. *Witches, Midwives And Nurses: A History Of Women Healers*. Writers and Readers Publishing Cooperative, London.

Francke, Linda Bird. 1978. *The Ambivalence Of Abortion*. Dell, New York.

Gordon, Linda. 1976. *Woman's Body, Woman's Right: A Social History Of Birth Control In America*. Grossman, New York.

Hansson, Carola and Karin Liden. 1983. *Moscow Women: Thirteen Interviews*. Pantheon, New York.

Knight, Hilary. 'Abortion Policy In U.S.S.R. Between 1917 And 1936.' Unpublished paper on file at the Women's Research and Resources Centre, London.

Lefkowitz, Mary R. and Maureen B. Fant. 1982. *Women's Life In Greece And Rome*. Johns Hopkins University Press, Baltimore, Maryland.

Margolis, Alan J., MD and Sadja Goldsmith, MD. 1973. 'Techniques for Early Abortion.' In Osofsky, Joy D., Ph.D., and Howard Osofsky, MD, eds. *The Abortion Experience: Psychological And Medical Impact*. Harper & Row, Hagerstown, Maryland: 436–46.

Mohr, James C. 1978. *Abortion In America: The Origins And Evolution Of National Policy*. Oxford University Press, New York.

Mosher, Stephen W. 1983. *Broken Earth: The Rural Chinese*. Free Press, New York.

*Off Our Backs*. June 1983. 'Britain: Woman-Hating Abortion Clinic.' XIII (6): 10.

Osofsky, Joy D., Ph.D. and Howard Osofsky, MD. 1973. *The Abortion Experience: Psychological And Medical Impact*. Harper & Row, Hagerstown, Maryland.

Potts, Malcolm, Peter Diggory and John Peel. 1977. *Abortion*. Cambridge University Press, Cambridge, Great Britain.

Roberts, Helen, ed. 1981. *Women, Health And Reproduction*. Routledge & Kegan Paul, London and Boston.

Rothman, Lorraine and Laura Punnett. 1978. 'Menstrual Extraction.' *Quest*, 4(3): 44–60.

Spender, Dale. 1982. *Women Of Ideas And What Men Have Done To Them: From Aphra Behn To Adrienne Rich*. Routledge & Kegan Paul, London.

Spender, Dale. 1983. *There's Always Been A Women's Movement This Century*. Pandora Press, London.

Taussig, Frederick J., MD. 1936. *Abortion, Spontaneous And Induced: Medical And Social Aspects*. C. V. Mosby, St. Louis, Missouri.

Williams, Jean Morton and Keith Hindell. 1972. *Abortion And Contraception: A Study Of Patients' Attitudes*. P.E.P., London. Pamphlet also on file at Women's Research and Resources Centre, London.

Woodhouse, Ann. 1980. 'The Sexual Politics Of Contraception.' Unpublished master's thesis on file at Women's Research and Resources Centre, London.

# IF YOU WOULD BE THE MOTHER OF A SON

# TECHNOLOGY AND PRENATAL FEMICIDE

Betty B. Hoskins and
Helen Bequaert Holmes

Choosing the sex of their children appeals to many people worldwide, and boys are usually favored. In this chapter, the biological technologies in development and in use are described. Then the authors present arguments for and against the use of these techniques, from a feminist perspective on values. Finally, their hope for a caring, gynandrous world is envisioned.

## INTRODUCTION

Worldwide, most people say they want 'balanced' families, that is, equal numbers of boys and girls.[1] On the surface this sounds fine, even egalitarian. But the data also reveal that those who specify unequal numbers of boys and girls almost always want to choose more boys than girls, and *nearly everyone* would choose a firstborn boy.[2] In some countries, girls are virtually unwanted (Chacko, 1982). Now, with current medical technologies, sex selection may indeed be possible.

International medical research is directed, performed, and funded by men (despite the presence of some women in science and industry). A key target of manipulation is women's power of reproduction. The awesome ability to grow and give life is an object of men's envy; and they often respond to this envy by trying to regulate and control.

In this chapter, first, we survey several present and developing technologies of sex choice. Then we consider whether these technologies are in the best interests of humanity in our present patriarchal society. Our arguments, both for and against sex preselection, are structured within a feminist cluster of values. Finally we present a vision of a gynandrous, caring society.

## SEX CHOICE TECHNOLOGIES

Some techniques *select* sex before conception; others *detect* sex of a developing embryo, for possible elimination. Although at present few of these techniques have been fully investigated, sex preselection or detection might become possible at any of the stages of development. These stages, all of which could be available to manipulation, are: sperm or egg; fertilization (whether by intercourse, artificial insemination, or in vitro procedures); early embryo (when cells divide to form inner cell mass and pre-placenta); late embryo (when organ rudiments or organs are present); and fetus (after two months in uterus).

### Selection of embryo sex
#### 1 Sperm separation
In people, sex is determined at the time of fertilization. As a man produces sperm, the cell divisions distribute either an X- *or* a Y-chromosome, along with one member of each other chromosome pair, to each sperm. In a woman, one X and one member of each other chromosome pair distribute to each egg. The sperm with an X- or a Y-chromosome fertilizes an egg with an X, starting, respectively, a female (XX) or a male (XY) offspring. (Were humans like birds, butterflies or the African clawed toad, in which the female is the sex determiner, sex choice procedures would be different!) Attempts to separate the X- from the Y-chromosome-containing sperm (here to be called X- and Y-sperm) have received much research attention. Separated sperm, inserted into the vagina, it is claimed, should increase the probability that the child will be of the desired sex.

Attempts at sperm separation have been made, based on differences in surface characteristics, such as antigen proteins. Though the work is only beginning, 'vaccination' against X- or Y-sperm may become possible.

Techniques further along in development attempt

physical separation by weight and motility. The two kinds of sperm are slightly different, perhaps partly because the X- and Y-chromosomes have different weights. When a sperm specimen is centrifuged in a density gradient (increasingly thick layers of a solution such as serum albumin), heavier cells settle into the thicker layers. Such centrifugation, which concentrates Y-sperm to approximately 70 percent of the specimen, was first tried in the USA for cattle breeding, then to concentrate the motile sperm of subfertile men with low sperm counts (Ericsson, 1973; 1977). Ericsson's technique is now used in at least seven US clinics advertised 'for sex selection (male) and male infertility.' In April of 1982, using data pooled from five of these clinics, Beernink and Ericsson (1982) reported that, after fertilization with Y-enriched sperm samples, 75 percent of the children from ninety-one deliveries were male. Ericsson has publicized his technique in women's magazines, such as *Good Housekeeping*, and in a new book (Glass and Ericsson, 1982).[3] However, independent observers without a vested interest in the technology have never, to our knowledge, confirmed the clinical results.

In another physical technique for sperm separation, Steeno et al. (1975) of Belgium pour a sample of sperm cells through a column of the resin Sephadex, after suspension in a balanced salt solution. Motile sperm are concentrated. The X-sperm are isolated in a separate fraction with over 90 percent purity reported. Why, then, do we hear of no clinics for female preselection? Indeed, Steeno's technique could be used to choose for female fetuses in families carrying a sex-linked disease. (Almost always, it is males who are affected by such diseases.) Have clinical tests been unsuccessful? Or has it been impossible to find an experimental population of parents who seek girl babies?

Some German investigators reported the Sephadex technique as unsuitable: X-sperm were not always in high proportion in the first fractions extracted (Schilling et al., 1978). On the other hand, Adimoelja et al. (1977) from Indonesia, working in Steeno's laboratory, reported an enrichment of X-sperm to 96.0 percent from an initial concentration of 62.8 percent. Comparing the Ericsson and

Steeno techniques in California, Quinlivan et al. (1982) found that sperm from different men responded differently to each technique; they speculated that clinically both procedures may be needed.[4]

## 2 Fertilization timing

Several years ago the intercourse timing techniques of Shettles received considerable public attention in the USA (Rorvik and Shettles, 1970; 1977). However, the timing, position, and acid/alkaline conditions that might favor a boy or a girl are not reliably clear. Guttentag and Secord (1983) believe that additional factors, such as sperm count and frequency of intercourse, may be important.

A significant increase in the proportion of male births has been correlated with high sperm counts after several days of male abstinence from both intercourse and masturbation. According to the Talmudic Code, a male Orthodox Jew must abstain during his wife's menstrual period and seven days afterwards until she has her ritual bath (Guttentag and Secord, 1983: 98). In Eastern European Orthodox Jewish communities, a preponderance of sons is found, generation after generation. Sometimes there are only sixty to seventy women per hundred men.

Harlap (1979), studying Orthodox Jewish women in Israel, found that more male (65 percent) babies were born when intercourse was resumed two days *after* ovulation. She estimated that ovulation occurred on day fourteen of the menstrual cycle. Guerrero (1974) of Columbia found a different result: intercourse *before* ovulation seemed to facilitate the conception of boys. Using pregnancy outcome data and basal body temperature charts kept by 875 women in family planning clinics in the USA, France, Canada, Mauritius Island, and Colombia, he estimated ovulation from the recorded temperature rise. However, when he studied the temperature charts of 443 women who conceived by artificial insemination, he found reverse results: slightly more males were conceived from fertilizations after ovulation. The point is that different researchers, using somewhat different approaches, obtained opposite results.

## 3  Diet

Desire for a personally controlled, low-technology way to choose sex of offspring has led to repeated claims that diet can affect the selection of sperm for conception. Such methods have never been found reliable, yet the attempts continue. Recently, Stolkowski and Choukroun (1981) in France have reported another diet, one that allegedly influences selective fertilization by altering the ionic balance. To conceive a boy, the potential mother should eat, for the preceding six weeks, foods high in sodium and potassium: sausage, meat, potatoes, beans, artichokes, bananas, peaches, apricots. For a girl, the mother should eat, they say, foods high in calcium and magnesium (alkaline earth elements), including dairy products, eggs, and greens. Their forty-seven experiments (sic) between 1970 and 1980 resulted in twenty-two chosen males, seventeen chosen females, and one set of boy/girl twins, plus only seven 'failures' – six of them girls instead of boys. In the USA their method was reported in *People* magazine (Johnson, 1982) and in a poular book (Langendoen and Proctor, 1982).

## 4  Parthenogenesis and egg fusion

Let us not neglect the possibility of selecting the egg, without using sperm. Amphibian eggs can begin to divide without the entrance of a sperm. Pricking with a bloody needle, treating with an antibiotic that releases calcium and magnesium stored in the egg, and treating with ions – all begin cell division. Aphids, flatworms, rotifers, certain arthropods, and some lizards routinely develop from unfertilized eggs (parthenogenesis).[5] And, since two body cells can be fused in tissue culture, it should also be possible to fuse two eggs. If either of these techniques could be done with humans, the embryo could only be female, for each egg has only an X-chromosome.

## Detection of embryo or fetal sex

### 1  Y-specific DNA detection after chorionic biopsy

Sex detection using new DNA biotechnologies has recently been reported. A tiny portion of the chorionic part of the placenta in a pregnant woman can be removed (biopsied) via the cervix. In Scotland, Gosden et al. (1982) used the procedure with thirteen patients at six to thirteen weeks gestation, who had given informed consent and who had requested abortions. After extraction of DNA from the placental cells, Y-specific DNA fragments were detected in cells from male fetuses; in every case sex was predicted correctly.[6]

## 2 Maternal hormone level measurement

The testis of a male embryo produces androgens such as testosterone, which cross into the woman's blood. Testosterone measurements in maternal blood and maternal saliva, to date, seem no more predictive than guessing. For example, Glass and Klein (1981) at the Walter Reed Hospital in Washington, DC, measured maternal blood testosterone levels in eighty-three pregnant women; the fetuses were four to twenty weeks old. Hormone concentration was not a good indicator of sex. Held et al. (1981) in Hamburg tested women at eighteen to thirty-two weeks of pregnancy for the presence of androgens in their saliva and then checked the chromosomes of the fetus. Results predicting boys were accurate in 40.7 percent of the cases; those predicting girls matched the chromosome test in 56.5 percent of the cases. In Austria another saliva study after twenty weeks of pregnancy (Loewit et al., 1982) was correct 52 percent of the time, 76 percent with non-morning saliva.

## 3 Fetal cell analysis

Some investigators report fetal blood cells in maternal blood beginning at ten weeks. Schröder of Finland has concentrated Y-containing cells by fluorescent cell sorting (Herzenberg et al., 1979). In Belgium, Kirsch-Volders et al. (1980) looked for male fetal lymphocytes (a type of white blood cell) in cultures of blood of eighteen pregnant women. Comparison of results with sex of newborn showed 83 percent *or* 89 percent accuracy, depending on the scoring method.

## 4 Fetal hormone measurement

Measuring testosterone in samples of amniotic fluid taken from fetuses at fifteen to thirty-two weeks, Méan et al. (1981) of Switzerland found a wide range of levels of this hormone, with a statistically significant difference between the *averages* from male and female fetuses. However, they found so much of an overlap of testosterone levels that in 30 percent of the cases sex could not be determined. Furthermore, use of such a method would necessitate late abortions of fetuses of undesired sex.

### 5 Mid-pregnancy chromosome analysis

Around the globe, amniocentesis is used in the second trimester to monitor pregnancies at risk for birth defects, particularly pregnancies of older women and of women in families known to carry undesired genetic diseases. A small sample of amniotic fluid is removed by a hollow needle guided through the mother's abdomen into the amniotic sac. Cells from this fluid are grown in tissue culture until enough of them are present for a chromosome analysis. At the same time that certain chromosome or enzyme abnormalities can be detected, sex can be ascertained with almost 100 percent accuracy. Usually male, not female, fetuses are at risk of expressed X-linked diseases. There has been much debate about whether to tell the sex to the woman tested, when an X-linked disease is not at issue.

### 6 Ultrasonic visualization

Another late-pregnancy method is ultrasonic viewing of penis or vulva. In a report from Australia, these body parts were 'seen' in 66 percent of 137 fetuses scanned at twenty-four to forty weeks, with only a 2 percent error (deCrespigny and Robinson, 1981). In Sweden, diagnoses could be made in 74 percent of 101 fetuses at thirty-two weeks, with 3 percent error (Weldner, 1981). This, of course, is midway in the third trimester.

Some of the techniques surveyed above are already in use; others are under intense development; still others are being explored. Will these technologies become part of a beautiful dream come true or will they add to the nightmares of our world? Next let us look at how we think women can choose what *should* be done.

## VALUE ANALYSIS

Why is sex preselection desired? By whom? What standard societal values are involved? What women-centered values are pertinent?

### Patriarchal values
In the medical literature we find the following expressions:

> (USA) There are definite medical reasons for ensuring that a new born infant is of a particular sex. (Some) 200 sex-linked genetic diseases have been described. These include Cooley's anemia, hemophilia . . . several types of muscular dystrophy . . . (which) could be prevented if the child was of the unaffected sex. (Quinlivan et al., 1982: 104).

> (Indonesia; Belgium) Especially the second half of this century, since the whole world shows an imminent population explosion, experiments to predetermine the sex of a child become more alive. . . . [T]here is no doubt that the determination or method to have a child with the predetermined desired sex will support family planning and life welfare. (Adimoelja et al., 1977: 289).

> (France) Man has always wanted to select his children's sex. . . . (Stolkowski and Choukroun, 1981: 1061).

> (Sweden) (The) main use (of fetal sex detection by ultrasound) has been to satisfy the curiosity of parents (Weldner, 1981: 333).

Primary values in this scientific and medical literature are: disease prevention, population limitation, family welfare, knowledge, and control over nature.[7]

### Feminist values
Although ordinary women wrestle with and settle ethical dilemmas throughout our daily lives, our methods do not fit neatly into the various categories of patriarchal philosophy, such as utilitarian and deontological ethics. Carol Gilligan, in her excellent study on how women's ethics and values develop differently from men's, has called women's moral

reasoning an 'ethic of care' that 'rests on the premise of nonviolence – that no one should be hurt.' (Gilligan, 1982: 174) Women's ethical vision seems focussed within a network, with responsibility to various commitments. It appears as if we women sense a connection to the members of our families, to our friends and neighbors, to children in general, to women and men; and, as if this sense of connectedness extends to other countries, to the poor and hungry, to other living creatures, and to the rest of the living and non-living Earth. A feminist analysis suggests that women operate within clusters of values, excluding neither individual nor social considerations. Similar expressions of feminist ethics can be found in writings by Gray (1981; 1982), Hoskins (1980), Culpepper (1981), and Holmes (1981).

Often when facing moral dilemmas, many women reason in this way: if a problem seems to be solvable only by ranking values hierarchically and regarding some as less important, we may refuse to choose. Instead, we continue to reframe the problem until a question can be asked whose answer will incorporate all of the pertinent values. Although this mode of ethical reasoning has received little attention, we believe that it is common among women and pertinent to the question of sex preselection.

## FEMINIST VALUES: A CASE *FOR* SEX PRESELECTION?

Are there any arguments that speak for sex selection? Bill and Diane Allen in Arizona used the Ericsson sperm separation technique. Bill stated on the PBS *Hard Choices* video program 'Boy or girl' (1981: p. 20) that he sees nothing wrong with sex selection. 'It's simply a more sophisticated form of family planning. And why shouldn't we have the right, if the opportunity is available to us, to do that sort of planning?' Bill Allen's argument for individual rights has an important truth between its lines. Any legal restriction on practices in family planning clinics may also jeopardize other aspects of women's currently precarious reproductive freedom.

Suppose a woman believes she can raise, wants to raise, a

family of all girls, or a family of all boys, or a mixed-sex family with a particular birth order. She may believe that *this* she can do well, and that people in her circle of commitments will benefit. And what of the family that simply does not wish to raise a boy or a girl? Should not every effort be made to spare a child that degree of unwantedness? Should we allow each other this 'choice'?

Imagine another woman who can stay married only if she produces a son. To survive economically she may need to be married; socially she may need the status that production of a son will give her. Since each woman's responsibilities to herself and to others are unique, can we generalize? Or judge?

To the child, there may be advantages if sex was chosen. A chosen girl would grow up aware that she had been wanted and chosen as a girl – a strong basis for self-confidence. Many a woman today is affected by childhood knowledge that one or both parents had wanted her to be a boy. If sex choice were universally used, then each girl would know that she was wanted as a girl.

And the present society without preselection is not a paragon. Sally Miller Gearhart (1982) has fantasized a population structure with 90 percent females in the essay, 'The future – if there is one – is female.' Examining our present militaristic, competitive society in which male values and male bonding play so large a part, she asserts that with men in charge our world order clearly is not viable, and that it is about time to give women a chance to set things right. Without killing any male adults or fetuses, she suggests a technology like egg fusion to bring about her utopian society.

## FEMINIST VALUES AND THE CASE *AGAINST* SEX PRESELECTION

Then why not proceed with sex preselection, since we see with Gearhart that the survival of all humankind is in jeopardy? A contributing factor could be that too many policies have been determined by too many firstborn males. However, sex selection seems likely to yield more firstborn males: would not it exacerbate international misbehaviors? Then sex selection endangers the entire global community.

If sex selection technologies were widely used in our present patriarchal world, it is likely that males would predominate. Guttentag and Secord (1983)[8] have studied the effects of sex ratios in many historical situations and on several continents. In societies with a preponderance of males, they find more male commitment to wives and children. Typically, strong constraints on female behaviour are present, such as dire penalties for nonvirginity before marriage, and tight control by men over their daughters and wives. Female infanticide and neglect often occur. In India, with ninety-six women to every hundred men, girl babies often have been and still are unwanted. Currently the modern technology of amniocentesis followed by selective abortion, although not state-condoned, is a frequent practice (Chacko, 1982).

Even if we were to imagine that sex preselection were to be used to produce a society with a plurality of women, the characteristics that Guttentag and Secord (1983) have reported from such communities – in our patriarchal world – are just as dreary:

> [Men] can negotiate exchanges that are most favorable to them. . . . Men are more reluctant to make a commitment to any one woman, and if they make it, it is a weaker one, and is more apt to be broken. . . . Women are more apt to feel exploited, because even when they meet a male partner's demands, he may break off the relationship. . . . This feeling of being exploited generates attempts by women to redefine male and female roles in a relationship, to reject a male partner, and/or to reduce their dependency by becoming more independent. (Guttentag and Secord, 1983: 190)

Furthermore, we and members of other disadvantaged groups should be alarmed to learn that some population planners advocate male sex selection as a means to control overpopulation. Clare Boothe Luce (1978) urged the invention of 'pills to make most babies male.' Her logic is simple: fewer wombs will produce fewer babies. Luce further reasoned that any sex selection method would be enthusiastically received because of strong worldwide preferences for male progeny. Calling the problem 'overpopulation' and identifying it primarily as a problem of non-white, Third World populations, mask deep-rooted economic, social, and racial injustices.

Desires for boys and desires for girls often mean that parents have sex role ideologies. Treating people according to the sex role we envision, instead of according to their individuality, is sexism. What is more sexist than to *create* a person to fit a sex role ideology? Powledge (1981) has called this 'the original sexist sin.' Markle (PBS, 1981: 18) calls it 'the ultimate form of sex discrimination.' Markle further argues that, when people are asked why they want a firstborn son, the reasons given reflect male supremist values and sexual prejudice (such as carrying on the family name).

And what benefit does a daughter have in her 'wantedness' if she is wanted only as a second child? Steinbacher (1983) has observed:

> The psychological ramifications subsequent to the discovery that one was chosen-to-be-second are immeasurable but predictably negative. Inferiority, now societally dictated for women as a class, would be further internalized and externalized as 'big brother, little sister' became institutionalized. . . . (A)n increase in the number of male firstborns . . . could not only sharply reduce the number of females born, but could relegate those born to powerlessness.

And, what about the mistakes? Suppose a daughter is born after 'failure' of a technique. If someone went to expense and trouble to procure a son, would not the resulting daughter suffer much more psychological (if not physical) abuse than if she had arrived by 'reproductive roulette'? Unwanted sons would suffer equally.

Sons, even chosen sons, also may be abused by patriarchy. They may be ruthlessly driven, by others' ambitions, to succeed. The hierarchical, competitive actions of daily society can damage self-esteem and stifle creativity. Even more, sons who try to escape patriarchal behaviors may find little place in the feminist *or* the general society.

## AND IN A GYNANDROUS WORLD?

A gynandrous[9] world, free of patriarchal habits, might require us to take into account very few of the previous considerations. In such a world, we envision, each child would be planned – as a child – and welcomed at birth as herself or himself. Roles would not be expected or applied. Technology would be appropriate, using as little energy and machinery as suitable, maintaining the dignity of persons and the Earth. High technology would be reserved for crucial interventions, and the participation of those affected would be sought and fully used in the decision process.

In a profound sense, fewer choices would be made. Many of our present troubles result from needless Western dualisms, such as whether the mind is 'better than' the body, whether professionals are more valuable than laborers, whether 'man must rule over the earth,' whether male power-concept is preferable to female empowerment ideals. Thus we believe that feminists should act in ways that avoid unnecessary choices. We conclude that a reasonable stance, in the case of sex preselection, would be *not* to choose a girl or a boy, a boy or a girl, but to welcome each *child*.

What can we do now? Clearly, attempts at sex selection and sex detection abound in clinics and laboratories. Technology has brought the age-old patriarchal 'dream' of selecting children's sex very close to fulfillment. The sum total of individual action on that dream, the world over, could be disastrous not only to women but to everyone. Under the guise of providing 'choice,' such technologies could exacerbate sexist oppression, negate struggles to prevent wars, and eliminate ethnic and racial groups. We must encourage more feminist women to become scientists and physicians, and to work toward making science more humane. We must affirm and extol the gentler, caring traits of personality in all people. We must inform men and women about the ramifications of these technologies and urge them to think carefully whether choosing children's sex is desirable after all. We must continue to expose unexamined assumptions and hidden agendas of the developers and promoters of reproductive technologies. Let us change the patriarchal mindset and stop the momentum of technological experimentation that could lead us relentlessly to prenatal femicide.

## ACKNOWLEDGMENTS

We thank Diana Axelsen, Roberta Beeson, Jalna Hanmer, Francis Holmes, Arthur Mange, Roberta Steinbacher, and Margaret Werry for valuable discussions and suggestions on various versions of this paper. The ideas and interpretations in the final paper, of course, are the responsibility of the authors.

HBH was supported in this research by the National Science Foundation (Grant No. ISP82-09516) and the National Endowment for the Humanities. The views expressed are those of the authors and do not necessarily reflect the views of NSF or NEH.

To date there are two multi-author, interdisciplinary analyses of sex preselection: the book *Sex Selection of Children*, edited by Neil G. Bennett (1983, New York, Academic Press); and a feminist collection, the section 'Sex Preselection' edited by Janice Raymond (1981), in *The Custom-Made Child? Women-Centered Perspectives*. Also, Nancy Williamson (1976; 1978) has ably and thoroughly discussed the literature from many disciplines.

## NOTES

1 For citations to the voluminous literature on parents' and potential parents' preferences for sex of offspring, see the bibliographies in Williamson (1976; 1978), Steinbacher (1983), and Gray et al. (1983).
2 See notes 1 and 3; also Pebley and Westoff (1982); Stinner and Mader (1975).
3 Nan Chico, a sociologist in Hayward, California, is analyzing for her Ph.D. dissertation sex preferences expressed in letters written

to Dr Ericsson. She finds that 85.9 percent of 1,583 couples who described their wishes for sex distribution in their children wanted balanced families. However, she has a very select sample because the Ericsson method is advertised only as a technique for male selection; 64.3 percent of the group said that they already had at least one girl and want a boy to balance their families (personal communication to HBH).

4  Should sperm separation technologies be perfected, they might in combination with the new technology of IVF (in vitro fertilization), open a new dimension for sex selection. Selected sperm might then be placed on a human egg in the laboratory for a sex-determined conception. (As is now done with untreated sperm samples, separated sperm could be frozen or freeze-dried until needed.)

5  At Harvard, *Time* magazine reports, current studies of lizards – several species of which never have males, and which rub each other, apparently to facilitate ovulation and embryo development – so intrigue some Harvard scientists that they are treating lizard eggs with hormones to transsexualize them to males! ('Detection of embryo or fetus sex', *Time*, 115(7): 50, February 18, 1980).

6  The accuracy of chromosome analysis used in conjunction with IVF technology, we speculate, could permit choice of sex before implanting an embryo. First an unneeded cell would be removed from a 'test-tube' embryo to have its chromosomes checked to determine sex. The embryo might be frozen to arrest its development until the results were back from the laboratory.

7  For an analysis of patriarchal values in the development and deployment of technologies in reproductive medicine, see Holmes, 1981. Salient values identified there are: technology infatuation, domination, objectification, exploitation of nature, hierarchism, and profit.

8  Guttentag and Secord (1983) provide an excellent and fascinating analysis of sex ratio imbalances and their effect on sex roles. These authors do not intend to be sexist – in fact, quite the contrary – but they fail to recognize some heterosexist assumptions. Also, they use the standard terminology of sex ratio demography, which reflects omnipresent patriarchal biases: ratios are stated with males first; the value-positive term 'high' is used for a sex ratio with more males than females.

9  'Gynandry' means (in our linear language, which expresses choice by putting the male *andros* or the female *gynos* first) that we favor women-associated traits. 'Androgyny' could imply desire for aggressive, world-conquering, nature-dominating traits so prevalent now.

# REFERENCES

Adimoelja, A., R. Hariadi, I. G. B. Amitaba, P. Adisetya and Soeharno. 1977. 'The separation of X- and Y-spermatozoa with regard to the possible clinical application by means of artificial insemination.' *andrologia*, 9(3): 289–92.

Beernink, F. J. and R. J. Ericsson. 1982. 'Male sex preselection through sperm isolation.' *Fertility and Sterility*, 38(4): 493–5.

Chacko, Arun. 1982. 'Too many daughters? India's drastic cure.' *World Paper* (November): 8–9.

deCrespigny, Lachlan Ch. and Hugh P. Robinson. 1981. 'Determination of fetal sex with ultrasound.' *Medical Journal of Australia*, 2 (July 25): 98–100.

Culpepper, Emily E. 1981. 'Uncovering patriarchal agendas and exploring woman-oriented values.' In Holmes, Helen B., Betty B. Hoskins and Michael Gross, eds. *The Custom-Made Child? Women-Centered Perspectives*. Humana Press, Clifton, NJ: 301–10.

Ericsson, Ronald J., C. N. Langevin and M. Nishino. 1973. 'Isolation of fractions rich in human Y sperm.' *Nature*, 246: 421–2.

Ericsson, Ronald J. 1977. 'Isolation and storage of progressively motile human sperm.' *andrologia*, 9(1): 111–14.

Gearhart, Sally Miller. 1982. 'The future – if there is one – is female.' In McAllister, Pam, ed. *Reweaving the Web of Life: Feminism and Nonviolence*. New Society Publishers, Philadelphia: 266–84.

Gilligan, Carol. 1982. *In a Different Voice: Psychological Theory and Women's Development*. Harvard University Press, Cambridge, MA.

Glass, Allan R. and Thomas Klein. 1981. 'Changes in maternal serum total and free androgen levels in early pregnancy: Lack of correlation with fetal sex.' *American Journal of Obstetrics and Gynecology*, 140: 656–60.

Glass, Robert H. and Ronald J. Ericsson. 1982. *Getting Pregnant in the 1980s: New Advances in Infertility Treatment and Sex Preselection*. University of California Press, Berkeley.

Gosden, J. R., A. R. Mitchell, C. M. Gosden, C. H. Rodeck, and J. M. Morsman. 1982. 'Direct vision chorion biopsy and chromosome-specific DNA probes for determination of fetal sex in first-trimester prenatal diagnosis.' *Lancet*, 2 (December 25): 1416–19.

Gould, Carol, ed. 1983. *Beyond Domination: New Perspectives on Women and Philosophy*. Littlefield, Adams, Totowa, NJ.

Gray, Elizabeth D. 1981. *Green Paradise Revisited*. Roundtable Press, Wellesley, Massachusetts.

Gray, Elizabeth D. 1982. *Patriarchy as a Conceptual Trap*. Roundtable Press, Wellesley, Massachusetts.

Gray, Elmer, Valina K. Hurt and S. O. Oyewole. 1983. 'Desired family size and sex of children in Nigeria.' *Journal of Heredity*, 74: 204–6.

Guerrero, Rodrigo. 1974. 'Association of the type and time of insemination within the menstrual cycle with the human sex ratio at birth.' *New England Journal of Medicine*, 291(20): 1056–9.

Guttentag, Marcia and Paul F. Secord. 1983. *Too Many Women? The Sex Ratio Question*. Sage Publications, Beverly Hills.

Harlap, Susan. 1979. 'Gender of infants conceived on different days of the menstrual cycle.' *New England Journal of Medicine*, 300(26): 1445–8.

Held, K. R., U. Burck and Th. Koske-Westphal. 1981. 'Pränatale Geschlechtsbestimmung durch den GBN-Speicheltest. Ein Vergleich mit den Ergebnissen der pränatalen Chromosomendiagnostik.' *Geburtshilfe und Frauenheilkunde*, 41: 619–21.

Herzenberg, L. A., D. W. Bianchi, J. Schröder, H. M. Cann and G. M. Iverson. 1979. 'Fetal cells in the blood of pregnant women: Detection and enrichment by fluorescence-activated cell sorting.' Proceedings of the National Academy of Science (USA), 76: 1453–5.

Holmes, Helen B. 1981. 'Reproductive technologies: The birth of a women-centered analysis.' In Holmes, Helen B., Betty B. Hoskins and Michael Gross, eds. *The Custom-Made Child? Women-Centered Perspectives*. Humana Press, Clifton, NJ: 1–18.

Holmes, Helen B., Betty B. Hoskins and Michael Gross, eds. 1981. *The Custom-Made Child? Women-Centered Perspectives*. Humana Press, Clifton, NJ.

Hoskins, Betty B. 1980. 'Feminist thought and reproductive technology: The circle and the ladder.' Paper presented at Universalist/Unitarian Collegium, September, Craigville, Massachusetts.

Johnson, Bonnie. 1982. 'Move over, Mother Nature! A new diet may help moms select their babies' sex.' *People* 18(8) (August 23): 49–51.

Kirsch-Volders, M., E. Lissens-Van Assche and C. Susanne. 1980. 'Increase in the amount of fetal lympocytes in maternal blood during pregnancy.' *Journal of Medical Genetics*, 17: 267–72.

Langendoen, Sally and William Proctor. 1982. *The Preconception Gender Diet*. Evans, M. & Co, New York.

Loewit, K. von, H. G. Kraft and W. Brabec. 1982. 'Zur Geschlechtsbestimmung des Fetus aus dem Speichel der Mutter.' *Wiener klinische Wochenschrift*, 94(8) (April 16): 223–6.

Luce, Clare Boothe. 1978. 'Next: Pills to make most babies male.' *Washington Star* (July 9): C-1; C-4.

McAllister, Pam, ed. 1982. *Reweaving the Web of Life: Feminism and Nonviolence*. New Society Publishers, Philadelphia.

Méan, M., G. Pescia, D. Vajda, J. B. Pelber and G. Magrini. 1981. 'Amniotic fluid testosterone in prenatal sex determination.' *Journal de Génétique humaine*, 29(4): 441–7.

PBS (Public Broadcasting System). 1981. 'Boy or girl? Should the choice be ours?' First broadcast January 2 in series *Hard Choices*. Transcripts available from PTV Publications, P.O. Box 701, Kent, OH 44240.

Pebley, A. R. and C. F. Westoff. 1982. 'Women's sex preference in the United States: 1970 to 1975.' *Demography*, 19(2): 177–89.

Powledge, Tabitha. 1981. 'Unnatural selection: On choosing children's sex.' In Holmes, Helen B., Betty B. Hoskins and Michael Gross, eds. *The Custom-Made Child? Women-Centered Perspectives*. Humana Press, Clifton, NJ: 193–9.

Quinlivan, W. L., K. Preciado, T. L. Long and H. Sullivan. 1982. 'Separation of human X and Y spermatozoa by albumin gradients and Sephadex chromatography.' *Fertility and Sterility*, 37(1): 104–7.

Raymond, Janice, section ed. 1981. 'Sex Preselection.' In Holmes, Helen B., Betty B. Hoskins and Michael Gross, eds. *The Custom-Made Child? Women-Centered Perspectives*. Humana Press, Clifton, NJ: 177–224.

Rorvik, David and Landrum B. Shettles. 1970. 'How to choose your baby's sex.' *Look*, 24 (April): 88–98.

Rorvik, David and Landrum B. Shettles. 1977. *Choose Your Baby's Sex*. Dodd, Mead & Co, New York.

Schilling, E., R. Lafrenz and F. Klobasa. 1978. 'Failure to separate human X- and Y-chromosome bearing spermatozoa by sephadex gel-filtration.' *andrologia*, 10: 215–17.

Steeno, O., A. Adimoelja and J. Steeno. 1975. 'Separation of X- and Y-bearing human spermatozoa with the Sephadex gel-filtration method.' *andrologia*, 7: 95–7.

Steinbacher, Roberta. 1983. 'Sex preselection: From here to fraternity.' In Gould, Carol, ed. *Beyond Domination: New Perspectives on Women and Philosophy*. Littlefield, Adams, Totowa, NJ.

Stinner, W. F. and P. D. Mader. 1975. 'Sons, daughters or both. An analysis of family sex composition preference in the Philippines.' *Demography*, 12: 67–80.

Stolkowski, J. and J. Choukroun. 1981. 'Preconception selection of sex in man.' *Israel Journal of Medical Sciences*, 17: 1061–7.

*Time*. 1980. 'Detection of embryo or fetus sex', 115(7): 50. February 18.

Weldner, E.-M. 1981. 'Accuracy of fetal sex determination by ultrasound.' *Acta Obstetricia et Gynecologia Scandinavica*, 60: 333–4.

Williamson, Nancy E. 1976. 'Sex preferences, sex control, and the status of women.' *Signs: Journal of Women in Culture and Society*, 1: 847–62.

Williamson, Nancy E. 1978. *Boys or Girls? Parents' Preferences and Sex Control*. Population Bulletin. Population Reference Bureau, Washington, DC.

# IF YOU WOULD BE THE MOTHER OF A SON

## Kumkum Sangari

This poem literally describes the things men and women do before, during, and after conception in the hope of having a son. The social, religious and economic importance of sons in India is well known. The desire to have sons is an aspect of patriarchy and is part and parcel of the oppression, devaluation and exploitation of Indian women. This piece draws its data from two sources – ancient rites surrounding conception, and interviews with contemporary, middle-class urban women. The potency and persistence of the belief that parents can determine the sex of their child, the religious, mystical and symbolic nature of the methods used, and the fact that this is little more than an initial foray into a sparsely documented area, made me feel that a historical, sociological or medical analysis may be premature. In search of a more 'expressive' and descriptive form I have chosen verse.

Part I of the poem describes *garbhādhāna* and *pumsavana*, the two rituals prescribed in ancient literature for the conception of a male child, and is practically a quotation from Pandurang Vaman Kane's *History of the Dharamśāstra: Ancient and Medieval Religious and Civil Law*, vol. II, part 1, Government Oriental Series: Class B, no. 6 (Poona; Bhandarkar Oriental Research Institute, 1941: 188–221).

Part II attempts to counterpoise the contradictory ideas of free will and fate which coexist in this lore. Part IV shows the survival of the ancient practices described in Part I in contemporary India. Dr Samar Sen's *Gharelu Ilaaj* is a popular collection of 'Home Remedies' (Delhi, Subodh Pocket Books, 1976: 187). Parts III and V are based on

contemporary accounts, and Part VI describes the
'symptoms' which are popularly believed to indicate that
the woman is pregnant with a boy child.

I
Woman, it is
the *samskāras* contain
the rites and actions that render
the mind and body fit to attain
maturity and *brahma*.
Said Manu, the all-knowing lawgiver,
this human frame is justified only
by the generation of sons.
Man must procreate
according to the practices of *garbhādhāna*,
and by the rites of *pumsavana*
ordain the *garbha* to become male.

In order to perform *garbhādhāna*,
woman, bathe three days after menstruation.
Husband, after she has thus bathed
get her to pound rice, and boil it
and eat it, with various other things,
according as you desire
a fair son, a dark or brown son, a learned son
(or a learned daughter).
Near the morning hour make offerings
of *ghee*, little by little,
to the holy fire
saying
'This is for Agni, *svāhā*
this for Anumati, *svāhā*
this for the divine Savitṛ, the true creator, *svāhā*.'
Take out then the rest of the rice,
eat it, and having eaten,
give a portion to your wife.
Cleanse your hands, fill a jar,
sprinkle her thrice with water
saying
'Arise, O Viśvāvasu,

seek another blooming girl,
a wife with her husband.'
Embrace her, saying
'I am Ama, thou art Sā.
Thou art Sā, I am Ama.
I am the Sāman, thou art the Ṛk.
I am the sky, thou art the earth.
Come, let us strive that a man child be begotten.'

Remember on *cathurthīkarma*
to chant this verse:
'May a male embryo enter thy womb
as an arrow into the quiver.
May a man be born here,
a son, at ten months end.'

Remember
each of the even nights from fourth to the sixteenth
after the commencement of the monthly illness
are more and more conducive
for the excellence of male offspring.

Remember
Manu, the *Yājñavalkyāsmṛiti*, the
   *Vaikhānasa-smārta-sūtrā*
all pronounce that a man desirous
of male issue should cohabit
only on the even days from the fourth
day after the commencement of the monthly illness.
Says the *Vaikhānasa*
a woman in her unclean days
should bathe on the fourth day,
wear white,
anoint herself with unguents.
Besides, she must hold no converse
with another woman or a *śūdra*,
must see nobody save her husband
since the baby to be born
becomes like the man
the woman looks at after her *ritūsnāna*.

And then, under the constellation Tiṣya,
you shall perform *puṁsavana*
by virtue of which performance
a male child is born.
In the third month after conception
after she has fasted rigorously on
the preceding Punarvasu configuration
give her thrice to eat in the curds
of a cow that has a calf of like colour
two beans and one grain of barley
for each handful of curds.
When you ask the woman
'What dost thou drink?
what dost thou drink?'
she must thrice reply
'*Puṁsavana, puṁsavana, puṁsavana.*'
In this way make her take
three mouthfuls of curds with two beans
and one grain of barley, or
instead, bring a shoot of the branch
of a *nyagrodha* tree, a tree which
points east or north, a tree
which has two fruits,
fruits that resemble testicles.
Get a pre-pubescent girl to pound
the shoots and fruits between two
upper stones of two several grinding mills
with water. While your wife lies facing
east but to the west of the fire
insert into her right nostril
with your thumb the pounded
substance, saying '*Puṁsavanani-asi*'
and pour the bile of a tortoise into her lap.

Woman, your rightful place
is on your husband's left.
Stay on your back for some time,
then return to your right side,
the male side, for the son you desire.

II
Do you know King Dasaratha performed
a *puttreshṭi yagya* and Ram was born?
Don't you know Jijabai willed herself
to have a warrior son – *chattrapati* Śivājī?
Woman, with the force of your will
you can determine the gender
of your child, up to the third month.

But the astrologer said
there is no son ordained for you,
your stars deny it.
You will have to borrow one
from your last life or your next
by praying to Shantinatha bhagwan,
by worshipping the silver snake
for nine months, by giving away
a golden snake when your boy is born.

In any case, if your first period came
in the days of the waxing moon
your first child will be a boy.

III
If you want a son read the *Sūryā Purana*
worship the sun, make offerings of water
to him, for nine months let his light
warm and quicken your abdomen
after you think you have conceived.

If you wish for a son, fast
on every *purnamāsi*.
Conceive under the full moon.

First time pregnant woman
look up to the full moon,
drink a glass of water and pray
that a boy as beautiful as the moon
be born unto you.

If you desire a son
worship the banana tree
pray to Shiva
offer at the shrine of Kali
pay obeisance at the shrine of Lolarak Baba
visit Baba Balaknathji's hut
take a vow to perform *mundān*
at the shrine of the god who grants a son.
Find the lonely temple of a goddess
enshrined outside the city
for twenty-five years at the least.
Offer her holy water,
water mixed with milk, rice and *batasa*,
water stored in a copper pot.
Catch the drops that trickle down
catch them in a vessel
drink them twice a day
drink them for twenty-one days in the
first month, then drink for nine days
every month. Drink in the faith that
a male child shall be yours.


IV
After *ritūsnāna* peel a grain of barley
swallow it with water for eight days
on an empty stomach.
That is what mother said.
But the homeopath says
eat a grain of barley every day
till the child turns around in the womb.


Dr Samar Sen says in *Gharelu Ilaaj*
four days after *ritūsnāna* grind
into a powder three grams *gorochan*,
ten grams *gajpipal*, ten grams *asagandha*.
Use the concoction for five days
before *garbhādhāna*.
You must know
the old *grānthas* were written
on the bark of the *bhojapatra* tree.

Take a piece of bark,
write it over with a pomegranate pen
dipped in saffron.
Write the *gāyatrī mantra*, the *mahāmṛituñjaya mantra*,
write under the stars, under the Puṣyanakṣhatra.
While you are still in your first month
wash the bark every day in holy water
and drink the water.

Hold a *puta*, a phallus-like pestle
swaddled in cloth in your lap
when you sit to eat at *saptamrita*.
At *sadh*, women and children will come
to ceremonial feast bearing gifts
when you sit to eat the food you like,
the food you crave for,
and a boy child will sit on your lap.

V
Keep, expectant mother, the
picture of the infant Krishna
or a beautiful boychild in your room.
Put your right foot first on the ground
when you leave your bed in the morning.

Stick the seed of a coconut
the feather of a peacock
in a piece of jaggery.
Eat it when you are three months gone.

Eat the small white flower
inside the green, unripe coconut
for three days on a hungry morning
stomach in the second month.
Eat it and you shall have a boy.

Eat the last-born leaves,
leaves not quite leaves
of a *bar* tree. Eat them once
with unbroken *urad* grains and curds

and other things.
Eat them in the third month, said the *vaidji*,
eat nothing else for twenty-four hours
and you shall have a boy.

Take this pill first thing in the morning
when you think you have conceived,
said the holy man.
Gulp it down with the uncooked milk
of a cow with a newborn calf
a male calf.

Come and stay in my house, young women,
who are three months gone, said
the old aunt.
I will give a potion in milk and rice
pudding, keep you in a room for twenty-four
hours, where you will not see the face
of girl or woman
and you will have a boy.

Catch with courage a droning bee
wrap it wriggling in a twist of dough
and swallow it.

VI
Thus, pregnant woman, do you
crave for fish, sweets, mutton,
feel active and alert,
look plain and awful,
look plain beautiful?
Do you have a flatly swelling tummy
a crooked line above and below your navel?
Is your right foot heavier than the left?
Does your waist hurt
and your nose shine?
Why, then, you will surely
have a boy.

## GLOSSARY

Agni   god of fire

Ama   this; strength, power

Anumati   a goddess

asagandha   *witharia somnifera*

Baba Balaknathji   a local saint

baṛ   banyan tree

batasa   a semi-spherical crisp and spongy sugar cake

bhojapatra   a tree

brahma   God, the eternal spirit, knowledge

cathurthīkarma   a part of the marriage rite prescribed in
  the *Sāṅkyāyana-gṛhya-sūtrā* (c. 800 BC–400 BC) which is
  performed on the fourth night after marriage and culmin-
  ates in intercourse

chattrapati   king or ruler

gajpipal   a root

garbha   child in the womb

garbhādhāna   insemination, Vedic ritual for impregnation

gāyatrī mantra   a verse of great sanctity addressed to the
  god Saviṭra in the *Ṛg Veda*

*Gharelu Ilaaj*   'Home Remedies'

ghee   clarified butter

gorochan   a paste

grānth   book

Jijabai   queen and mother of seventeenth-century Marāthā
  chief, Śivājī

Lolarak Baba   a local saint with shrine near Benaras

mahāmṛituṅjaya mantra   a sacred verse with magical
  powers to overcome death

Manu   author of *Manusmṛti* (c. 200 BC–200 AD)

mundān   ceremony involving the first shaving of the hair on
  a child's head

nyagrodha   a tree mentioned in the *Āpastamba-gṛhya-sūtrā*
  (c. 600 BC–300 BC)

puṁsavana   generation of a male, ceremony performed
  during the third month of pregnancy

Punarvasu   a constellation of stars

purnamāsi   full moon day

Pusyanakshatra   a constellation of stars

puta   the word for pestle in East Bengal/Bangladesh. In Hindi 'pu:t' means son. Here the pestle becomes a surrogate for a male child

puttreshṭi yagya   an ancient sacrifice performed for the sake of begetting a son

ritūsnāna   ritual bath and hair bath after menstruation

Ṛk   one verse of the *Ṛg Veda*

Sā   she; giving, bestowing, granting

sadh   Bengali ceremony performed in the ninth month of pregnancy

Sāman   one verse of the *Sāmaveda*

samskāra   sacrament, rite, purification, improvement, refinement; ritual believed to be necessary for unfolding the latent capacities of human beings

saptamrita   Bengali ceremony performed in the seventh month of pregnancy

Savitṛ   old solar god

Shantinath bhagwan   a local god

śūdra   low caste person

svāhā   word pronounced at the time of offering oblation

Tiṣya   a constellation of stars

uṛad   black gram, horse-bean

vaidji   Ayurvedic physician

*Vaikhānasa-smārta-sūtra*   *c.* 200 AD–500 AD

Viśvāvasu   a group of deities

*Yājñavalkyāsmṛiti*   *c.* 100 AD–300 AD

# ABORTION OF A SPECIAL KIND: MALE SEX SELECTION IN INDIA

Viola Roggencamp

Viola Roggencamp interviews an Indian woman who went for a sex-identification test to the Bhandari clinic run by a business-minded husband-wife team of gynecologists and who, when the test said 'female,' had an abortion. The desperation of this woman who is already the mother of three girls and could not bear the thought of a fourth one reflects the worldwide devaluation of women and points to the many painful contradictions inherent in the availability of reproductive technologies as long as we live in a world in which men oppress, exploit and hate women.

In Amritsar, sacred city in the state of Punjab in Northern India, two doctors — husband and wife — run an abortion clinic of a special kind: general practitioner Singh Bhandari and gynecologist Kanan Bhandari work towards the systematic eradication of women through practice of selective abortion of female fetuses:

> It is now possible to find the sex of your child in early pregnancy before it is born with the aid of the latest sophisticated imported electronic equipments and established scientific techniques. For details contact or write: Antenatal Sex Determination Clinic M/s. New Bhandari Hospital (Regd.) 2638 Chowk Moni (1/8 Chatiwind Gate), Amritsar. phone 32 500.

This was the ad that appeared in March 1981 in a number of Indian newspapers and journals — just in time for the opening of the Bhandari Clinic in Amritsar. The message spread quickly across the whole country, flyers were distributed on trains and stuck on housewalls, it appeared in large print on state and private buses and was even shown as a commercial in cinemas. No one seemed to mind: 'Plan your family. Get over financial worries. Know the sex of your child before it is born. At a nominal cost.' In addition, the business-minded couple sent publicity letters to their medical colleagues:

> Most prospective clients in quest of a male child, as the social set-up in India demands, keep on giving birth to a number of female children, which in a way not only enhances the increasing population (sic) but leads to a chain reaction of many social, economic and mental stresses on these families . . . antenatal sex determination has come to our rescue and can help in keeping some check over the population as well as giving relief to the couples requiring male children.

Each medical doctor who sends a client to the New Bhandari Hospital in Amritsar receives a premium of 100 rupees.[1] In its first year of existence the clinic carried out over 500 sex determinations. 'The tests,' as the Bhandaris state without hesitation 'are a boon for mothers harassed by family members for having too many daughters.'

In summer 1982, six women's organizations from within political parties, the trade unions and the autonomous women's movement held a joint public meeting. Sushila Gopalan, member of parliament, said:

> We are living in a country with a strong sex bias against women. In Uttar Pradesh, in Bihar and Rajasthan baby girls continue to be killed after birth, many more women and girls die from malnutrition and lack of medical care, and now killing female fetuses has become big business.[2]

Vimala Ranadive, trade union activist, concurred:

> Female infanticide is one reason for the sharp decline in India's sex ratio; from 972 female births for every 1000 male births in 1901 to 930 in 1971 before rising slightly to 935 in the 1981 census. It is like the Nazi's 'final solution' to exterminate Jews and it only adds a touch of sophistication to the brutal practice.

And Anjali Deshpande, speaking for autonomous feminists, declared:

> In the good old days women were tied hand and foot and thrown on to the funeral pyres of their husbands. Nowadays people seem to be in more of a hurry to burn them – they are killed or driven to suicide while their husbands are still alive. And now there comes an even quicker and less cumbersome method of getting rid of a female child, by a modern technique known as amniocentesis.

Amniocentesis was first practised in India in 1974 at the Human Cytogenetics Unit of New Delhi's All India Institute of Medical Sciences (AIIMS). The intent was to detect severe mental and bodily disabilities of the fetus. However, a 'by-product' of the test is the determination of the sex of the fetus. After this knowledge had spread more widely, sex determination became *illegal* in all state hospitals: it had become evident that more and more wives were being forced by their husbands into having an abortion when the test-result said 'a healthy fetus – a girl.'

However, after its prohibition in state hospitals, the test's secrets were quickly passed on to medical colleagues in private clinics. After all there was money to be made. Once the necessary skills have been acquired it is not too difficult to carry out amniocentesis. Take a syringe and remove a few cells of the fetus which are free floating in the amniotic fluid in which it develops. After the cells are grown in culture in the laboratory, chromosome analysis can be done to determine the sex of the fetus. The lab equipment does cost a couple of hundred thousand rupees, but they'll be earned back soon. It is said the husband-wife team from Amritsar made almost 300,000 rupees in their clinic's first year.

Not surprisingly in a male-dominated society, the official decision to make sex determination illegal is neither observed nor enforced. Amniocentesis continues to be carried out for the purpose of sex-selection. The result is the systematic abortion of female fetuses. And, as a female doctor, Ms Kucheria from the Human Cytogenetic Unit at AIIMS, says: 'How do you police a backyard laboratory?'[3]

In order to avoid being accused of 'female fetuscide,' the Bhandaris keep a few deformed fetuses in a glass jar. But among them are a pair of 'normal' female twins. Gynecologist Dr Kanan Bhandari explains: 'We have preserved it because it is a good medical specimen of twins with one placenta.' And husband and wife go on, emotionless and rather bragging: 'Moreover we have faltered in only one out of the many cases carried out so far.' Indeed, the Bhandaris have many thank-you letters to show. They come from all parts of India: Kerala, Rajasthan, Gujarat, Jammu, Kashmir and Madhya Pradesh. In the words of Mr K. K. Loomba, pathologist at the New Bhandari Hospital: 'A couple who has a daughter has a right to opt for a son!' 'But what a tragedy,' as Dr Kripal Kaur, head of the Obstetrics and Gynecology Department of the Government Victoria Jubilee Hospital, said to me, 'when the test result is wrong, that is, when the aborted fetus turns out to be male and not female.' 'Immense psychological traumas' were her words to describe the women's responses when they heard about the mistake. And who would want to blame them, for a son, for sure, would have made their life much worthier – in the eyes of society.

That women are oppressed, exploited, mistreated, raped and in general discriminated against is a truth that applies to all countries. But there are some specific dimensions to women's oppression in India as there are specific dimensions to many other phenomena. India's size equals the whole of Europe. It has 700 million inhabitants, 80 percent of whom, despite constant migration into urban areas, continue to live in rural areas where, for example, only one-fifth of all the villages are supplied with electricity. Almost 90 percent of the 300 million Indian women are illiterate. About 600 million of Indian women and men are followers of Hinduism, a religion which – not very different from any other religion – regulates the social and sexual interaction of its followers; that is, Hinduism is a social movement as much as a religious philosophy.

There are four major castes with 3000 sub-castes. Being born into a low caste means that you remain in it and that your family and children will be members of the same caste. For the individual man things might improve in his next life.

For the individual woman only if she will be reborn as a man. At the bottom of the four castes are those who do not have a caste, the Harijans – the untouchables. The Hindu caste system condemns them to do all the shitwork that no higher-caste Hindu would do: draining the sewer, cleaning the latrines, removing dead animals. Sixty million Indian women are untouchables. As all other religions, Hinduism also determines the social position of women. Of course, in favour of males. Man equals god. To serve a man is to serve god. As a daughter the girl belongs to her father, as a wife to her husband, her father-in-law and her brother-in-law. As a widow she belongs to her son(s). Thus the birth of a daughter implies bad luck because she isn't a 'real' member of the family. She already belongs to the family of her future husband. And although officially illegal, marriage contracts between 2–3-year-old girls and 6–10-year-old boys continue to be made.

The bride's family pays a dowry to the bridegroom's family; in other words, in order to get rid of one's daughter one has to pay. In 1919, an average dowry was around 500 rupees, in 1970 it was up to 22,000 rupees. These figures apply to marriages in rural areas; in cities, the prices are three to four times higher depending on caste, standard of living and above all on the bridegroom's demands.

It is not unusual for the bride's parents to finance the bridegroom's studies or professional training. When the marriage takes place the bride's parents provide new clothes for the bridegroom's whole family. And a fridge, a scooter, a radio, a TV are today's 'ordinary' presents – from the bride to the bridegroom. Many, indeed very many, families get enormously indebted because of the dowry pressure and the debt is often carried on to the next generation. Too dreadful to imagine that it is not only one, but three or four daughters, who need to be 'provided' for – sold, to put it a bit more crudely. To have an unmarried daughter, however, is a social stigma for any family.

In the last ten years, more and more cases of 'dowry deaths' became public. And about four to five years ago, hesitantly at first, newspapers started to report these incidents. While the official version mentions 'accidents in the kitchen' or 'suicides' the reality is that husbands pour kerosene (the fuel which is used in all Indian kitchens) over their wives and set them on fire. They burn to death while still alive. The reason: a wife's dowry wasn't high enough. The husband had further desires. But the woman didn't want to ask her parents for still more money. So, all of a sudden her sari was on fire. Small problem for the mourning widower. He will soon find a new wife – with a new dowry. In New Delhi, to give one example, there are 400 to 500 dowry deaths each year.

According to the law, all of this is, of course, totally illegal: the burning of widows (sati), prostitution, child marriages, trade in women, the selling of girls to brothels, and the institution of having to provide a dowry. But 'paper is patient' – the real world takes little note of such laws. Some parts of society may be uneasy, perhaps even complaining about these incidents. But for many that is as far as their protest will go. After all, criminal as the husband's behaviour to his wife may appear, she is his wife, his property. No action is taken. Small wonder then that for a large number of Indians it seems easier to eradicate 'the problem' – girl fetuses, that is – before it arises.

So how can a mother be happy about the birth of her daughter when her husband and family turn away from her in disappointment, discontent and anger? How, in fact, can women avoid projecting society's contempt of women onto other women – including their own daughters? ·

On August 8, 1982, at Rajindra hospital, a mother refused to accept her baby – it was a girl. She maintained that a week ago she had given birth to a son. Apparently, Mrs Nachattar Kau had been told by hospital personnel that she had given birth to a son. Upon this happy news the relatives had donated the usual monetary gifts to celebrate the birth of an heir. But then she was brought a girl. . . . A confusion, however, was out of the question: on that very day only girls had been born. The director of the clinic asked her husband to see him. Apparently not to his satisfaction: Mrs Kaur left the hospital without her child (but returned after four hours). It is now assumed that because of a sex determination test the couple had expected the birth of a son. 'Who would want to go on giving birth to daughters in the hope of delivering the desired son?' This is what a young doctor, a mother of two daughters, said to me. And as she continued she herself would go for an amniocentesis 'before trying a third time.'

'It is better to spend 500 rupees now, than to spend *lakhs*[4] later,' says the young wife of a man who owns a transportation business. She had just undergone an amniocentesis test in the Bhandari Clinic at Amritsar and was waiting with her husband and their whole family for the test result. It is difficult to describe the young woman's state of nervousness and tenseness as she awaited the result. And it is even less possible to give an account of the triumph when the doctor announced 'It is a boy, congratulations!' The future parents were adorned with flower garlands – the parents of the couple wept with joy and relief.

For Sharkuntala, 25 years of age, mother of three girls, married to a businessman from Ahmedabad in Gujarat when she was 18 years old, it was less joyful: she had an abortion when she heard the result of her sex-determination test – a girl. The following is the transcript of our conversation (with the help of an interpreter):[5]

*Question*:   You went to the New Bhandari Hospital in Amritsar.
*Sharkuntala*:   Yes, three weeks ago.
*Question*:   Why did you go there?
*S*:   My husband and his family wanted it.
*Q*:   What was it that they wanted?
*S*:   Well, I have already three girls.
*Q*:   You mean that three children are enough? Is this why you chose to abort the fourth?
*S*:   Yes . . . that is, actually no. We want a son. My husband wants a son so much. And I am his wife, so I have to give him a son.
*Q*:   And not a fourth girl?
*S*:   Exactly. Really, we have enough girls. And when we heard about this test to find out what sex the child will be. . . .
*Q*:   But the test is actually to find out whether the baby – girl or boy – is healthy.

*S*: Really? All I know is that the test can tell whether it's going to be a girl or a boy.

*Q*: When did you have the abortion?

*S*: Well, we saw the ad about the clinic in a newspaper when I was in my fourth month.

*Q*: Did you read the ad?

*S*: Yes. . . . no, my husband did.

*Q*: Can you read and write?

*S*: No.

*Q*: Why did you have an abortion?

*S*: Because they said it was going to be a girl.

*Q*: So, it was because it was going to be a girl that you had an abortion?

*S*: Yes.

*Q*: What did they do?

*S*: They punctured my belly with a huge needle.

*Q*: And the abortion?

*S*: We did that in Ahmedabad. That's where we live. But I don't want to talk about it.

*Q*: Was it so terrible?

*S*: I don't want to talk . . . (crying) each child is sent by God.

*Q*: Do you think God makes a difference between boys and girls?

*S*: I really don't know. But why doesn't he give me a son? Will he never give me a son? How shall it continue? Maybe I will never have a son? Maybe it is my fault? Who knows. Only God does. But what do I have to do? What should I do? I am so afraid. Do you think it will have to continue like that?

*Q*: You mean test, again and again . . . abortions, again and again.

*S*: Yes, that's what I mean. . . . But I will do it if only my body will take it. And I am afraid that my husband will divorce me and take a new wife who will give him sons.

*Q*: When your husband suggested the test to you, did you immediately agree?

*S*: Yes.

*Q*: But weren't you afraid?

*S*: He is the man. He has a right to a son.

*Q:* Is it really that simple?

*S:* I shall do anything to give him a son.

*Q:* If you'd already had three sons – instead of three girls – would you also have had the test done in order to get a girl?

*S:* I don't understand.

*Q:* Would you have done all these things in order to get a girl? Would you have the fourth and fifth son aborted to ensure that your fourth child will be a girl?

*S:* (hesitates) Well, I don't know . . . but if I know it will be a son how can I possibly think of aborting him?

*Q:* But with a girl you can?

*S:* You just don't know what I've been going through in the last seven years because all I gave birth to were girls! Again and again it is a girl. I carry her for nine months. The family prays to God, the priest pays a visit, the family undertakes *puja* (a religious ceremony). Then the day arrives, the labour starts. Then finally the birth. And again – nothing. After my second and third delivery all they did was to send my little brother-in-law to see me at the hospital. It would be so much easier for me with a son. My husband and his family would respect me much more.

The Bhandari Clinic at Amritsar set an example throughout India. Today there are similar clinics in New Delhi, Bombay, Jullundur, Kanpur and Meerut. Even the governmentalized Sir Hurkisondas Nurrotamdas Hospital and the King George's Medical College in the industrial town Lucknow perform the sex determination test and thus enable the selective abortion of female fetuses. A private clinic in Bombay carries out the test on a large scale for other towns. As Dr Kucheria of AIIMS says, from New Delhi alone more than fifty gynecologists send their cell samples to the Bombay clinic for analysis. Gynecologists have started to run advertisements in which they encourage women to have the test done – at the price of $100.00, which is 1,000 rupees or one-and-a-half times the monthly salary of a schoolteacher. To make 'quick money' the test results are delivered after only one day. The method used in this test is much less reliable than the usual one which takes two to three weeks.

In July 1982, Indian feminists asked Indira Gandhi's government to sue the doctors and declare the test to be illegal. They demanded of the Indian Medical Council to take away the license from the accused medical doctors. So far nothing has happened. Dr Kaur thinks that 'It is for the government to stop it,' but when the Union health minister B. Shankaranand was asked what was being done, he declared emotionlessly, trivializing the matter: 'Only some private doctors were encouraging pregnant women to take these tests for female fetuside.' (*India Today* 1982). He agreed that this was unethical but it became clear that he did not plan on taking action against these doctors or to legally prohibit the test.

Because, really, with the exception of feminists no one sees much wrong in all of this. For many men – and for many women – the possibility to determine the sex of the unborn baby constitutes the solution to the problem of overpopulation. Hasn't 'family planning' been encouraged for many years? As the majority of the Indian people are illiterate, the government has designed an optical sign: a red triangle and four heads – father, mother, son and daughter. To curtail the enormous population increase, many more women than men were made infertile.[7]

'In any case,' explained an Indian doctor quite calmly to me 'in India women are discriminated against a lot. The question is really only whether they get killed in their mother's wombs or whether they are burnt by their in-laws.' And the *Indian Express* (1982), which prides itself to be one of India's most progressive daily newspapers, asks: 'And who is at fault? The women themselves. Women, especially Indian women, are crazy for a son.' And the conservative *Times of India* (1982) echoes: 'Women, after all, are the worst enemies of women.'

It appears as if the Indian public in general goes along with the opinion of the Bhandaris, who say: 'If the parents decide to have an abortion once they know the test results, it is, after all, their own affair.' An 'affair' which, if they go to a state hospital will not cost them anything (after they initially spent 500 rupees for the amniocentesis). Abortion on social or medical grounds is free; in private clinics it costs between 70 and 700 rupees, depending on comfort. There is not the shadow of a doubt that all doctors – male and female – acknowledge the test result 'female fetus' as good enough a reason to have a free abortion. As in all other countries, women in India have had to fight to make abortion legal. In 1972 the Medical Termination of Pregnancy Act – the MTP Act – was introduced and put an end to illegal abortions, which up to that time cost between 100 and 1,000 rupees. 'Now is this facility to be used specifically against unborn women,' writes the political magazine *India Today* (1982), 'because the MTP Act has no provision against selective killings of female fetuses.'

This is very true and it holds for all countries which have made abortion legal by introducing special laws, including European countries and the USA. It seems as if there are no boundaries to mechanisms enforcing men's oppressive brutality against women. Feminists worldwide need to organize and to expose – and resist – the systematic eradication of women. For you don't know who's going to be next . . . . you can never tell!

## NOTES

1  15.15 rupees are approximately £1. Ten rupees are approximately $1.
2  Uttar Pradesh, Bihar and Rajasthan are three Indian states with about 100 million, 60 million and 30 million inhabitants respectively.
3  I am indebted to an Indian woman who provided invaluable help in my research on sex-selection. She prefers to remain anonymous. To her and the many other Indian feminists who gave me their time and information go my profound thanks.
4  *Lakh* is an Indian unit of measurement. One lakh means 100,000 (of anything).
5  I conducted the interview in Amritsar in November 1982.
6  All the quotations from Indian newspapers and magazines in this article are from 1982. At the time I write this in Germany, the material is stored in Candolim/Goa and it is therefore impossible for me to insert publication dates.
7  Indian men do not like having a vasectomy. They are afraid of becoming impotent; also they believe it attacks their honour – and

why should they have to do it in the first place? A sentiment they share with men worldwide. It must be noted, however, that many poor men were sterilized under a government scheme.

This chapter was translated from German by Renate Duelli Klein.

# A LONG OVERDUE FEMINIST ISSUE: DISABILITY AND MOTHERHOOD

# CLAIMING *ALL* OF OUR BODIES: REPRODUCTIVE RIGHTS AND DISABILITY[1,2]

Anne Finger

Both the disability rights movement and the feminist movement are rooted in the rights of people to have control over their own bodies; and yet a wide gulf often seems to separate these two movements. This paper merges a disability rights perspective with a reproductive rights analysis, telling the history of the eugenics movement and sterilization abuse and detailing ways in which the abortion rights movement has exploited fears and stereotypes of disability. It urges the reproductive rights movement to incorporate the demands of disabled people for access, sexual freedom, parental rights and rights to safe and effective birth control.

I can't remember a time of my life when I wasn't a feminist, just as I can't remember not believing in disability rights. From the time I was a very young child, I understood that I was more 'handicapped' by people's perceptions and attitudes towards me than I was by my disability (I had polio shortly before my third birthday). Although as a child I didn't have the word 'disability,' never mind 'oppression' or 'attitudinal barriers' to describe my experience, what I *did* have was the example of the Black civil rights movement, then beginning in the South. From about the age of five or six, I used to think, 'People are prejudiced against me the same way that they are against Negroes.'

While increased understanding has led me to see the differences as well as the similarities between Black experiences and my own, my belief that disability in and of itself was much less of a problem than social structures and attitudes towards disability has never changed. In part

281

because I was exempted from traditional feminine roles – *no one* ever mentioned the possibility of my having babies when I grew up – I was also a feminist, at least in some incipient form, as far back as I can remember.

But it has not always been easy building a politics that connects these two parts of my experience. The feminist movement – the movement which has been my home for most of my adult life – has by and large acted as if disabled women did not exist. For instance, the 1976 edition of *Our Bodies, Ourselves* mentions disability only twice – both times speaking of fetuses with potentially disabling conditions, not disabled women. (Boston Women's Health Book Collective, 1976)* In the early years of the feminist movement I heard constantly about how women were sex objects – I could see that that was true for a lot of my abled sisters, but there were no voices saying that being stereotyped as asexual was also oppressive – and also was part of our female experience. More recently, the disability rights movement and the women's movement have seemed to be at loggerheads with each other over issues of reproductive technologies, genetics, and fetal and neonatal disabilities. I hope this article will be a step towards helping us to claim *all* of our selves.

Most discussions of disability begin with a laundry list of disabling conditions. Disability, we are told, does not just mean being in a wheelchair. It also includes a variety of conditions, both invisible and visible. These include being deaf or blind, having a heart condition, being developmentally disabled or being 'mentally ill.' While this is necessary to an understanding of disability, thinking about disability only in medical or quasi-medical terms limits our understanding: disability is largely a social construct.

Women, like disabled people, can be defined in terms of physical characteristics that make us different from males (only women menstruate; only women get pregnant). We can also be defined socially. A social description would include the above physical characteristics, but would emphasize

---

* Editors' note: the subsequent edition (1984) of *Our Bodies, Ourselves* was written with assistance from an advisory committee of feminist activists in the disabilities rights movement.

that, in our society, we are paid far less than men; we are less likely to vote Republican; and more likely to be emotional and empathetic.

In the same manner, when we start looking at disability socially, we see not only the medically defined conditions that I have described, but also the fact that white disabled women earn 24 cents for every dollar that white abled men earn (for Black disabled women, the fraction is far smaller).[3] Media images almost always portray us as being either lonely and pitiful or one-dimensional heroes (or, occasionally, heroines) who struggle valiantly to 'overcome' our 'handicaps.' Many of us are still being denied 'the free public education' that all American children supposedly receive; and we have a (largely unknown) history of fighting for our rights that stretches back at least to the mid-nineteenth century (and probably further). To understand that disability is socially constructed means understanding that the economic, political, and social forces which now restrict our lives can (and will) change.

## THE EUGENICS MOVEMENT AND STERILIZATION ABUSE

The reproductive rights movement has, by and large, failed to address the ways that sterilization abuse has affected disabled people. Compulsory and coerced sterilization of the disabled began in the late nineteenth century. The eugenics movement provided the ideological basis for these actions (as well as providing a similar rationale for racist actions).

The term 'eugenics' was coined by Sir Francis Galton; the *Oxford English Dictionary* defines the word as 'pertaining or adapted to the production of fine offspring, esp. in the human race.' The aim of this movement was to apply the same principles of improving 'stock' that were used for horses and vegetables to human beings. Obviously, this movement has strong roots in Social Darwinism – the idea that life is a struggle between the fit and the unfit. The unfit – which included the 'feeble minded, insane, epileptic, diseased, blind, deaf (and), deformed (including the crippled)' were to be bred out of existence, according to the Harry Laughlin Law (Bajema, 1976).

Based on the mistaken notion that all disabilities are inherited (most, of course, are not), there were several factors that contributed to the growth of the eugenics movement at this period. One factor was the prevalent assumption of nineteenth-century science that human perfection could be achieved through a combination of technological and social manipulation, an increased understanding of heredity, and the fact that surgical techniques for sterilization had become available. But any discussion of the eugenics movement which leaves out the changing social role of disabled people at this period fails to grasp the true nature of this movement.

As America industrialized, there was less room for those who had physical or mental limitations to adapt their work environment to their needs. Our history as disabled people has yet to be written. But from what I have been able to glean, I believe that in rural societies disabled people had far more of a social role than they have had in the more urban and industrialized world. The fact that folk tales and rhymes refer to 'the simple'; that 'the village idiot' was a stock figure; that blind and other disabled people appear in the myths and legends of many places, all indicate that in the past, disabled people had more of a daily presence in the world.

As work became more structured and formalized, people who 'fit' into the standardized factories were needed. Industrializing America not only forbade the immigration of disabled people from abroad, it shut the ones already here away in institutions. The growth of social welfare organizations and charities which 'helped' those with disabilities did provide jobs for a certain segment of the middle class; and volunteer charity work fitted in with the Victorian notion of women's duties and sphere.

This change in attitudes towards disabled people can be traced in language. The word *defective*, for instance, was originally an adjective meaning faulty or imperfect: it described one aspect of a person, rather than defining that person totally. By the 1880s, it had become a noun: people were considered not merely to have a defective sense of vision or a defective gait – they had become totally defined by their limitations, and had become *defectives*. A similar transformation took place a few decades later with the word *unfit*, which also moved from being an adjective to being a noun. The word 'normal,' which comes from the Latin word *norma*, square, until the 1830s meant standing at a right angle to the ground. During the 1840s, it came to designate conformity to a common type. By the 1880s, in America, it had come to apply to people as well as things. (Illich, 1976)

Close on the heels of the rise of institutions for disabled people was an increase in forced and coerced sterilization. Adele Clarke has pointed out that

the intentional breeding of plants and animals is almost exclusively undertaken to improve the products . . . (to increase) profitability from the products, whether they be Arabian horses or more easily transportable tomatoes or peaches. Eugenics applies, I believe, the same profit motive to the breeding of people. (Clarke, unpublished paper (a))

Since disabled people were of little or no use to the profit-makers, and since they were thought likely to become burdens on the state coffers, they were to be stopped from producing others like themselves.

Compulsory sterilization laws were passed in the early 1900s. By the 1930s, in addition to sterilization laws, forty-one states had laws which prohibited the marriage of the 'insane and feeble-minded,' seventeen prohibited the marriage of people with epilepsy; four outlawed marriage for 'confirmed drunkards.' More than twenty states still have eugenics laws on their books. (Clarke, unpublished paper (b))

Coerced sterilization is still very much a reality, especially among the developmentally disabled. 'Voluntary' sterilizations are sometimes a condition for being released from an institution; there has been at least one recent case of a 'voluntary' sterilization being performed on a six-year-old boy. (Friedman, 1976)

It is important to understand the connections between sterilization abuse of disabled people and of Third World people. The US Senate Committee on Nutrition and Human Needs reported in 1974 that between 75 percent and 85 percent of the 'mentally defective and retarded children' who are born each year are born into families with incomes below the poverty line. This means that a large number of those who are labeled as 'retarded' are people of color. The vast majority of people who are diagnosed as being mentally retarded have no definite, identifiable cause for their retardation: they are called the 'mildly retarded,' the 'educable,' and those with 'cultural-familial' retardation. The same IQ tests which 'prove' that Black people as a whole are less intelligent than whites label a far greater percentage of individual Black children as 'retarded.' (Chase, 1980).

**The eugenics movement in Nazi Germany.**
The Model Sterilization Law of Harry Laughlin, which I cited earlier, was never passed in its totality by any state in this country; however, a version of it was adopted in Nazi Germany. American eugenicists were often enthusiastic supporters of Hitler's attempt to rid Germany of 'defectives.'

Nazi ideology stressed purity, fear of disease, and the importance of heredity, intertwining these concepts with racism. In *Mein Kampf*, Hitler calls syphilis 'the Jewish disease'; Jewish people (and other 'sub-humans') are portrayed as being weak, sickly, and degenerate, in contrast with healthy blond Aryans. Before the start of World War II, Nazi eugenics courts had forced hundreds of thousands of disabled people to be sterilized. This forced sterilization helped to pave the way for the wartime genocide of Germany's disabled population. (Chase, 1980).

## THE REPRODUCTIVE RIGHTS MOVEMENT

Many disabled women find involvement in the reproductive rights movement problematic. Not only have many activists in this movement talked about the issues raised by disabled fetuses in ways that are highly exploitative and prey upon fears about disability, the movement also has, by and large, failed to address the denial of reproductive rights to disabled women and men. It has also failed to make itself physically accessible to disabled women.

I often hear an argument in favour of abortion rights that says, 'The right-wing would even force us to give birth to a child who was deformed.' ('Deformed' is mild in this context. I've heard 'defective,' 'grossly malformed,' and 'hideously deformed.') This attitude has become so widespread that at a recent conference on reproductive rights I heard disabled infants referred to as 'bad babies.' *Off Our Backs* parodied a conversation between Nathanson and Hatch on 'the joys of having a (sic) mongoloid child.'[4] (Thorne, 1981)

No woman should be forced to bear a child, abled or disabled; and no progressive social movement should exploit an oppressed group to further its ends. We do not need, as Michelle Fine and Adrienne Asch point out, to list conditions – such as the presence of a fetus with a disability – under which abortion is acceptable. The right to abortion is not dependent on certain circumstances: it is our absolute and essential right to have control over our bodies. (Fine and Asch, 1982) We do not need to use ableist arguments to bolster our demands. There are racist and classist arguments that can be made for abortion: to argue against them does not compromise our insistence on abortion rights. The analogy is obvious.

## Issues raised by fetal diagnosis

When we first fought for and won abortion rights, we focused on the situation of the *woman* herself. Most women who choose abortion do so early on in pregnancy, having made the decision that they do not want a child, any child, at the time. Now, however, the availability of techniques for diagnosis of fetal disabilities (such as amniocentesis, ultra-sonography, and fetoscopy) means that women can now choose not to give birth to a *particular* fetus. This is a radical shift, one which raises profound and difficult questions. Perhaps some of the kneejerk reactions to the issues of disabled fetuses reflect our unwillingness to fully explore these hard issues.

It is a little too pat to say that decisions about whether to have amniocentesis or to abort a disabled fetus are personal ones. Ultimately, of course, they are and must remain so. But we need to have a feminist, political language and ways of thinking about this issue to aid us in making those personal decisions and discussing these issues.

One thing that feminists should push for is good amniocentesis counseling. I have heard that some of this counseling is extremely negative and frightening about disability. Much of this may stem from doctors' attitudes towards physical impairment. One woman did an informal survey in which she asked doctors, 'What things would be worse than death?' They answered, being paraplegic, or being deaf, or partially sighted or not having both arms. (Carlton, 1981) (I think having attitudes like that is a fate worse than death.) Too often, people with attitudes like these are counseling women following amniocentesis. Are women who are told they are carrying a Down Syndrome fetus told that, due to deinstitutionalization and better educational methods, some people with Down Syndrome now go to school in regular classrooms, live in their own apartments and hold jobs? Are they told that 95 percent of Down Syndrome people have moderate to mild retardation? Are they told that if they chose to bear their child, but not to raise her or him, the child can be adopted immediately – usually within twenty-four hours? (Ganz, 1983) Do they have anything more to go on than fear, shame, and their own prejudices combined with those of doctors? Women who are considering aborting a disabled fetus should have the opportunity to talk to disabled people and the parents of disabled children.

Women considering whether or not to give birth to a disabled child have few, if any, positive role models. Mothers of disabled children (who remain the primary caregivers) are seen as being either self-sacrificing saints or bitter, rejecting women. These popular images get carried into the 'objective' scientific literature. Wendy Carlton reviewed the studies done on mothers of disabled children: they were seen as either being 'rejecting' or 'overprotecting'; they denied the child's condition or had unrealistic expectations; they are 'unconcerned or overinvolved.' (Carlton, 1981) No matter what they did, they couldn't seem to get it right. One in every twenty children is born with some sort of disability (a quarter of a million children a year). In addition, many become disabled during childhood. There are millions of mothers of disabled children, most of whom, I am sure, manage to do a halfway decent job of childrearing, despite stereotypes, cutbacks, and the nuclear family.

## Dealing with fears

This article grew out of a talk that I gave to a reproductive rights group on this issue. In the discussion that followed, I was very disappointed that women in the audience never once addressed the reproductive rights of disabled women and men, despite extensive presentation of such issues. Instead, the discussion focused on disabled infants and, more specifically, on women's fears of having a disabled child. The women I talked to are hardly alone.

For instance, Sheila Kitzinger, fairly well-regarded in the alternative birth movement, has a chapter on 'The Psychology of Pregnancy' in her book *The Experience of Childbirth* (1975). In the subsection entitled 'Fear that the baby will be malformed,' she states:

> Any time after about the fifth month of pregnancy, when the child begins to move and becomes a reality to the mother, she may start to think about her baby as possibly deformed. . . . What if this thing I am nourishing and cherishing within my own body, around which my whole life is built now, whose pulse beats fast deep within me – what if this child should prove to be *a hideous deformed creature, sub-human, a thing I should be able to love, but which I should shudder to see?* (emphasis added) (Kitzinger, 1975: 62)

Kitzinger deals with this issue solely on the level of a neurotic fear, never once discussing what happens when a child is actually born with a disability.

The deeply-rooted fears that many women have of giving birth to a disabled child extends to our politics. They need to be worked through. But please don't expect disabled women to sit there and listen to you while you do so.

## Killing babies, left and right

Infanticide of the disabled has gone on for at least as long as history has been recorded. (Although the Reagan administration would like us to believe that it has gotten worse in the past ten years – *i.e.*, since the legalization of abortion.) Killing of disabled infants continues today – sometimes through denial of nutrition, more often through withholding of medical treatment. It is far more common in England than here – where three out of four spina bifida children go untreated (one out of twenty are untreated in the US).

'Baby Doe' is probably the best-known case. A Down syndrome infant, born with a blocked esophagus, his parents and the doctors involved decided to deny him standard life-saving surgery, resulting in his death by starvation. This happened despite the fact that child welfare workers went to court to try to get an injunction to force the surgery to be performed, and despite the fact that there were twelve families ready to adopt the child, and a surgeon willing to perform the surgery for free. (Ganz, 1983) (Nearly all Down syndrome children, up to about the age of five, are now adoptable – thanks in large part to legal abortion and the increased number of single women who keep their children.)

I believe that it is inconsistent with feminism for us to say that human beings should be killed (or allowed to die) because they do not fit into oppressive social structures. 'Anatomy is destiny' is a right-wing idea. It is right-wing whether it is applied to women or whether it is applied to disabled children by the people I usually think of as my sisters and brothers.

So-called 'right-to-lifers' are among the loudest voices heard in defense of these children's lives, and I have heard the argument made that it is dangerous for us to sound like we are on 'their' side. If we fail to call for full rights for *all* disabled people, we will have allowed right-wing, anti-feminist forces to totally define the terrain on which we struggle. And we can distinguish ourselves from the right on this issue, by standing for full rights for disabled people – not just the right to live so that we can, in the words of anti-abortionist Nathanson, 'evoke pity and compassion' from the abled.

## Sexuality, birth control, and parental rights

Occasionally, reproductive rights groups (and other women's groups) make a token mention of disabled women. When we are included, it usually at the end of a long list. But our particular needs and concerns are rarely addressed, much less fought for. One reproductive rights activist said to me, 'We always used to talk about the rights of disabled women, but I was never sure exactly what that meant.' Lack of access to our offices, newsletters, demonstrations and meetings remains a barrier, preventing many disabled women from being physically present within the movement to voice their concerns.

Part of this problem lies in the pervasive stereotype of disabled women as being asexual. Disabled women have been asked, 'What do you need birth control for?' or 'How did *you* get pregnant?' In 1976, SIECUS, the Sex Information and Education Council of the United States, which is a quite respectable organization, prepared a booklet on 'Sexuality and the Handicapped,' which was sent to the 1976 White House Conference on the Handicapped – and promptly rejected as 'inappropriate.' (Calderone, 1981)

At least some of this prevalent stereotype of asexuality stems from seeing disabled people as eternal children. Telethons and other charitable activities have played a large role in creating this image. They portray us as being wan, pathetic, pitiful. The Jerry Lewis telethon even showed a series of film clips of adult disabled people saying, 'I'm forty-seven years old and I'm one of Jerry's kids,' 'I'm fifty-five years old and I'm one of Jerry's kids.' (I won't go into the way that children's sexuality is treated in this society.)

This asexual image is often prevalent among doctors and counselors as well. Women who have had spinal cord injury report that when they asked questions about their sexual functioning, they were given the information that they could still have children – and nothing more. Or else they received sexist and heterosexist information, typified by the following:

A female paraplegic can have intercourse more easily than a male paraplegic, since she does not have to participate actively. Although some such women have no subjective feeling of orgasm (as opposed to an objective feeling of orgasm?) they are perfectly capable of satisfying their husbands. (Becker, 1978) (parentheses added)

All human bodies are sexual. People without genital sensation (which is a fairly common occurrence following spinal cord injury) can have orgasms through the stimulation of other parts of their bodies, such as their breasts, earlobes, or necks. One measure of the rigid structure which the medical profession imposes on our bodies is that these non-genital orgasms are sometimes referred to by clinicians as 'phantom orgasms': these are not genuine, medically approved orgasms – they only *feel* like the real thing.

There is an opposite stereotype (in some ways, this is similar to the madonna-whore dichotomy which women face). Disabled people (particularly men, although also women) are sometimes seen being filled with diseased lusts. Lewis Terman, one of the early authorities on what was then called 'feeble-mindedness' said that all developmentally disabled women were 'potential prostitutes' since moral values could not 'flower' without full intelligence. Media images portray disabled men – whether they are physically disabled or 'escaped mental patients' – as rapists and potential rapists. (The chilling realities about rape of disabled people, particularly within institutions, has been largely ignored both by the public at large and within the women's movement.)

## Birth control

The stereotype of asexuality persists in information that comes from the women's health movement. I have never seen a discussion of birth control methods – no matter how exten-sive – that talks about how a particular method works for a woman who is blind, or has cerebral palsy, or is develop-mentally disabled. *Our Bodies, Ourselves* (1976), for instance, warns that the pill should not be taken by women who have any 'disease or condition associated with poor blood circulation,' without mentioning what those diseases or conditions are (see editors' note, p. 282). Unfortunately, many of us with disabilities are far from fully informed about our medical conditions. I had no idea (and neither, apparently, did any of the gynecologists I saw) that, due to my disability, taking birth control pills put me at great risk of thrombo-embolism.

When we work for improved birth control, we need to remember that there are many disabled women for whom there is *no* method that comes close to being safe and effective. The pill is contraindicated for most women in wheelchairs because of circulation problems; many women who have paralysis cannot insert a diaphragm; and these same women may have problems with an IUD, especially if they do not have uterine sensation (and cannot be warned by pain and cramping of infection or uterine perforation).

The 1983 hearings in Washington about the possible licensing of Depo-Provera highlight another area of contraceptive abuse of which feminists must be aware. Depo-Provera is an injectable contraceptive. Because it is not user-controlled, it is often recommended for women who have developmental disabilities. (It also has the 'beneficial' side effect of doing away with menstruation; for developmentally disabled women, this is supposed to be a special plus, since it is more 'hygienic.')

Part of the problem with this use of Depo is that many of those who are considered severely or profoundly retarded also have physical disabilities. One study found that users of Depo 'are several times as likely to undergo thromboembolic (blood clotting) disease without evident cause as non users.' (Duffy, 1981) It seems likely that their physical disabilities would put them at increased risk.

Depo-Provera, because of the many side effects that have occurred with its use, is only licensed for use as a treatment for cancer. However, individual doctors can prescribe Depo for any reason they chose; and developmentally disabled women are probably receiving it now, with no method of reporting the side effects and other problems they experience. *Toward Intimacy,* (Task Force on Concerns of Physically Disabled Women, 1978) an otherwise excellent booklet about contraception for disabled women, lists only a few of the known side effects associated with Depo, and candidly notes: 'Available only through private physicians until FDA approval is obtained for Depo-Provera's use as a contraceptive. Family planning clinics can often refer you to private physicians if you are interested in this method.'

## Parenting, custody issues, and adoption

In preparing this article, I looked for, but was unable to find, any statistics about the number or percentage of disabled people who have children. I did find lots of anecdotal information about disabled people told they *shouldn't* have children, and heard some chilling stories from disabled women about being pressured into having abortions. There is almost no public image of disabled people as parents, and I do not know of a single book about being a disabled parent – although there are probably hundreds about having a disabled child.

There have been two fairly well-known cases in which a disabled parent fought to win or keep custody of a child. One of these concerned a single mother who had been born without arms or legs: welfare workers attempted to take her child away from her. After demonstrating to a judge that she was able to care for her child's needs herself, she won the right to custody. In the second case, a divorced quadriplegic father won custody of his sons.

It is particularly important that we in the women's movement take up these issues, since too often they are ignored when demands for disability rights are raised. The American Civil Liberties Union puts out a handbook called, *The Rights of Handicapped People*, which contains no mention of parental rights, sexual rights, rights to adoption, or rights to safe and effective birth control.

The many political issues around adoption are too complex for me to delve into here. We do need to be sure that people are not denied the right to adopt on the basis of their disability. This has a special importance for two reasons: a small percentage of people with disabilities are unable to become biological parents. In addition, there is a growing tendency for disabled people to adopt children with disabilities, so that they can be raised within our community.

Because both the reproductive rights movement and the disability rights movement are rooted in our rights to control our bodies and our lives, there are strong links between the two. Just as there needs to be a realization within the disabled rights movement that the rights of disabled women must be fought for, so there needs to be an awareness within the reproductive rights movement that those of us who are disabled can no longer be exploited and ignored.

## NOTES

1  I would like to thank Adele Clarke, Judy Heumann, Susan Hansel, Jean Miller, Kim Marshall, Carla Schick, Lisa Manning, Susan Dambroff, and Sex Education for Disabled People in Oakland, California, for their assistance in preparing this article.

2  This article first appeared, in a different form, in *Off Our Backs* (October 1983).

3  According to 1980 census data, for the age range 45–55, comparable qualified disabled white women earned only 24 cents for every dollar earned by a non-disabled white man. For disabled Black women, it was a shocking 12 cents on the dollar (Grothaus, 1982).

4  The term 'mongoloid' to describe children with the chromosomal disorder now termed 'Down syndrome' originated in the mid-nineteenth century. It was thought that the birth of these children to white parents was a 'hereditary throwback' to the 'lower race' of Mongols (Asians) from which the white race had ascended. (See Gould, 1981.)

## REFERENCES

Bajema, Carl. 1976. *Eugenics Then and Now*. Benchmark Papers in Genetics, 15. Dowden, Hutchinson & Ross, Stroudsburg, Pennsylvania.

Becker, Elle F. 1978. *Female Sexuality Following Spinal Cord Injury*. Accent Special Publications, Bloomington, Indiana.

Boston Women's Health Book Collective. 1976. *Our Bodies, Ourselves*. Simon & Schuster, New York.

Calderone, Mary S. 1981. 'Sexuality and disability in the United States.' In David G. Bullard and Susan E. Knight, eds. *Sexuality and Physical Disability: Personal Perspectives*. C. V. Mosby, St. Louis, Missouri.

Carlton, Wendy. 1981. 'Perfectability and the Neonate: The Burden of Expectations on Mothers and their Health Providers'. In

Holmes, B., Hoskins B. and Gross, M. (eds). *The Custom-Made Child*. Humana Press, Clifton, N.J.

Chase, Allan. 1980. *The Legacy of Malthus*. University of Illinois Press, Urbana, Illinois.

Clarke, Adele. Unpublished paper (a). 'Compulsory sterilization: past, present, and future.'

Clarke, Adele. Unpublished paper (b). 'The double-life of eugenics 1900–1930: pseudo-science and social movement.'

Duffy, Yvonne. 1981. *All Things Are Possible*. A. J. Garvin. Ann Arbor, Michigan. Compilation of questionnaire responses and interviews with women who are orthopedically disabled.

Fine, Michelle and Adrienne Asch. 1982. 'The question of disability: no easy answers for the women's movement.' *Reproductive Rights Newsletter*, Fall. Excellent article which discusses the exploitation of the disabled fetus issue by the abortion rights movement.

Friedman, Paul. 1976. *The Rights of the Mentally Retarded*. Avon Books, New York. Discusses sterilization abuse, parental rights and rights to sexual expression.

Ganz, Mary. 1983. 'Retarded boy's right to live: who decides.' *Sunday San Franciso Examiner and Chronicle*, January 30.

Gould, Steven Jay. 1981. *The Mismeasure of Man*. W. W. Norton, New York.

Grothaus, Rebecca. 1982. *CSCD Voice* (Community Service Center for the Disabled), 6(4):13.

Illich, Ivan. 1976. *Medical Nemesis: The Expropriation of Health*. Pantheon, New York.

Kitzinger, Sheila. 1975. *The Experience of Childbirth*. Pelican, Middlesex.

*The Rights of Handicapped People*. 1979. American Civil Liberties Union handbook. Kent-Hull City, Avon Books.

Thorne, Becky. 1981. 'Abortion battle intensified over Hatch's amendment'. *Off Our Backs*. November.

## FURTHER READING

Bullard, David G. and Susan E. Knight. 1981. *Sexuality and Physical Disability: Personal Perspectives*. C. V. Mosby, St. Louis, Missouri. Excellent collection of articles, most of which are written by people with physical disabilities. Deals with a broad range of disabilities from differing perspectives.

Califia, Pat. 1980. *Sapphistry: The Book of Lesbian Sexuality*. Naiad Press, Tallahassee, Florida. Very good chapter on disabled lesbians.

Campling, Jo. 1981. *Images of Ourselves: Women with Disabilities*

*Talking*. Routledge & Kegan Paul, London. While not specifically focused on sexuality or reproductive rights, offers insights into lives of disabled women.

Sex Information and Education Council of the US. 1978. *Sexuality and Disability: A Bibliography of Resources Available for Purchase*. SIECUS, New York. Annotated list covering general works and information on specific disabilities. (Available from SIECUS, 80 Fifth Avenue, New York, NY 10011 for $1.00 and a stamped, self-addressed business envelope.)

Task Force on Concerns of Physically Disabled Women. 1978. *Toward Intimacy: Family Planning and Sexuality Concerns of Physically Disabled Women*. Human Sciences Press, New York. Includes drawings of disabled people making love.

Task Force on Concerns of Physically Disabled Women. 1978. *Within Reach: Providing Family Planning Services to Physically Disabled Women*. Human Sciences Press, New York. Both of these books are informative and written from the perspective of disabled women.

# BORN AND UNBORN: THE IMPLICATIONS OF REPRODUCTIVE TECHNOLOGIES FOR PEOPLE WITH DISABILITIES

## Marsha Saxton

This chapter discusses issues surrounding the current practice of prenatal genetic screening with intent to abort those fetuses affected by genetic or other kinds of disability. The author explores some of the stereotypic attitudes and myths about disabled persons and how these attitudes influence parents and medical practitioners in the decision-making process regarding abortion. The discussion is illustrated with personal anecdotes of the author's own experiences as a disabled adolescent, and then as an adult woman considering pregnancy and confronting the prospects of reproductive technologies.

Some time in the first month after my conception, a disruption occurred in the growth of my lower spine, and the nerves coursing through my bladder and down to my lower legs and feet, the 'perineal' tract, did not develop normally. About two out of a thousand babies are effected by this 'neural tube defect' or 'NTD,' the second most common birth difference after cerebral palsy. The range of disability varies considerably from 'spina bifida occulta' (or a slight niche in the spine of which the individual may be unaware, or experience back pain) to myelomeningacele like mine, but sometimes characterized by paraplegia and including hydrocephalus (fluid on the brain). Some babies are born with such severe NTD they have no brain and die soon after birth.

I have been told many times how 'lucky' I am to be only moderately disabled, 'It could have been much worse,' they say, an attitude which perplexes me. I have never been told how unlucky I am to be disabled at all. In my view I am not lucky or unlucky, I'm just disabled. On occasion I've wondered what might have been different had I not grown up with a disability, the doctors, the hospital, and surgeries, the funny attitudes and behaviors displayed to me, a child who wore leg braces until age twelve. The pitying stares, the smiling condescension mostly from the adults, for as a young child I had early on learned to present such a matter-of-fact explanation about my leg braces to my peers that I was rarely teased.

Now, at thirty-two, I have a slight limp, and somewhat skinny legs lined with pale incisions. I catheterize myself three or four times a day. It takes me about as long as another woman would to urinate and it can be done in any restroom.

I have always planned and looked forward to becoming a mother. The varying statistics from doctors or books over the years about the possibility of my having a baby with my disability had not caused me to reconsider this goal. I knew though, that I wanted to learn as much as I could about the risks both to my own body and to my baby. And what technologies had been developed to address these risks?

My gynecologist referred me to many specialists: a urologist, neurologist, and a genetics counselor. I learned from the first two that, though my body had differences and limitations, these are apparently not likely to cause difficulties in pregnancy and delivery. However, neither physician had ever encountered a pregnancy by a woman with spina bifida. A medical literature search revealed only a handful of somewhat relevant cases of unusual pregnancies: spinal cord injured women, women with illeostomy (rerouteing of the ureters to a bag for urine collection) or other bladder conditions. No one like my case. It appeared that there just aren't that many women with spina bifida who've had babies. I knew of only one other woman. Is this perhaps because most spina bifida women are more severely disabled than I? (About 75 percent have hydrocephalus.) Unexplained as yet, spina bifida is about twice as common in females. My husband and I together went to the genetics counselor to learn about some new technologies and how I could use them. The counselor, a woman physician and pediatrician impressed me as direct and knowledgeable. She asked us about ancestral origin and family history of disability. Spina bifida is apparently more prevalent among populations with Irish as well as Native American ancestry, explaining the myth I'd heard ('Don't eat potatoes during pregnancy.') She explained what is known about how the genetics of spina bifida works. There 'appears' to be a genetic component, in that a mother producing one child with spina bifida has an increased likelihood of her subsequent children having the condition too, though no spina bifida gene has been identified. There also appears to be a nutritional component in that studies have shown that nutritional supplements, particularly the B vitamin, folic acid, considerably reduced the expected incidence.[1] There may be other as yet unidentified factors. My own mother described the period of her life which included my first month of gestation when spina bifida occurs as 'one of the most upsetting times in my life.' There may be no spina bifida gene but perhaps a genetic tendency for the mother to over-absorb the available B vitamin, leaving an inadequate supply for fetal development.

Eventually, the counselor told us that I had a 3–5 percent *increased* chance of having a baby with NTD. However, as these figures were derived from mothers who have already had one child with spina bifida, they seemed relevant only for a secondborn child. Therefore these statistics were not really helpful in my decision-making. The counselor went on to explain the various reproductive technological tests available to me. One of them is the alpha-feto protein test: 'AFP' is a chemical produced by the fetus and present in the mother's blood. Over the nine-month gestational period the AFP level in the maternal blood is known to gradually build up, peak, and decline. The mother's blood sample is taken between the fourteenth and twentieth weeks. Elevated AFP levels can be associated with the presence of NTD (but may also indicate twins or simply that the gestational age was estimated incorrectly). Also there are differing views on what exactly is an elevated range. I know of a mother who was told by one physician that her level was high, and, by another, that it was within the normal range. At any rate, to confirm the AFP test, I could choose to have an amniocentesis. This is more conclusive than tests of maternal blood, as the extracted fluid can be analyzed for protein and enzymes or

the fetal fibroblast cells which are normally shed into the
amniotic fluid. These can be cultured and the chromosomal
composition determined. Amniocentesis is also used to detect
or confirm a number of chromosomal disorders, including
Down syndrome, Patau's syndrome, Edward's syndrome, and
blood diseases such as Tay Sach's disease.

I was told that amniocentesis carries a 0.05 risk of mid-
trimester miscarriage. My counselor stated that this is
commonly regarded as negligible. 'With such a slight risk
why not just go ahead and have it done?' many doctors tell
women. However, to the women to whom miscarriage does
occur, that statistic is not negligible. An ultra sound scan
(sonogram) is often used in conjunction with amniocentesis to
locate the site of fluid extraction. It reveals the visible outline
of the fetus and would show the characteristic bump on the
spine of a spina bifida fetus. As yet, it is not known whether
the sonogram endangers fetus or mother. Techniques to
surgically repair NTD in utero are in the experimental stage.
(Kolata, 1983)

My options were several: I could choose the AFP test and,
if elevated, proceed with amniocentesis and ultra sound.
I could use only the AFP test or only the ultra sound, and if
the tests indicated a disabled fetus, I could then choose
abortion.

The counselor asked me, if I were to learn that my fetus
was abnormal, would I choose to abort?

I remembered the spina bifida newsletter[2] when I first
read about the AFP test available to detect spina bifida and
other neural tube defects. I remember having mixed feelings.
Could I choose to abort a baby with my own disability, end the
life of someone somehow an even closer kin to me than my
own child? But then could I choose to continue the life of
someone possibly destined to endure some of the same treatments I had experienced? Another thought emerged: if this
test had been available to my mother I might never have been
born.

How can I, a disabled person myself, as well as a woman
planning pregnancy, regard this option to end the life of
another one disabled? The rationale for prenatal screening is
provided by the assumption that the life of an affected fetus

should be ended. I feel this issue has received remarkably little attention given its implications.

As a feminist I have supported the pro-choice position on the question of abortion. I feel a woman must be able to choose or reject motherhood and exert control over her own body. I view abortion as a stop-gap measure which women must maintain to counteract the oppressive forces that limit women's control over our lives, which include poor access to, and harmful birth control methods. Because of the emotional and social costs of abortion to the individual mother, the fetus, and society, I cannot view abortion as another form of birth control. The debate, 'at what age does the fetus constitute a human life?' in my estimation, can never be satisfactorily resolved. Indeed, such an argument misses the point of the true issues at hand, namely, the real resources, financial, social, and emotional of the parents and the community to welcome the child.

It is on this basis that I question the practice of systematically ending the life of a fetus *because it is disabled*. Real 'choice' involves an understanding of all the options and the opportunity for flexible decision-making for the individual woman in her own situation based on an accurate assessment of her available resources. It also necessitates closely scrutinizing society's view of 'ablebodiedness.' We need to better understand disability and our relationship to it. In particular,

1  How does society define and treat disability?
2  What are the implications of prenatal technology in relation to societal oppression of disabled persons?
3  How are disabled women affected by the new technologies and the attitudes surrounding them?
4  How can both consumers and health care professionals more rationally consider these issues and act in humanly responsible ways?

Disability triggers much fear in our culture. Some of the recent media coverage on the topic has begun to challenge the widespread ignorance in this area, but the old attitudes persist. Perhaps from prehistoric times, disability must have appeared to humans as some mysterious force leaving many human beings with physical limitation, loss of body functions, constant pain, disfigurement, and sometimes early death. It is no wonder that we have feelings of powerlessness about disability. It forces us to confront our own vulnerability.

We, especially in the US, live in a culture obsessed with health and well-being. We value rugged self-reliance, athletic prowess, and rigid standards of beauty. We incessantly pursue eternal youth, and the treatment of our elders attests to an ingrained denial, fear and even hate of our own aging and accompanying physical limitation. The disabled person in our society is the target of attitudes and behaviors from the able-bodied world, ranging from gawking to avoidance, pity to resentment, or from vastly lower expectations to awe. Along with these attitudes disabled persons confront a variety of tangible barriers: architectural inaccessibility, lack of sign language interpreters for deaf people, insufficient taped or brailled materials for blind persons. In addition, disabled persons confront less tangible barriers: discrimination in employment, second-class education, and restricted opportunities for full participation in the life of the community.[3]

A common assumption is that disabled people are asexual either because they are incapable of sexual function or because they 'just shouldn't want it.' These assumptions stem from simple-minded myths, including:

disabled people are 'childlike' and sex is for adults;
disability may be contagious and being sexual is getting too close;
sex is somehow like a rare comodity and should be reserved for a highly valued people, i.e. attractive able-bodied people.

Disabled persons, whether they are re-entering the mainstream of the community after an injury or an illness, or whether theirs is a long-standing or congenital disability, have to struggle with these attitudinal barriers to their sexual fulfillment.

Many of the cultural assumptions about sexuality are particularly hurtful to disabled women:

sex shouldn't be discussed or planned, it should be
spontaneous';
sexual intercourse and orgasm are the only 'real thing'.

Such assumptions lead to a sense of failure for women
with physical limitations requiring adaptations, planning, or
assistance. These myths interfere with the realization that
sexuality is not limited to specific 'acts' or 'behaviors.' Indeed,
disabled women are the target of a 'double handicap' in the
patriarchal, able-bodied world. As recent studies document,
the vast majority of research about disability has focused on
disabled men. Virtually no attention has been paid to sexual
and/or reproductive health care needs of women with disabilities or chronic illness (Zwerner, 1983).

Disabled women who choose parenthood are often
targeted by assumptions both by medical professionals and
the larger community. Many medical professionals assume
disabled persons cannot cope with the responsibility and role
of parenting. Of the disabled parents I know, a common
reaction they hear is that the child they are with could not
have been their own and 'should they really be babysitting in
their condition?' It may well be that persons who were
parents before incurring a traumatic injury or chronic
disease must perhaps develop compensatory resources to
assist in caring for their children. However, the assumptions
they have to face are that they are more likely to fail as
parents.

Increasingly, severely disabled women are considering
parenthood. I am acquainted with several dozen disabled
mothers whose lives, and mother-child relationships, apart
from the provision of physical assistance by an attendant, do
not differ from those of able-bodied women I know. The
Independent Living Movement is enabling severely disabled
persons to function in virtually all activities that able-bodied
persons do. As of yet, the medical community in general has
not displayed its awareness of these resources.

Pregnancy or parenthood – clear sign of the adult sexual
potential of a disabled woman – triggers alarm, ridicule or
disgust in many. This is worse for women with congenital or
genetically inherited disabilities. The assumption which we

often hear is 'you have no business getting pregnant – how terrible to make another one like you.' This may even be said to women where there is no likelihood of them producing a child with their own disability. Just because they are disabled it is often assumed that the child will be too.[4]

I found myself the target of such attitudes. When I was thirteen I decided to ask a doctor about my sexuality. I was raised to regard myself as 'normal,' but because of my birth differences I wasn't sure what to expect. I wasn't sure if the teenage magazines, the scenes at the movies, the clandestine discussions with other girls about sex really applied to me.

Could I have children? Could I enjoy sex? I had never masturbated, largely because my own responsibility for the genital area of my body had fairly well been taken over by the doctors, nurses, and my mother who, when I was two, had learned how to catheterize me when it was discovered that my bladder wasn't working well. They always washed their hands or wore sterile gloves. Germs. I was afraid to risk infection for pleasure. Or perhaps the clinical treatment that part of my body received did not define it to me as a positive source of comfort or pleasant sensation. The doctor I chose to ask, one I never met before, was 'an expert' in the field. Knowledgeable I expected. I went to see him about the condition of my bladder in the light of my developing female body. I had begun to menstruate the year before. The crassness of his replies stunned me: he indicated that if I were to marry I shouldn't be concerned about my own sensation, my vagina would work well enough to please a husband, but I shouldn't consider pregnancy for I might produce another one like me.

I left there numbly reeling, so impressionable, so vulnerable, a thirteen-year-old girl. The effects of that insult and others like it are still with me, but substantially mitigated by the saving grace of a strong will: I knew he was wrong. Today in my counseling practice though, I have met many disabled women who were given the same messages, and who heard them so consistently they began to believe they were true.

Where do these attitudes come from? Many women are familiar with the ongoing and widespread practice of the physician's advice to parents who give birth to a disabled child, to 'put him away in a home with others like himself.' Institutionalization is an outgrowth of the assumption that neither the parents nor the community could cope with the child at home. Such an assumption becomes a self-fulfilling prophecy: the family, friends, and community are never exposed to the child and its actual needs, so dreaded fantasies reinforce stereotypes. The child, as a result of being institutionalized, does indeed become a social outcast, ill-prepared to cope with community life, exhibiting many of the social behaviors and extreme dependencies which the parents had feared.[5]

From the youth and beauty-oriented culture we are beset with messages to buy products which hide or disguise our differences and body functions, and strive to achieve rigid standards of appearance. Such standards are particularly harsh on disabled women whose appearance or body function may be further from 'acceptable.' My experiences as a teenager attest to this pressure. I was ashamed of my skinny incision-lined legs and for years never wore clothing that revealed them. All the disabled women I know confirmed my experience, but so do many non-disabled women.

There is tremendous pressure upon us to have 'perfect babies.' Do we want a world of 'perfect people'? I really wonder what are the human costs of attempts to control our differences, our vulnerability. I believe that if women are to maintain our 'choice' we must include *the choice to have a disabled child*.

How do the oppressive attitudes about disability affect the woman facing prenatal screening? Very often prospective parents have never considered the issue of disability until it is raised in relation to testing. But what is it that comes to most prospective parents' minds at the mention of the term 'birth defects'? Our exposure to disabled children has been so limited by their isolation that most people have only stereotyped views which include telethons, displays in drugstore counters depicting attractive 'crippled' youngsters soliciting our pity and loose change. The image of a child with Down syndrome elicits an even more intense assumption of eternal parental burden.[6]

Related to the question of 'burden' is the fact that the

oppression of women as the sole and often isolated caretakers of children affects the resources of many mothers in caring for their disabled children. Many factors in our culture, such as the weakening of the extended family, contribute to the isolation and overwhelming feelings of the mother. Such issues are typically ignored, again placing the blame of 'burden' on the disabled child.

Another of the myths affecting prospective mothers is about the 'suffering of the disabled.' In speaking to a group of rehabilitation graduate students, I mentioned that I'm considering pregnancy and also that I have a statistically increased change of producing a baby with my disability. One student blurted out, 'But how could you go ahead and have a baby knowing it might *suffer*?' Her question led to a discussion which, with some probing, revealed a set of broad assumptions about disabled people. In reaction to the ideas 'genetic transmission' and 'birth defect' this student had conjured up images of a miserable, sickly person on life support machines, eternally dependent, lonely, isolated. Her assumption was that life must be too painful for a disabled person, not worth living. When I asked her if I was included in her view of disabled people she replied, no of course not, because here I was, teaching!

Earlier in this paper I pondered what would life have been like were I not disabled. It is clear to me that the most painful and scarring parts of growing up disabled were the unnecessarily long and unnecessarily frightening separations from my parents when I was hospitalized in a charity hospital, and the patronizing, pitying and invalidating remarks from others. Having a body with physical limitations is a snap compared to dealing with those experiences. The *oppression*, as I have heard many other disabled people say, in one way or another, is what's disabling about disability.

There is no doubt that there are disabled people who 'suffer' from their physical conditions. There are even those who may choose to end their lives rather than continue in pain or with severe limitations, but is this not obviously as true for non-disabled people who suffer from emotional pain and limitation of resource? As a group, people with disabilities do not 'suffer' any more than any other group or category of humans. Our limitations may be more outwardly visible, our need for help more apparent, but, like anybody else, the 'suffering' we may experience is a result of not enough human caring, acceptance, and respect.

How do women typically learn about their options about prenatal testing? 'Choice' requires that information be presented in an unbiased way. Most physicians will indicate their intention to adhere to a 'nondirective' philosophy where decisions are left up to the patient. However, not just in my childhood, but recently when I have mentioned to medical professionals my intention to get pregnant, I have encountered a wide array of emotional responses. An orthopedic surgeon to whom I indicated a desire to minimize the use of X-ray while I was trying to conceive blurted out, 'You're going to get pregnant? I hope you'll get an amniocentesis.'

The consumers of medical services tend to put considerable faith in their physicians and assume that they are acting in their best interest. Few of us are made aware that while some medical procedures may be necessary and life-sustaining, many are also in the financial interest of the health-care industry. Ninety-five percent of all amniocenteses performed indicate no anomalies, and thus their only function consists of reassuring parents that their baby is fine. I think that the value of such an invasive, risky and expensive procedure must be questioned. As my genetics counselor stated, screening is 'sometimes used as a substitute for thinking.' On this basis the American College of Obstetrics and Gynecology, and the American Academy of Pediatrics oppose routine AFP screening.

The biggest challenge to professionals who are counseling both disabled and non-disabled prospective parents about options and the use of reproductive technologies is in presenting the information in understandable and non-biased ways.[7] Genetics professionals should take responsibility to learn about and teach more accurate pictures of disability. They need to examine their own values and fears about disability, and how these can influence their work. Ideally this process would begin early in the training programs, in the preclinical years when trainees are still fresh in their perspectives. Role modeling of clarity about disability and respectful interaction with disabled consumers must be demonstrated by senior staff.

Although most health care professionals are motivated by a sense of human caring, they are as much subject to confusion and prejudice as anyone else. They have a responsibility to present information in as unbiased a way as possible, but blaming them for not doing so does not advance the cause of the consumer. Regarding ourselves as hapless victims of an oppressive profit-motivated health-care system does nothing to enhance our power or to challenge the institutionalized pattern of the health-care industry. We as women consumers have to regard ourselves as powerful and assert our power in the face of continuing prejudice.

We must regard ourselves as the directors of our own needs. Health care professionals are available to us as educators and consultants. But we must be the ones to make the decisions. To do this we must take responsibility for obtaining the necessary information and we must trust our own thinking. We, more than any other, know of our own life circumstances, goals and capabilities. As disabled women, we have more frequent encounters with the medical system and thus are particularly vulnerable to feelings of powerlessness to challenge stereotyped and hurtful interactions with unaware professionals. An important goal for us as women and mothers is to make our decisions based on clarity about our values, adequate knowledge of the issues, and an accurate appraisal of available resources. One avenue toward obtaining that needed confidence is through meeting and sharing with other women. In this way we can gain safety, clarity, and strength. Peer groups are an excellent place to begin discussion about the issues raised here (Saxton, 1981).

What would I ask or tell another woman who considers having an amniocentesis with the intention to abort a disabled fetus? Did she think she had sufficient knowledge about disability, sufficient awareness of her own feelings, and did she feel confident in herself to make a rational choice? Did she personally know any disabled adults or children? What was it that she had been taught about disability by adults when she was young? Was she aware of the distorted picture of the lives of disabled people presented by advertisements, telethons, and stereotyped characters in the literature and media? I would also ask her to consider the personal and emotional cost that abortion could take. And to consider whether abortion of her disabled fetus seemed worth that cost?

So – do I think all disabled fetuses should be born into this world as it is now? Do I think parents should be forced to accept and care for a baby born disabled? No, I don't. I feel our priority should be to assess our own current capabilities, determine the realities of the situation, and make decisions that are workable for all concerned.

The questioning by disabled activists of abortion of disabled fetuses has been criticized by some feminists as 'too much like Right To Life.' I can understand this fear, for women's control over our own bodies and lives that access to abortion has provided is currently so much under attack that any challenge to abortion may feel threatening. But I feel that it's important to point out that the basis for choosing to abort a disabled fetus is the same basis for choosing to abort a fetus *because it is female* – a practice clearly denounced by the Women's Movement. But regardless of the logic of our current views as activists, we have a responsibility to persistently re-evaluate the implications of our positions and examine how they apply to individuals and specific populations.

At this point, if I became aware that the fetus I was carrying would be disabled, I would not choose to abort it. These are my reasons: I hope for and look forward to a time when all children can be welcomed to a world without oppression. I would like to exercise this view if only in my own personal world. I would like to welcome any child born to me. I believe I have the emotional, financial, and other resources to effectively care for a child. I know I can be a good mother and my husband a good father to any child, disabled or not. I hope that my children will be physically healthy and mentally able, but if they are not, I believe I can kindle in them the strength to challenge the social barriers they may meet, and reinforce in them the joy to be alive.

## NOTES

1 'Spina Bifida: Controversy Over Test Continues.' 1982. *Nature*, 300, December.
2 'AFP Screening Issues Still Drawing Attention.' 1979. *The Pipeline of the Spina Bifida Association of America*. May/June.
3 I choose not to use the term 'birth defect' because, consistent with the stereotypic attitudes about disability, it implies that our physical differences are 'bad', 'tragic,' or 'never should have been,' a view which is at best useless to someone for whom disability is a daily fact of life. The Disability Rights movement has generated a number of terms such as 'physically challenged,' 'other abled,' and 'physically different' which attempt to describe us in non-invalidating or non-condescending ways.
4 Only genetic counseling by a qualified professional can determine the mechanism of inheritance. A given gene trait might be determined not to be transmitted any further when both partners' traits are analyzed.
5 In 1978 a woman with spina bifida, my own age, unsuccessfully attempted to sue both her parents and the physician who at her birth diagnosed her as retarded and placed her in an institution where she stayed until age seven, when she was identified as having normal intelligence and placed out for adoption.
6 A contradiction to the stereotypic portrayal of disabled children as 'burdens' comes from such programs as 'Project Impact' in Massachusetts, where multiply-handicapped children are placed in adoptive families who *choose* disabled children. These parents readily attest to the pleasure and fulfillment their adoptive children bring them.
7 'Decision analysis' is one process whereby the parents' values and resources can systematically be incorporated into the decision-making. This tool has been applied to genetic counseling. (Pauker, Pauker, McNeil, 1982).

## REFERENCES

Dejanikus, Tacie. 1983. 'Report on the National Conference on Women and the Law.' *Off Our Backs*, XIII, 7: 27.

Kolata, Gina. 1983. 'Fetal Surgery for Neural Defects?' *Science*, July: 441.

Pauker, Stephen G., Susan P. Pauker and Barbara J. McNeil. 1982. 'Implications of Parental Attitudes on Alternative Policies for Prenatal Diagnosis' in *Critical Issues in Medical Technology*. Auburn House, Boston: 313–69.

Hubbard, Ruth, Debra Kaplan and Barbara Katz Rothman. 1983. 'From the Panel' in Letters. *Off Our Backs*, XIII, 8: 34.

Saxton, Marsha. 1981. 'A Peer Counseling Training Program for Disabled Women.' *Journal of Sociology and Social Welfare*, 8, 2: 334–5.

Zwerner, Janna. 1983 'Disabled Women and Reproductive Health Care.' Conference Proceedings of the Sixth World Congress of Sexology, May 22–7, Washington, DC.

# XYLO: A TRUE STORY

Rayna Rapp

'XYLO: A True Story' recounts the author's personal
experience with amniocentesis, and uses it to raise
questions about the social and political consequences of
this technology.

Mike called the fetus XYLO, X-Y for its unknown sex, LO for
the love we were pouring into it. Day by day we fantasized, as
newly, first-pregnant people do, about who this growing
cluster of cells might become. Would it have Mike's thinning
hair or my thick locks? My rubbery skin or his smooth com-
plexion? Day by day, we followed the growth process in the
myriad of books that surrounds modern pregnancy for the
over-35 baby boomlet. Products of our time and place, both
busy with engrossing work and political commitments, we
welcomed this potential child with excitement, fantasy, and
the rationality of scientific knowledge. As a women's movement activist, I had decided opinions about treating pregnancy
as a normal, not a diseased condition, and we were fortunate
that adequate health insurance and good connections netted
us a health care team – obstetrician, midwives, genetics counselor – who were eager to answer our questions, but believed,
as we did, that most pregnancies required little intervention.

The early months of the pregnancy passed in a blurr of exhaustion and nausea. Preoccupied with my own feelings, I lived in a perpetual underwater, slow-motion version of my prior life. As one friend put it, I was already operating on fetal time, tied to an unfamiliar regimen of enforced naps, loss of energy and rigid eating. Knowing the research on nutrition, on hormones, and on miscarriage rates among older pregnant women, I did whatever I could to stay comfortable, and relaxed. Neither romanticism nor rationalism would see us through these months – we just had to accept the major changes in my body and our lives that a late, desired pregnancy brings.

I was thirty-six when XYLO was conceived, and like many of my peers, I chose to have amniocentesis. Both Mike and I knew about prenatal diagnosis from our friends' experiences, and from reading about it in newspapers and magazines. Each year, more than 20,000 American women choose amniocentesis, and the number is growing rapidly. The test is performed between the sixteenth and twentieth weeks of pregnancy (counted from the last menstrual period). Most obstetricians, mine included, prefer to send their pregnant patients directly to hospital-associated genetics Centers, where counseling is provided, and the lab technicians are specialists in the procedure. This, of course, ups the already considerable cost of quality pregnancy care. Amniocentesis requires complex laboratory work, and is priced between $400 and $1000 in the state of New York, where my test was performed. In New York, medicaid covers the costs and the City lab, a model of its kind, has a sliding scale fee for women not covered by private or government health plans and outreach services in several languages. But since the Hyde amendment's cut-off of medicaid funds for abortion at the federal level, very few states still fund the procedure. And of those that fund abortion, even fewer fund amniocentesis for eligible, low-income women. So accessibility of the test varies widely throughout this country, depending on healthcare economics, state welfare law, and on the attitudes of obstetricians, who may or may not refer patients, depending on how current their knowledge of the literature is, and how they feel about genetics, genetic diseases, and the decision to abort an affected fetus. Given these mazeways of resources, medical services, and public health information, the majority of women undergoing amniocentesis are like me – consumers of expensive healthcare services, late childbearers, middle-class, and white. But we aren't the only group of women who need to know about the test.

Three groups of women are 'at risk' (to use the epidemiological language) of carrying genetically damaged fetuses, and might therefore want to seek out prenatal diagnosis. The first is women who've already borne a child with a genetic disease or birth defect, or have such children in their own or their partner's family. The second includes women and their partners from extended families or ethnically specific communities in which the incidence of certain inherited diseases is known to be relatively high. And the third is older women, or women with older partners since the risk of bearing a Down syndrome child increases with age. While prenatal diagnosis can only reveal a certain number of genetic diseases and fetal anomalies, not by any means all of the conditions known to occur, it can detect ones such as:

dominant gene conditions that affect one of the two parents, like a type of very serious inherited high cholesterol with a predisposition to heart disease;

recessive gene conditions in which parents are carriers but never manifest the problem themselves, such as thalassemia, Tay Sachs and sickle-cell anemia;

X-linked (sex-linked) diseases for which the woman is the carrier, and only male offspring are affected, like Duchenes's muscular dystrophy, and hemophilia (bleeders' disease) (in most X-linked conditions, there is no specific test for the disease, only for the sex of the fetus. So the parents must face the possibility that a male fetus is 50 percent likely to be affected, and 50 percent likely not);

neural tube defects such as anencephaly (a missing portion of the brain) and spina bifida (caused by a prenatal lesion in the neural tube, this disease may leave a person

differentially paralyzed, depending on where the lesion occurs);
chromosomal anomalies in which the 'wrong number' of chromosomes lead to a series of different conditions, like Turner's syndrome, Kleifelter's syndrome, and, most commonly, Down syndrome.

While all of these conditions are relatively rare, certain groups are at greater than average risk of having offsprings affected by them: neural tube defects are more likely among Anglo-Irish couples, Tay Sachs afflicts Ashkenazi Jews, sickle-cell anemia is most prevalent among people of African origin, and thalassemia is a Mediterranean disease. Down syndrome increases with the age of the pregnant woman and, to a lesser degree, with the age of her partner as well. At the age of thirty, a woman's chances of giving birth to a Down syndrome child are about one in 885; at thirty-five, they increase to one in 365, and at forty, they're about one in 109 (Hendin and Marks, 1979; Consensus Development Conference, 1979; President's Commission, 1983).

The increased risk of Down syndrome has something to do with aging. Perhaps we ovulate with more 'mistakes' during cell reproduction, perhaps accumulated environmental assaults affect relatively more of our eggs, perhaps our bodies become less able to 'slough off' genetically anomalous fetuses as early miscarriages. Men's semen is also affected by age, but their contribution to Down seems to go up much more slowly.

It was the fear of Down syndrome which sent us to seek prenatal diagnosis of XYLO. Down syndrome produces a characteristic physical appearance – short, stocky size, large tongues, puffy eyes with skin folds pointed upwards – and is a major cause of mental retardation, world-wide. People with Down syndrome are quite likely to have weak cardiovascular systems, gastrointestinal problems, and run a much higher risk of developing childhood leukemia. While the majority of Down syndrome infants used to die very young, a combination of antibiotics and infant surgery enables modern medicine to keep them alive. And programs of childhood physical-mental stimulation and cosmetic surgery may facilitate their assimilation. Down syndrome is caused by an extra chromosome, of the pair that geneticists label as number 21, and is sometimes called 'trisomy 21' for that reason. There is no cure for Down syndrome. A pregnant woman whose fetus is diagnosed as having the extra chromosome can either prepare to raise a mentally retarded and physically very vulnerable child, or decide to abort it.

Initially, in the mid-to-late 1960s, women over forty were counselled to have the test. Then, the age dropped to thirty-eight, and currently it's recommended for women who are thirty-five or older when they conceive. (President's Commission, 1983; Sadovnick & Baird, 1981) We're thus witnessing two social processes at work: the routinization of a frontier of medicine is being extended more deeply into the population at the same time that an increasing number of women are choosing to delay childbearing. As these two trends intersect, amniocentesis becomes a new pregnancy ritual among people like me, with great implications for our lives, and the lives of other women as well.

Some of these facts about chromosomes I could vaguely dredge up from a college course on the February morning when Mike and I arrived at a local medical center for genetic counseling, in my nineteenth week of pregnancy. Nancy Z., our social-work trained counselor, took a detailed pedigree (or family tree) from each of us, to discover any rare diseases or birth defects for which we could be tested. She then gave us an excellent genetics lesson, explained the amniocentesis procedure and the risks, both of amniocentesis, and of discovering a serious genetic defect. Less than 1 percent of pregnancies miscarry after amniocentesis. That's a low risk, but it isn't no-risk, and during pregnancy we all feel very concerned and vulnerable about anything that might cause damage or death to our fetuses. Most women feel fine after the test, but a certain percentage (perhaps 10 percent) experience uterine cramping or contractions, and are told by doctors to rest until they subside. Overall, about 98 percent of the women who go for amniocentesis will be told that no fetal defects or anomalies have been found. So the overall rate of genetic defect detection (about 2 percent) and of miscarriage following the procedure (less than 1 percent) are both very small, but also very similar.

After counseling, we descended to the testing area, where an all-female team of radiologist, obstetrician, nurses and staff assistants performed the tap. In skilled hands, and with the use of sonogram equipment, the tap is a rapid procedure. I spent perhaps five minutes on the table, belly attached to sonar electrodes, Mike holding my feet for encouragement. The radiologist flipped off 'polaroid' pictures of XYLO, and we went home with our first 'baby album' — grey blotches of a head and spine of our baby-in-waiting. The radiologist located the placenta, which enabled the obstetrician to successfully draw a small, clear sample of amniotic fluid (less than one-eighth of a cup). The tap felt like a crampier version of drawing blood. It wasn't particularly painful or traumatic. We marched the fluid back to the genetics lab where it would be cultured, and went home.

The waiting period for amniocentesis results is a long one, and I was very anxious. Cells must be cultured, then analyzed in intensive lab examination, and this process of karyotyping takes two to four weeks. While we are all told that 'no news is good news,' it's a hard period to endure. Caught between the late date at which sufficient amniotic fluid exists to be tapped (sixteen to twenty weeks), the experience of quickening, when the woman feels the fetus move (roughly, eighteen to twenty weeks), and the legal limits of abortion (few abortions are performed after twenty-four weeks in the USA), we all have terrible fantasies, and many of us report distressing dreams.

For the 98 percent of women whose amniotic fluid reveals no anomaly, reassurance arrives by phone, or, more likely, by mail, confirming a negative test. When Nancy called me twelve days after the tap, I began to scream as soon as I recognized her voice; in her lab, only positive results (very negative results, from a potential parent's point of view) are reported by phone. The image of myself, alone, screaming into a white plastic telephone is indelible. Although it only took twenty minutes to locate Mike and bring him and a close friend to my side, time is suspended in my memory, and I replay the call, and my screams echo for indefinite periods. Results are not formally communicated by phone, but with a bit of intervention from our midwives and obstetrician, we learned that a tentative diagnosis of a male Down syndrome fetus had been made. Our fantasies for XYLO, our five months' fetus, were completely shattered.

Mike and I had discussed what we would do if amniocentesis revealed a serious genetic condition long before the test. For us, the diagnosis of Down syndrome was reason to choose abortion. Our thinking was clear, if abstract, long before the concrete horror became reality. We were eager to have a child, and prepared to change our lives to make emotional, social, and economic resources available. But the realities of raising a child who could never grow to independence would call forth more than we could muster, unless one or both of us gave up our work, our political commitments, our social existence beyond the household. And despite a shared commitment to co-parenting, we both understood that, in this society, that one was likely to be the mother. When I thought about myself, I knew that in such a situation, I would transform myself to become the kind of twenty-four-hour-a-day advocate such a child would require. I'd do the best and most loving job I could, and I'd undoubtedly become an activist in support of the needs of disabled children. But even if we *did* totally transform our lives to raise a Down syndrome child, other stark realities confronted us: to keep a Down syndrome child alive through potentially lethal health problems is an act of love whose ultimate consequences are problematic. As we ourselves age, to whom would we leave the person XYLO would become? In a society where the state provides virtually no decent, humane services for the mentally retarded, how could we take responsibility for the future of our dependent Down syndrome child? In good conscience, we couldn't choose to raise a child who would become a ward of the state. The health care, schools, various therapies that Down syndrome children require are inadequately available, and horrendously expensive in America, and no single family can take the place that a decent health and social policy may someday extend to physically and mentally disabled people. In the meantime, while struggling for such a society, we did not choose to bring a child into this world who could never grow up to care for himself.

Other genetic diagnoses may present less, or more, clear choices to potential parents. If your fetus has Tay Sachs, it's a 100 percent childhood death sentence, while the disabilities associated with spina bifida range from quadraplegic, but mentally alert, to both much milder physical, and much harsher mental, diagnoses. A disease like sickle cell anemia is episodic, and ranges from life-threatening to livable, depending on severity. It nearly always involves intense bouts of pain. Diseases like hemophilia can now be medically managed to allow for livable, if restricted lives. The diagnosis of Down syndrome spells mental retardation, but the detection of an extra chromosome can't tell us if our specific Down syndrome fetus will grow up to have the mental age of three or seven, learn articulate speech or toilet training. So both the kind of genetic anomaly, and the range of its potential severity make the choices surrounding prenatal diagnosis a parental nightmare.

Most women who've opted for amniocentesis are prepared to face the question of abortion, and many of us *do* choose it, after a seriously disabling diagnosis is made. Perhaps 95 percent of Down syndrome pregnancies are terminated after test results are known. Reports on other diseases and conditions are harder to find, but, in one study, the diagnosis of spina bifida led to abortion about 90 percent of the time. These were all women who'd borne and raised a previous spina bifida child. (Hook, 1978a, 1978b; Brock, 1977; Lawrence and Morris, 1981).

In shock and grief, I learned from my obstetrician that two kinds of late second-trimester abortions were available. Most common are the 'installation procedures' – saline solution or urea is injected into the uterus prostaglandins are injected into the woman's veins to bring on labor, and sometimes pitocin, a labor-enhancing drug, is also used. The woman then goes through labor to deliver the dead fetus. 'Giving-birth-to-death' (as one woman who'd chosen an abortion after a Down syndrome diagnosis described the process) is emotionally draining on both the woman and her mate, who is often allowed to stay with her through the labor. Sedation may or may not be available. The second kind of mid-trimester abortion, and the one I chose, is a D and E – dilation and evacuation. Performed in the operating room of a hospital after the cervix has been dilated with laminaria (sterile seaweed sticks that absorb fluid, inserted twenty-four to forty-eight hours in advance), the D and E demands more active intervention from a doctor, who vacuums out the amniotic fluid, and then removes the dismembered fetus manually. A general anesthetic or heavy sedation is used. From the medical team's point of view, the D and E requires some intense, upsetting work, but it's over in about twenty minutes, without putting the woman through labor.

Either way, all the women I've spoken to found this a very tough abortion to endure. Like me, they'd wanted the pregnancy, or they would have ended it at a much earlier stage. Both forms of late abortion entail increasing maternal risks as the fetus grows – the later, the riskier, although both are still quite safe. But the psychological pain is enormous. Deciding to end the life of a fetus you've wanted and carried for most of five months is no easy matter. More than 90 percent of abortions in America are performed in the first trimester, long before fetal life is felt by the pregnant woman. The number of relatively late second-trimester abortions performed for genetic reasons is very small, perhaps about 400 a year in the USA. It's an almost inconsequential number, unless you happen to be one of them.

Making the medical arrangements, going back for counseling, the pretests, and, finally, the abortion, was the most difficult period of my adult life. I was then twenty-one weeks pregnant, and had been proudly carrying my expanding belly. Telling everyone – friends, family, students, colleagues, neighbors – seemed an endless nightmare. But the rewards of making our decision public were very great. Friends streamed in from all over to teach my classes: I have scores of letters expressing concern, and the phone never stopped ringing for weeks. There were always flowers being delivered to our door, and everyone eased my return to work. Our community of friends was invaluable, reminding us that our lives were rich and filled with love despite this terrible loss. My parents flew a thousand miles to sit guard over my hospital bed, answer telephones, shop and cook. Filled with sorrow for the loss of their first grandchild, my mother told me of a conversation she'd had with my father. Despite their grief, they were deeply grateful for the test. After all, she reasoned, we were too young and active to be devastated like this; if the child had been born, she and my dad would have taken him to raise in their older years, so we could get on with raising other children. I can only respond with deep love and gratitude for the wellspring of compassion behind that conversation. But surely, no single woman, mother or grandmother, no single family, nuclear or extended, should have to bear all the burdens that raising a seriously disabled child entails. It points out, once again, the importance of providing decent, humane attention and services for other-than-fully-able children (and adults).

And, of course, parents of disabled children are quick to point out that the lives they've nurtured have been worth living. I honor their hard work and commitments, as well as their love, and I think that part of 'informed consent' to amniocentesis and selective abortion (as my experience is antiseptically called in medical jargon) should include information about groups for parents of Down syndrome children, and social services available to them, not just the individual, medical diagnosis of the problem. And even people who feel they could never choose a late abortion may none the less want amniocentesis so they'll have a few extra months to prepare themselves, other family members, friends, and special resources for the birth of a child with special, complex needs.

Recovering from the abortion took a long time. Friends, family, co-workers, students did everything they could to ease me through the experience. Even so, I yearned to talk with someone who'd 'been there.' Over the next few months, I used my personal and medical networks to locate and interview a handful of other women who'd opted for selective abortions, and in each case, I was the first person they'd ever met with a similar experience. The isolation of this decision and its consequences are intense. Hard as it is to break the barriers of privacy that surround sex, birth control, pregnancy and childbirth in our culture, the feminist in me ardently champions their demise. Only when women (and concerned men) speak of the experience of selective abortion as a tragic but chosen fetal death can we as a community offer the support, sort out the ethics, and give the compassionate attention that such a loss entails. I was fortunate, probably more fortunate than most women, to receive that kind of attentiveness throughout this experience.

For two weeks, Mike and I breathed as one person. His distress, loss, and concern were never one whit less than my own. But we were sometimes upset and angered by the unconscious cultural attitudes which precluded acknowledgment of his loss. He was expected to 'cope,' while I was nurtured through my 'need.' We've struggled for male responsibility in birth control, sexual mutuality, childbirth and childrearing, and I think we need to acknowledge that those men who do engage in such transformed practises have mourning rights during a pregnancy loss, as well.

And yet, having spent fifteen years arguing against biological determinism in my intellectual and political life, I'm compelled to recognize the material reality of this experience. Because it happened in my body, a woman's body, I recovered much more slowly than Mike did. By whatever mysterious process, he was able to damp back the pain, and throw himself back into work after several weeks. For me, it took months. As long as I had the 14 pounds of pregnancy weight to lose, as long as my aching breasts, filled with milk, couldn't squeeze into bras, as long as my tummy muscles protruded, I was confronted with the physical reality of being post-pregnant, without a child. Mike's support seemed inadequate; I was still in deep mourning while he seemed distant and cured. Only much later, when I began doing research on amniocentesis, did I find one small study of the stresses and strains selective abortion engenders. In a tiny sample, a high percentage of couples separated or divorced following this experience (Blumberg, Golbus and Hansen, 1975; Sorenson, 1974). Of course, the same holds true after couples face serious childhood disablement, and child death. Still, I had no idea that deep mourning for a fetus could be so disorienting. Abortion after prenatal diagnosis is so medicalized, so privatized, that there is no common fund of knowledge to alert us as individuals, as couples, as families, as friends, to the aftermath our 'freedom of choice' entails.

Which is why I've pierced my private pain to raise this issue. Amniocentesis raises many questions which women should be thinking about. We need to discuss this experience, analyze its ethics and politics, its social dimensions, its freedoms and responsibilities. We must not leave this discourse solely to medical technicians, health economists, bioethics experts, or the forces of rightwing politics which would outlaw genetic research and funding because, in its view, amniocentesis leads to abortion. As 'consumers' of this service, and as feminists concerned for the future and quality of women's reproductive freedom, we need to face amniocentesis, and discuss it in our own fashion, as we have discussed sexuality, birth control and abortion, pregnancy, childbearing and childrearing, which similarly get appropriated as 'technical,' or 'medical,' rather than fully social and political issues.

A beginning check-list of feminist questions about amniocentesis might include:

who gets the test, and under what conditions? The few studies we have of 'underutilization' by low-income women – often Black, Hispanic or Asian – suggest they'd use amniocentesis. In practise, however, the high cost of a test rarely covered by medicaid, rushed and sometimes insensitive prenatal care, lack of medical staff trained to use their languages and cultural categories when confronted with hard questions often get in the way. Health care in America is stratified in this, as in all other, experiences, by race and class as well as sex (Marion, Kassam et al., 1980; Sokal, Byrd et al., 1980; Hook, Schreinemachers and Cross, 1981);

what does 'informed consent' mean, and how can we expand and insure its use? A coercive referral for amniocentesis so that a doctor won't face a malpractise suit is *not* reproductive freedom. And the opposite problem – a doctor who doesn't offer information about the test to eligible women because he/she doesn't believe in abortion –

is also a curtailment of our right to decide for ourselves the
conditions under which we'll bear our children;
how can we insure that the availability of amniocentesis
doesn't conflict with our commitment to build a better
world for disabled people? The disability rights movement
has raised the question of eugenics, and the goal of making
it 'cheaper' and 'more acceptable' to screen for genetically
'perfect' fetuses than to support the services disabled
children need. While health economists may find
amniocentesis and abortion more 'cost effective' than
caring for special-needs children, as feminists we need to
acknowledge that such lives are worth living. At the same
time, we know that a woman needs access to abortion *for
whatever reason* she chooses not to bear a specific
pregnancy to term. Our commitment to abortion
goes hand-in-hand with an equally feminist commitment
to decent prenatal care, child care, education and health
services for the children women *do* bear. The same
connections must be made in support of disability rights.
*Any* woman may decide she will not bear a specific fetus,
once prenatal diagnosis reveals a serious disability she
does not want to live with. But *every* feminist should
support the rights, based on special needs, of disabled
children and adults;
how can women who opt for amniocentesis learn the social,
as well as the medical 'facts' of the diagnoses their fetuses
receive? Genetics counselors and doctors necessarily focus
their limited time and resources on explaining technical
and medical questions. But we as 'consumers' and potential
parents need to reach out and establish networks of
information so that a woman confronting the diagnosis of
Down syndrome or sickle-cell anemia, or any other serious
prenatal diagnosis, can meet other parents and children
living with these conditions, and learn realistically about
the quality, cost, and availability of the services that make
such lives better.[1] Such a network would socialize an
otherwise-too-private set of problems;
how can we make second trimester abortions less
devastating for the women who choose them? As feminist
health activists, we need to insure that abortion laborers

aren't placed on delivery floors with live-birthing mothers.
We also need to establish self-help networks of women
who've recovered from selective abortions and are willing
to speak with those undergoing the process. Again, public
discussion, not private misery, can benefit future users of
selective abortion;

how can we insure that accurate, up-to-date information
about prenatal diagnosis, explained in clear, non-jargon
language is available to women? As many feminists have
pointed out, the legal, medical, and ethical practises
surrounding childbearing and 'fetal rights' are usually out
of our control.

Our justified cynicism about the medical establishment
should not prevent us from obtaining, scrutinizing and using
the most accurate scientific information we can find. With
embryo transplants, test-tube babies, and cloning making
front-page headlines continuously, feminists desperately
need scientific literacy. What we don't know *can* hurt us. And
the solution is certainly not to leave such issues to the Right
to Life, which would defund fetal and genetic research since,
in their view, it leads to abortion. Medical professionals and
ethicists often counter this argument by pointing out that the
availability of selective abortion allows people who are at
risk for a serious disease, and might therefore never have
reproduced, to have children. This is a necessary, but hardly
a sufficient response from a feminist perspective. We need to
develop our own informed support for prenatal diagnosis
programs, beginning with the defense of abortion rights and
incorporating the kinds of questions whose surfaces I've
barely touched on here.

As feminists, we need to speak from our seemingly
private experiences toward a social and political agenda. I'm
suggesting we pierce the veil of privacy and professionalism
to explore issues of health care, abortion, and the right to
choose death, as well as life, for our genetically disabled
fetuses. If XYLO's story, a true story, has helped to make this
a compelling issue for more than one couple, then his five
short months of fetal life will have been a great gift.

## NOTES

1 Such networks of support and information are frequently mentioned by genetics counselors, but it is hard to track them down. Newsletters, such as *Down's Syndrome*, report the activities of parents' and advocates' groups. Local health departments often have listings of parents' groups. See, too, the list of resources in *Ms*, April 1984.

## REFERENCES

Blumberg, B. D., M. S. Golbus and K. H. Hansen. 1975. 'The Psychological Sequelae of Abortion Performed for Genetic Indication.' *American Journal of Obstetrics and Gynecology*, 122: 799–808.

Brock, D. J. H. 1977. 'Antenatal Diagnosis of Spina Bifida and Anencephaly.' In H. A. Lubs and F. de la Cruz, eds. *Genetic Counseling*. Raven Press, New York.

Consensus Development Conference. 1979. *Antenatal Diagnosis*. NICHHD Report; NIH pub. no. 79-1973.

Hendin, D. and J. Marks. 1979. *The Genetic Connection*. Signet, New York.

Hook, E. B. 1978a. 'Differences Between Rates of Trisomy 21 (DS) and Other Chromosomal Abnormalities Diagnosed in Live Births and in cells cultured after Second Trimester Amniocentesis.' *Birth Defects*, 14: 249–67.

Hook, E. B. 1978b. 'Spontaneous Deaths of Fetuses with Chromosomal Abnormalities Diagnosed Prenatally.' *New England Journal of Medicine*, 299: 1036–8.

Hook, E. B., D. M. Schreinemachers and P. K. Cross. 1981. 'Use of Prenatal Cytogenetic Diagnosis in NY State.' *New England Journal of Medicine*, 305: 1410–16.

Lawrence, K. M. and J. Morris. 1981. 'The Effect of the Introduction of Prenatal Diagnosis on the Reproductive History of Women at Increased Risk from NTD.' *Prenatal Diagnosis*, 1: 51–60.

Lipkin, M. and P. T. Rowley, eds. 1974. *Genetic Responsibility*. Plenum Press, New York.

Lubs, H. A. and F. de la Cruz, eds. 1977. *Genetic Counseling*. Raven Press, New York.

Marion, J., G. Kassam et al. 1980. 'Acceptance of amniocentesis by 100 low-income patients in an Urban Hospital.' *American Journal of Obstetrics and Gynecology*, 138: 11–15.

President's Commission for the Study of Ethical Problems in Medicine and Biomedical and Behavioral Research. 1983. *Screening and Counseling for Genetic Conditions*. US GPO 83-600502.

Sadovnick, A. D. and P. A. Baird. 1981. 'A Cost Benefit analysis of Prenatal detection of Down syndrome and Neural Tube Defects in Older Mothers.' *American Journal of Medical Genetics*, 10: 367–78.

Sokal, D. G., J. R. Byrd et al. 1980. 'Prenatal Chromosomal Diagnosis: Racial and Geographic Variation for Older Women in Georgia.' *Journal of the American Medical Association*, 244: 1355–7.

Sorenson, J. 1974. 'Genetic Counseling: Some Psychological Considerations.' In M. Lipkin and P. T. Rowley, eds. *Genetic Responsibility*. Plenum Press, New York.

# THE MOTHERHOOD
# MARKET

# PERSONAL COURAGE IS NOT ENOUGH: SOME HAZARDS OF CHILDBEARING IN THE 1980s

## Ruth Hubbard

In this chapter Ruth Hubbard examines the implications for women of some recent medical interventions in pregnancy. While these techniques may increase the range of options available to socially and economically privileged women, even for them, there are personal, social, and even legal costs. So, for example, the availability of prenatal diagnosis and fetal therapy has led physicians, attorneys, and judges to interpret pregnancy as a conflict of 'rights' between a fetus and the pregnant woman whose body sustains it. Instead of recognizing that the greatest problems and hazards of childbearing are due to the inadequate social supports that make it difficult for most women to live healthful and satisfying lives (and that make it exceedingly difficult to raise a disabled child), these experts point to the individual mother as the source of her child's illness or disability. Hence, they prescribe the ways in which women must behave so as to guarantee a fetus's 'right' to be born healthy.

In this chapter, I want to explore the implications of some of the new reproductive technologies for the experience of childbearing. Of course, I must immediately disembarrass myself of the notion that childbearing is a single, unique experience. No doubt, there are as many experiences as there are women bearing children and they range from bliss to agony, since they depend on the social and personal circumstances in which different women live. (For examples, see Davis, 1915; Emecheta, 1979; Kitzinger, 1979; McDonald, 1981; Rich, 1976; Wertz and Wertz, 1979.) However, the new technologies raise issues that can enter all these experiences, though they may affect different ones differently.

## CHILDBEARING – A SOCIAL CONSTRUCT

Before going any further, I want to clear up one point: I am *not* trying to distinguish between 'natural' and 'technological' childbearing practices (and by childbearing I mean the entire range of women's activities from conception through birth, and perhaps even lactation). This is because I do not believe that any human pregnancy or birth is simply 'natural.' All of us live in societies that define, order, circumscribe and interpret our activities and experiences. Just as our sexual practices from earliest childhood are socially constructed and not a natural unfolding of inborn instincts, so are the ways of structuring and experiencing pregnancy and birth. Whether a woman goes off to give birth by herself (as do Kung women in the Kalahari desert), calls in neighboring women and perhaps a midwife (as my grandmother did in a small town in eastern Europe), goes to a lying-in hospital (as I did in Boston some twenty-five years ago), or has a lay midwife come to assist her and her partner at home (as several of my friends have done in the last few years), all these are socially devised ways, sanctioned by one's community, even if sometimes not by the medical profession or the state. The question we as feminists need to ask is not which is more 'natural,' but to what extent the different constructs empower women or, alternatively, decrease our power to structure childbearing around our own needs and those of the people with whom we live our daily lives; to what extent we are compelled to accommodate to the convenience of 'authorities' who pretend to understand our needs and interests better than we do.

A recent blatant example of how the situation can be shaped entirely by medical 'experts' is a report issued by the Royal College of Obstetricians and Gynaecologists (1983) to regulate in Great Britain the practice of in vitro fertilization, embryo replacement and embryo transfer (see Glossary, p. 458).[1] According to this document, the practice is to be guided entirely by the clinical judgment and experience of the physician – though one must wonder what 'clinical experience' a physician can have with a new procedure whose benefits and risks are only beginning to be explored – as well as by 'his' risks from litigation (in the report the physician is always 'he'). Prospective parents are always referred to as patients and their needs and rights are evaluated entirely in a medical context. The report states explicitly that since physicians

> are taking part in the *formation* of the embryo . . . that role brings a special sense of responsibility for the welfare of the child thus conceived. . . . Therefore most practitioners will *intuitively* feel that IVF (in vitro fertilization) and ER (embryo replacement) should be performed in the *most* '*natural*' of family environments. (ibid.: 6; my emphases)

This line of argument then leads the authors to conclude that the physician has the 'natural' right to decide which of the women who would like to have IVF live in proper social and personal circumstances to make them fit parents.

This may be a drastic example, but what I am trying to show is that the realities of childbearing have changed not only for the relatively few women who are candidates for in vitro fertilization and embryo replacement or transfer. Other, more prevalent, technologies affect the experience. So, for example, in Britain and the US the 'check-ups' of many pregnant women include ultrasound visualization of the fetus. Indeed, some physicians have urged that this be made mandatory at least once or twice during pregnancy (Veitch, 1983). Real-time ultrasound recording allows women and their attendants to view a live image of the fetus in action, so to speak. Most women agree that the fetus becomes more real – more their 'baby' – when they see it that way and can take its picture home to show to relatives and friends. Yet for numbers of women (though for *whom*, at least in the US, depends more on social and economic circumstances than on health indicators), ultrasound visualization is followed by amniocentesis, which carries with it the possibilities of a second-trimester abortion. A few women become involved with further manipulations to modify and, hopefully, improve the health of the fetus by means of some of the new medical or surgical techniques that have come to be known as fetal therapy. (For a more detailed discussion, see Hubbard, 1982a.)

All these interventions, and indeed the mere possibility that they may occur, affect the way we look on our pregnancies. At the very least, we must decide whether to permit interventions and how far to go with them – something we can usually still do, though we may lose that choice (but more of that later). But whether we permit or refuse them, the decision affects how 'real' our fetus becomes for us and when we feel that it stops being 'a fetus' and becomes 'our baby.' Add to this that amniocentesis almost invariably implies that we may have to decide whether to abort this part-fetus/part-baby and you see that pregnancy now is very different from what it was only a decade ago when once we decided to become pregnant or to accept an accidental pregnancy, we did not confront further decisions about whether to carry that particular pregnancy to term.

Let me be clear. I completely support every woman's right to decide whether and when she wants to have a child and this requires that she have an unqualified right to abortion. Nor do I think (on the basis of my own and other people's experiences as pregnancy counsellors) that the decision to abort need be traumatic. This, too, depends on the social context in which the decision is made and implemented. But I believe that it is one thing to abort when we don't want to be pregnant and quite another to want a baby, but to decide to abort the particular fetus we are carrying in hopes of coming up with a 'better' one next time. In fact, the abortion itself may not be so bad once the decision is made, but friends who have had amniocentesis have told me about the stress of waiting the two or three weeks needed to culture and test the fetal cells before they get the results, knowing that they may end up deciding not to keep on with the pregnancy. This state of uncertainty can last till the twentieth week, so half-way through the pregnancy and several weeks after most pregnant women begin to feel the fetus move, by which time they may have come to look on it as very much 'their baby.' These stories agree with studies that are beginning to be published about the emotional impact of prenatal diagnosis and of abortions because of fetal abnormalities (Blumberg, Golbus and Hansen, 1975; Kenen, 1981; Neilsen, 1981). The ways in which ultrasound and amniocentesis are being used confront women with a major contradiction: ultrasound makes the fetus more our baby, while the possibility of abortion makes us want to keep our emotional distance in case the pregnancy isn't going to end up with a baby after all.

This particular problem may be relieved in the next few years, if the new technique of *chorionic villi* sampling which is currently being developed becomes generally available. In this procedure cells of fetal origin are withdrawn through a woman's cervix, something that can be done as early as the eighth to tenth week of pregnancy, and are examined immediately for chromosomal and some other genetic problems. The procedure was developed almost a decade ago in China in the context of sex selection (Department of Obstetrics and Gynecology, Tietung Hospital of Anshan Iron and Steel Company, Anshan, 1975) and is now being explored in Britain and the U.S. to help with prenatal screening for chromosomal and other inborn health problems (Rutenberg, 1983; *Science News*, 1983; Williamson et al., 1981). If it proves to be safe and acceptable, it will let women who have reason to be concerned about the health of their fetus, have tests for many of the problems for which they now have amniocentesis, in time for a first-trimester abortion, if they decide to terminate the pregnancy. However, though this new technique might help some women who have specific problems, it may make life harder for all other women. Having an easier (and safer) method to examine the fetus's characteristics early in pregnancy and thus to detect a 'wrong' fetus – possibly a *female* fetus? – may increase the pressure to screen every fetus as well as the pressure to abort 'wrong' ones.

## THE QUESTION OF CHOICE

Clearly this will eliminate or decrease some of the problems I have discussed; but it won't others because other important issues get into the question of our 'choice' of the kind of baby to have (see also Rothman, 1984a, 1984b). To sort them out, we need to put this new kind of decision into its historical context. Though women in most cultures and times have practiced some form of birth control (from contraceptive and abortifacient herbs and barrier methods to infanticide), only during the last century or so have the methods become sufficiently available and reliable that many socially and economically more privileged women can in fact decide whether to become pregnant and when. Until recent times, unwanted pregnancies, hazards of childbearing and high rates of infant and early childhood mortality made the reproductive lives also of economically more privileged women largely matters of chance and not choice. However, now the existence of this choice seems to be sliding over into the illusion that the more privileged of us can control not only whether and when to have children, but the kind and quality of children we 'choose' to have. As Barbara Katz Rothman (1984a, 1984b) points out, our consumer society encourages us to look upon children as products that we can or cannot 'afford.'[2] And we can easily, and realistically, come to see the prospect of raising a disabled child as quite beyond our means.

In this economy, children are expensive to bear and raise. If they are born with a disability, or later become disabled, in the US the expense can be overwhelming, which is why Americans often meet the challenge of disability with litigation in order to decrease the financial burden. Recent medical and social practices have made it possible to commodify our reproduction all down the line, making available for purchase eggs, sperm, embryos, surrogate mothers, and babies. (Some adoptive babies are for sale outright, though unofficially, on a 'black market.' And while the adoption agencies that mediate legal adoptions forbid cash payments, they are at pains to establish the financial 'soundness' of adoptive parents. So, even though money does not pass hands in agency adoptions, economic status is an important criterion for being considered a fit prospective parent.) And as Rothman (1984b) points out, once reproduction is seen as a form of commodity production, it is an easy step to require quality control, which is where genetic screening, ultrasound visualization and amniocentesis come in.

But we must realize that these techniques are not, and indeed cannot be, available for everyone. They are scarce resources that carry a price tag. Therefore, while women who can afford them are encouraged to view the new products and techniques as liberating advances that improve our lives, economically less privileged and socially more defenseless women continue to be deprived of the ability to reproduce by forced sterilization, often by means of hysterectomy (McDonald, 1981: 8–23; Rodriguez-Trias, 1982). Indeed, the present financial restrictions that limit the availability of abortions in the US are forcing pregnant women who want abortions, but cannot afford them, to 'choose' hysterectomies, because these are covered by social insurance.

The consumerist way of looking at reproduction creates the illusion that at least those of us who can afford the tests have the choice to have healthy babies. In reality, that choice exists only in a few circumscribed situations.[3] But before I say more about the limits on our ability to avoid the occasional birth of children with disabilities, I want to raise another point.

## TRADE-OFFS OF SCIENTIFIC 'PROGRESS'

Feminists have often portrayed medical interventions in pregnancy as part of an attempt by male physicians to control women's capacity to bear children. And though I agree with much in this analysis, I am bothered by the way it often downgrades, or even romanticizes, the pain and travail many women have experienced in childbearing. Bearing and rearing children *is* difficult under the conditions in which most women live. To take just one example, Ruth Perry (1979) has calculated that in eighteenth-century England a married woman who 'delivered six children (a not unusual number) . . . had at least a ten per cent chance of dying, and probably a much higher one.' Difficulties of childbearing also are described in many biographies and novels of the period and later. It is small wonder that many women have welcomed anesthetics and the other interventions physicians have introduced, believing that they would lessen the dangers and pain of pregnancy and birth.

Feminists have shown that these medical 'improvements' have taken their toll. For one thing, they often bring their own dangers; for another, they have given physicians (who in many parts of the world are predominantly men) authority and control over the ways women experience pregnancy and birth as well as over childrearing. (For accounts of these developments, see for example Ehrenreich and English, 1978; Rothman, 1982; Wertz and Wertz, 1979.) But given the limited choices most women have had and the very real risks of childbearing, it is not surprising that upper-class women in the nineteenth century used what little choice they had to opt for the 'improvements' their physicians promised them. Brack (1982) and Wertz and Wertz (1979), among others, have described how this virtually eliminated midwifery in the United States. In addition, Devitt (1979), Wertz (1983), and Wertz and Wertz (1979) have shown that the past two centuries' improvements in maternal and infant health are not to be credited to these medical interventions nor, in the United States, to the replacement of the services of midwives by physicians. Quite the contrary, both often contributed to the deterioration of health services and health outcomes rather than to their improvement.

However, despite this history, we are once again at a point where many women believe that the pregnancy interventions that have been introduced in the last ten years are increasing the range of positive reproductive choices and that they are therefore improving women's lives. The problem is that experiences of past generations of women are quickly erased as contemporary women find it impossible to imagine how they could live without the technologies that past women lacked, never missed, and often were better off without.

Take the Pill as just one example. Many women who became heterosexually active in the early 1960s seem to think that birth control was rare, if not unknown, for women earlier in the century. Yet many women of the pre-Pill era, by use of condoms and diaphragms (still much safer than the Pill or the IUD from a health viewpoint), planned their pregnancies as consciously and successfully as women who use the newer products do. True, the older methods have their problems and inconveniences, but though they are different, it is far from clear that they are greater than those of the newer methods.

Another example are pregnancies of older women – and in this context, 'older' is being used to denote younger and younger women as time goes on. It used to be over forty; in the US now it is over thirty-five; I suppose thirty-two and thirty are next. This seems strange to me who had children some twenty-five years ago, when I was between thirty-five and forty. I did not think that was anything to worry about since I and my partner were in good health. Yet women that age now tell me earnestly that only because they can have amniocentesis are they able to consider having a child. And it is true that now that it has been hammered into the present generation of 'older' women that the risks of bearing a child with chromosomal abnormalities such as Down syndrome increase dramatically after thirty-five, few will refuse amniocentesis and just hope for the best, when this test can reassure them by the twentieth week of pregnancy (as it usually does). However, partly because we have this technological fix and partly because the medical profession downgrades epidemiological research, the reasons why chromosomal abnormalities occur have not been properly analyzed. What environmental, occupational and socio-economic hazards are there? How relevant are the health histories of both partners? And so forth. In the midst of this ignorance, the mother's, and to a lesser extent, the father's age are put forward as the only relevant factor.

I have a not so sci-fi fantasy in which a woman five or ten years hence tells me that she could not possibly risk having a child by 'in body' fertilization. Only the existence of in vitro fertilization and embryo replacement make childbearing

possible, she will say. Her reason, that by then it has become
standard practice to fertilize eggs in vitro and allow the
embryos to develop until they contain six or eight cells. At
this point, two of the cells are removed and put through a
battery of genetic and metabolic tests, while the rest of the
embryo is quick-frozen and placed in cold-storage (something
that is already now being done in Australia (Duboudin, 1983;
Royal College of Obstetricians and Gynaecologists, 1983:
10–11)). If the tests are satisfactory, the embryo can be
thawed when convenient and implanted in the mother's (or
some other carrier's) womb whenever she 'chooses.'

How will I be able to explain my many objections to this
by then routine procedure? We will live in different
universes. I in one where I want to interfere as little as
possible with the delicate and complicated processes of fertilization and embryonic development *and* where I look upon
childbearing as a healthy, normal function that can sometimes go wrong, as can all biological functions, but that
usually doesn't. She in a world where the ability to control
her reproduction means the opportunity to use all available
medical techniques to avoid the possibility of biological
malfunctioning. I will tell her that the procedures introduce
unknown and unpredictable risks, cannot assure her of
having a healthy baby, and pervert childbearing into a Brave
New World activity. She will tell me that I am opting for
ignorance and stemming progress. But what worries me most
is that at that point 'in-body fertilization' will not only have
come to seem old-fashioned and quaint, but downright
foolhardy, unhealthful and unsafe. And it will seem that way
to the women who are 'choosing' to have babies in the new
way as well as to the physicians who pioneer the
'improvements.'

In fact, of course, some women over thirty-five are
refusing to have amniocentesis and other, usually poor and/
or Third World women, don't even know it exists. Thus, only a
minority of women of any age are being screened. But this is
largely because access to all costly resources is uneven in this
society and not because physicians feel the need to be
cautious about exposing women to these techniques. Rather,
to be cautious to them means to use all the available

technology (however little we can yet know about its long-term consequences) to avoid all manner of inborn 'defects.'

One of the reasons I am concerned about the widespread use of genetic screening is because it focuses our attention on our genes at a time when environmental hazards are on the increase and need much more attention than they are getting (see also Hubbard, 1982b; Hubbard and Henifin, 1984). The reason I worry about many of the other prenatal manipulations, including amniocentesis, is because usually at some point they involve the use of ultrasound (Bolsen, 1982). It took twenty to thirty years before epidemiological studies linked prenatal X-ray examinations to the production of leukemias and cancers. No reason to think that the health effects of irradiation with ultrasound can be evaluated more quickly. There is no question that exposure to higher doses of ultrasound than are usually used for diagnostic purposes can damage chromosomes, cells and tissues. As with other forms of radiation, the question is whether there is a threshold dose below which there are no destructive effects.[4] If there are risks, they clearly are long-term and they may be subtle. Is it really a progressive health measure to expose large numbers of healthy women and fetuses to unnecessary ultrasound examinations in the hope of detecting a relatively small number of problem pregnancies? Some people have reason to be concerned that their fetus may have a health problem because of the family, personal or environmental health history of either partner. To some of them it may seem preferable, on balance, to undergo examinations by means of ultrasound and perhaps further tests, such as amniocentesis. Yet at present, ultrasound has become such a widely used tool in obstetrics that it is used as though it were known to be safe. Indeed, it forms the technical basis of the newly designated specialty of 'fetal medicine.'

## DISABILITIES – A SOCIAL PROBLEM

And what all shall be termed a 'defect' and for what range of 'defects' shall a fetus be treated in utero or aborted? Down syndrome? Spina bifida? Wrong sex? For most inborn disabilities we cannot predict how serious the 'defect' will be and just how it will express itself – in other words, what kind of a person the child will be. To some people, and in some circumstances, the prospect of having a child with Down syndrome, no matter how mild – and as I just said, the degree usually cannot be predicted – is intolerable. Ten years ago when there were no tests, they might have taken the risk to have a child when they were over thirty-five. But now that tests exist they will, of course, have them. (They probably will not even be told that there may be a risk associated with the use of ultrasound since most practitioners have become so dependent on using it that they have convinced themselves that it is safe.) The problem for me is that the same thing can be said for parents who have a strong sex preference (Fletcher, 1979; but see also Powledge, 1980). In fact, though many feminists have argued against sex selection (Hanmer, 1981; Powledge, 1981), some feminists favor it as a way to give women who want it the option of being sure to have a daughter. Personally, I have problems with such so-called choices, and that because of the intrinsic unpredictabilities of bearing and raising children. No matter how hard we try, we cannot know what kind of children we will have, whether they will be healthy and able-bodied and remain so, and what sort of people they will grow up to be. No amount of prenatal testing can guarantee any of that. Having children is risky. To try to be sure we'll have the 'right' kind (and be clear in our minds what the 'right' kind is), in fact, is likely to increase the chances that we'll go wrong. I truly believe that we have the best chance of successful parenthood if we are prepared to accept our children, whoever they are, and do the best we can to help them accept themselves, and, hopefully, us as well.

People with disabilities have begun to speak out about this. They say – and I agree – that all children should be welcome, and that it is short-sighted to think that we can circumvent the uncertainties of childbearing and rearing by aborting 'defective' or 'wrong' fetuses. Furthermore, the focus on preventing the birth of disabled children is increasing the unfair stigma to which people with disabilities, as well as their parents, are exposed.

Another, quite different, issue that we must be aware of

is that the increasing emphasis on prenatal testing reinforces this society's unfortunate tendency to individualize people's problems: disability becomes a personal problem to be dealt with by individual parents (see also Rothman, 1984a). Yet parents on their own cannot possibly provide for a disabled child who may outlive them by decades. The logical solution: don't have one! Logical, maybe, but not practicable because, as I have said before, many inborn disabilities cannot be predicted or prevented and the incidence of disabilities resulting from accidents or exposure to chemicals or radiation is likely to increase rather than decrease in the near future. Therefore it makes better sense to see people's mental and physical disabilities as social, not personal, issues. Many of them – whether inborn or acquired later in life – are the result of social circumstances: accidents, inadequate living conditions, chronic poisoning by heavy metals or drugs, and so forth. They cannot be dealt with by victim-blaming individualizations, but require social measures.

As the world around us becomes more hazardous and threatens us and our children with social disintegration, pollution, accidents and, above all, nuclear war, it seems as though we seek shelter among the hazards that we are told lurk within us, perhaps hoping that we may have at least some control over them. And so we applaud the scientists and physicians who tell us that our problems lie in our genes or in our womb and who propose technological fixes to surmount them. As I write this, the daily paper carries a story under the headline 'Schizophrenia linked to changes in brain cells before birth' (*Boston Globe*, 1983). It starts with the portentous words: 'The devastating mental disorder of paranoid schizophrenia seems to have roots in the womb.' The rest of the story, of course, shows nothing of the sort. Rather, on the basis of the flimsiest of evidence gathered by examining the brains of '10 deceased schizophrenics ages 25 to 67' and 'eight nonpsychotic subjects used as controls' two researches at the University of California's Brain Research Institute in Los Angeles extrapolate the origins of schizophrenia back to 'the first few months of pregnancy' and suggest that 'These abnormalities (in the brain) someday may allow doctors to identify children who have a high risk of becoming paranoid schizophrenics.' This is but one of the many messages women get that say that our children's troubles originate in our womb (or our genes). (And what will it do for our own or our children's mental health to be told that they have a 'high risk' of becoming schizophrenic? And how can we scientifically test that prediction?)

The fact is that prenatal screening and diagnosis can help a relatively small number of women solve their individual problems and therefore can make a few lives better. But they are wrong signposts to what ails us. Prenatal interventions can prevent births of some disabled babies. Most of them will continue to be born. Yet, people are beginning to assume that disabilities can now be prevented, and so they feel that if you have a disabled child, it must be your fault. Not only that, but parents of disabled children and the children themselves (usually through their guardians) are beginning to litigate disabilities. Parents sue physicians claiming that they should have been warned more forcefully about all the possible risks of disability and told about all the available resources for prenatal detection (*Ob/Gyn News*, 1982). And a child who is born with a health problem that might have been detected and improved prenatally can probably sue the mother if she refused to be tested while pregnant (Robertson, 1983: 442, 448). And not only that. The state may be able to mandate prenatal screening 'with criminal penalties for the woman who fails to obtain it.' (Robertson, 1983: 449)

## FETAL 'RIGHTS'

More than ten years ago, Bentley Glass (1971: 28), in a speech he made as retiring president of the American Association for the Advancement of Science, said:

In a world where each pair must be limited, on the average, to two offspring and no more, the right that must become paramount is . . . the right of every child to be born with a sound physical and mental constitution, based on a sound genotype. No parents will in that future time have a right to burden society with a malformed or a mentally incompetent child.

More recently, the theologian, Joseph Fletcher (1980: 133), has written that 'we ought to recognize that children are often abused preconceptively and prenatally – not only by their mothers drinking alcohol, smoking, and using drugs non-medicinally but also by their *knowingly* passing on or risking passing on genetic diseases.' This language of 'rights' of 'the unborn' – which immediately translate into obligations of 'the born,' and especially of women – has now become even more explicitly one of social control. Margery Shaw, an attorney, reviewing the area of 'prenatal torts' argues as follows (Shaw, 1980: 228):

[O]nce a pregnant woman has abandoned her right to abort and has decided to carry her fetus to term, she incurs a 'conditional prospective liability' for negligent acts toward her fetus if it should be born alive. These acts could be considered negligent fetal abuse resulting in an injured child. A decision to carry a genetically defective fetus to term would be an example. Abuse of alcohol or drugs during pregnancy could lead to fetal alcohol syndrome or drug addiction in the infant, resulting in an assertion that he (sic) had been harmed by his mother's acts. Withholding of necessary prenatal care, improper nutrition, exposure to mutagens and teratogens, or even exposure to the mother's defective intrauterine environment caused by her genotype . . . could all result in an injured infant who might claim that his right to be born physically and mentally sound had been invaded.

And she urges (ibid.: 229):

[C]ourts and legislatures . . . should . . . take all reasonable steps to insure that fetuses destined to be born alive are not handicapped mentally and physically by the negligent acts or omissions of others.

Of course, one of the big problems with this line of

argument is that it not only posits that a fetus has rights, but that these 'rights' are different from, and indeed opposed to, those of the mother whose body keeps it alive (and who will most likely be the person who cares for it once it is born). Furthermore, it places the burden of implementing these 'rights' of fetuses squarely on the individual woman. Shaw does not ever suggest that the 'reasonable steps' that she urges 'courts and legislatures' to take include making sure that women have access to good nutrition, housing, education and work so that they are able to provide that 'proper nutrition' and prevent that 'exposure to mutagens and teratogens' that, according to her, every fetus has the 'right' to. This language of 'rights' is not one that argues for social improvements that could benefit women, children, everyone. It is a language of social control. This control is argued perhaps most clearly by John Robertson (1983), professor of law at the University of Texas. His basic proposition is this:

The mother has, if she conceives and chooses not to abort, a legal and moral duty to bring the child into the world as healthy as is reasonably possible. She has a duty to avoid actions or omissions that will damage the fetus. . . . In terms of fetal rights, a fetus has no right to be conceived — or, once conceived, to be carried to viability. But once the mother decides not to terminate the pregnancy, the viable fetus acquires rights to have the mother conduct her life in ways that will not injure it. (ibid.: 438)

This being so, 'Laws that prohibited pregnant women from obtaining or using alcohol, tobacco, or drugs likely to damage the fetus would be constitutional,' (ibid.: 442) and 'statutes excluding pregnant women from workplaces inimical to fetal health . . . would be valid.' (ibid.: 443). Thus:

The behavioral restrictions on pregnant women and the arguments for mandating fetal therapy and prenatal screening illustrate an important limit on a woman's freedom to control her body during pregnancy. She is free not to conceive, and free also to abort after conception and before viability. But once she chooses to carry the child to term, she acquires obligations to assure its wellbeing.

These obligations may require her to avoid work, recreation, and medical care choices that are hazardous to the fetus. They also obligate her to preserve her health for the fetus' sake or even allow established therapies to be performed on an affected fetus. Finally, they require that she undergo prenatal screening where there is reason to believe that this screening may identify congenital defects correctable with available therapies. (ibid.: 450)

This analysis gets women into an interesting predicament, though one with a long history. The same Professor Robertson is also a member of a panel that has proposed a model statute to guarantee a person's right to refuse treatment (Legal Advisors Committee, Concern for Dying, 1983). The first proposition in this statute states: 'A competent person has the right to refuse any medical procedure or treatment.' However, we have just seen that a woman loses this right when she becomes pregnant and decides to carry the fetus to term. Hence, at that point she ceases to be a 'competent person' and comes entirely under the control of physicians and judges.

Thus, by setting up pregnancy as a conflict of rights between a woman and her fetus, attorneys and judges (predominantly male, of course) have injected themselves into the experience of pregnancy where they have appointed themselves advocates for the fetus. Judging by other precedents, this new mechanism of social control could be used against us not only when we are pregnant, but could be expanded to cover all women of childbearing age by invoking 'rights' not just of the fetus we are carrying, but of a 'potential' fetus – the one we may become pregnant with at some future date. As Stellman and Henifin (1982) have shown, the concept of 'potential' pregnancy already has been used by some industries to exclude women from more prestigious and higher-paying employment.

To present pregnancy as a conflict of rights is even more inappropriate than to regard it as a disease. At least, some women do experience pregnancy as disabling. The problem with the disease metaphor is that it does not recognize that the needs of different women are different. Instead, the special needs of some of us are turned into the norm for us all.[5] But the rights metaphor does not at all represent women's experience of a wanted (or accepted) pregnancy – and the above arguments are addressed specifically to accepted pregnancies that will be carried to term. A wanted (or accepted) fetus is as much part of us as any part of our body. And, of course, women should have the means to take proper care of it as part of caring for ourselves, but a fetus does not have separable 'rights' until it is a separate person. We will have to fight this novel attempt to control women, just as we have fought the attempts to control us by defining our ability to bear children as a disease.

## FETAL THERAPY

At present, the status of 'fetal therapy' is somewhat equivocal. After an initial rush of surgical operations on fetuses (see, for example, Birnholz and Frigoletto, 1981; Harrison et al., 1982a) that were hailed in news and feature articles in the press (for example, Boston Globe 1981a, 1981b; Henig, 1982; Hollister, 1983), some of the physicians who pioneered so-called fetal therapy in the US recently issued a warning to go slow (Harrison et al., 1982b). Cynically interpreted, the warning says: 'We have begun to gain experience using these procedures at a few, prestigious teaching hospitals. Let us continue to do them here and don't anybody else get into the act.' For these 'fetal therapists' are far from restrained in their other writings. On the contrary, they wax eloquent – and even poetic – over the prospect of treating fetuses. For example, one of them, Michael R. Harrison, MD (1982), writes in a historical review, entitled 'Unborn: Historical perspective of the fetus as patient' (ibid.: 19):

> The fetus could not be taken seriously as long as he (sic) remained a medical recluse in an opaque womb; and it was not until the last half of this century that the prying eye of the ultrasonogram (that is, ultrasound visualization) rendered the once opaque womb transparent, stripping the veil of mystery from the dark inner sanctum, and letting

the light of scientific observation fall on the shy and secretive fetus. . . . Sonography can accurately delineate normal and abnormal fetal anatomy with astounding detail. It can produce not only static images of the intact fetus, but real-time 'live' moving pictures. And, unlike all previous techniques, ultrasonic imaging appears to have no harmful effects on mother or fetus. The sonographic voyeur, spying on the unwary fetus, finds him or her a surprisingly active little creature, and not at all the passive parasite we had imagined.

Who is 'we'? And Harrison concludes (ibid.: 23, 24):

The fetus has come a long way – from biblical 'seed' and mystical 'homunculus' to an individual with medical problems that can be diagnosed and treated, that is, a patient. Although he (!) cannot make an appointment and seldom even complains, this patient will at times need a physician. . . . Treatment of the unborn has had a long and painstaking gestation; the date of confinement is still questionable and viability uncertain. But there is promise that the fetus may become a 'born again' patient.

Frederic Frigoletto, MD, chief in the new speciality of 'Maternal and Fetal Medicine' at Boston's Brigham and Women's Hospital and another pioneer in 'fetal therapy,' is quoted as follows in an interview in *Patient Care*, a magazine for physicians (Labson, 1983: 105):

[R]eal-time ultrasound – which is now widely available – allows us to develop a composite picture of fetal state; it's almost like going to a nursery school to watch behavior of 3-year-olds. Eventually, we may be able to establish normative behavior for the fetus at various gestational stages. That will help us identify abnormal fetal development, perhaps early enough to be able to correct the environment to treat the fetus in utero.

Considering the personal and social problems that have been created when scientists have tried to establish norms, such as IQ, for real, live people, I can only shudder at the prospect of physicians coming up with norms for fetal 'behavior.' And note that the 'environment' of which Dr Frigoletto speaks happens to be a woman's body; but of course obstetricians for a long time have referred to pregnant women as the 'maternal environment.'

So, the fetus is on its way to becoming a person by virtue of becoming a legitimate patient. And, once the fetus becomes a patient with rights to medical attention, the pregnant woman, as we have seen, may lose her rights to refuse treatment. Not long ago, the same Dr Michael Harrison, with colleagues (Harrison, Golbus and Filly, 1981: 774), wrote in a medical article: 'When the neonate [newborn] will require highly specialized services, transporting the fetus in situ (maternal transport) may be preferable to postnatal transport of the fragile newborn.' So, the woman is not even the 'environment' or 'maternal environment,' but 'the fetus in situ' (*in situ* is Latin for 'in place' and a relatively common expression in scientific writing) – the vessel that can be viewed, poked, moved, medicated, punctured and cut in the interest of the fetus who is the ideal patient – one who does not protest or talk back.

## AND WHAT ABOUT US?

Much as this insults and degrades women, the problem I want to come back to and stress is that many – perhaps most – pregnant women probably will accept these intrusions and will even do so gratefully. For, as long as childbearing is privatized as women's individual responsibility and as long as bearing a disabled child is viewed as a personal failure for which parents (and especially mothers) feel shame and guilt, pregnant women are virtually forced to hail medical 'advances' that promise to lessen the social and financial burdens of bearing a disabled child (however rare and unlikely it may be that any particular one of us will do so). The very availability of the new techniques, however uncertain and unexplored they may be, increases women's isolation by playing on our sense of individual responsibility to produce healthy children. But who is to say what is a healthy child in the face of ever-lengthening lists of metabolic and physical 'defects'? (As of this week's unsubstantiated claims, anorexia nervosa as well as schizophrenia starts in the womb, *Boston Globe*, 1983.) The point I want to stress once more is that even with all conceivable methods of prenatal screening and fetal 'therapy', having children and raising them will continue to be a gamble. And our decision to have them will continue to need to be based on that peculiar mix of unpredictability and planning that makes childbearing and rearing often joyful, often painful and always chancy.

The important agenda for feminist research and activism is not to engage in, and support, expensive and often futile efforts to forestall the unpredictable, but to construct and implement alternatives to the social isolation in which most women in contemporary industrialized and industrializing societies bear and raise children. We have ample descriptions and analyses of what makes these activities difficult. The task now is to work for feasible, positive changes. I firmly believe that the reason many women readily accept untested (or insufficiently tested) technological interventions in their pregnancies is that it is becoming more and more difficult to be a responsible childbearer and mother. We get lots of 'expert' advice, but little or no comradely support. And unless our social conditions and supports improve, women will continue to be lured by every new will o' the wisp that promises to relieve our responsibility for the many different ways in which childbearing and rearing can, and sometimes do, go wrong.

## NOTES

1 I want to thank Renate Duelli Klein for calling my attention to this report and for making a copy of it available to me.
2 I want to thank Barbara Katz Rothman for letting me read the manuscript of her chapter in this collection (Rothman, 1984a) and the proposal for her forthcoming book (Rothman, 1984b).
3 I have written elsewhere about the biological and social limitations that restrict the usefulness of prenatal screening (Hubbard and Henifin, 1984). Tests can inform prospective parents only if they have reason to worry that they may have a child with a particular disability, and only about whether the

fetus in question has that specific health problem, not about its health in general.

4 At the end of a recent review of the effects of ultrasound, two senior members of the Acoustic Radiation Branch at the Bureau of Radiological Health of the US Food and Drug Administration, summarized the situation as follows (Stratmeyer and Christman, 1982: 78):

> Although there is presently no evidence to indicate that diagnostic ultrasound involves a significant risk, the evidence is insufficient to justify an unqualified acceptance of safety. The potential for acute adverse effects has not been systematically explored, and the potential for delayed effects has been virtually ignored. . . . (I)t is unreasonable to expect that in the near future, the degree of risk, if any, will be clearly defined for diagnostic ultrasound. . . . In the meantime, a prudent public health policy calls for judicious use of diagnostic ultrasound, using it only when diagnostic benefits to patients are indicated, and keeping any exposure to diagnostic ultrasound as low as practicable, consistent with its intended purposes.

5 It's as though because some men over fifty get strokes or heart attacks when they are under stress, all men that age were to be barred from positions of responsibility. (Perhaps not such a bad idea?)

# REFERENCES

Arditti, Rita, Renate Duelli Klein and Shelley Minden, eds. 1984. *Test-tube Women – What Future for Motherhood?* Pandora Press, London and Boston.

Birnholz, Jason C. and Frederic D. Frigoletto. 1981. 'Antenatal Treatment of Hydrocephalus.' *New England Journal of Medicine*, 303: 1021–3.

Blumberg, Bruce D., Mitchell S. Golbus and Karl H. Hansen. 1975. 'The psychological sequelae of abortion performed for a genetic indication.' *American Journal of Obstetrics and Gynecology*, 122: 799–808.

Bolsen, Barbara. 1982. 'Question of risk still hovers over routine prenatal use of ultrasound.' *Journal of the American Medical Association*, 247: 2195–7.

*Boston Globe*. 1981a. 'Gains cited in surgery on fetuses.' July 28.

*Boston Globe*. 1981b. 'Human fetus survives surgery, return to womb.' Nov. 15.

*Boston Globe*, 1983. 'Schizophrenia linked to changes in brain cells before birth.' June 7.

Brack, Datha Clapper. 1982. 'Displaced – The Midwife by the Male Physician.' In Hubbard, Ruth, Mary Sue Henifin and Barbara Fried, eds. *Biological Woman – The Convenient Myth*. Schenkman, Cambridge, MA: 207–26.

Davis, Margaret Llewelyn, ed. 1915. *Maternity: Letters from Working Women*. G. Bell, London. Reprinted 1978 by W. W. Norton, New York.

Department of Obstetrics and Gynecology, Tietung Hospital of Anshan Iron and Steel Company, Anshan. 1975. 'Fetal Sex Prediction by sex Chromatin and Chorionic Villi Cells During Early Pregnancy.' *Chinese Medical Journal*, 1: 117–26.

Devitt, Neal. 1979. 'The Statistical Case for Elimination of the Midwife: Facts versus Prejudice, 1890–1935.' *Feminist Studies*. 4: 81–96, 169–85.

Duboudin, Tony. 1983. 'Frozen embryo team defends methods.' *The Times* (London), May 5.

Ehrenreich, Barbara and Deirdre English. 1978. *For Her Own Good*. Anchor Press, New York.

Emecheta, Buchi. 1979. *The Joys of Motherhood*. Braziller, New York.

Fletcher, John C. 1979. 'Ethics and Amniocentesis for Fetal Sex Identification.' *New England Journal of Medicine*, 301: 550–3.

Fletcher, Joseph F. 1980. 'Knowledge, Risk, and The Right to Reproduce: A Limiting Principle.' In Milunsky, Aubrey and George J. Annas, eds. *Genetics and the Law II*. Plenum Press, New York: 131–5.

Glass, Bentley. 1971. 'Science: Endless Horizons or Golden Age?' *Science*, 171: 23–9.

Hanmer, Jalna. 1981. 'Sex predetermination, artificial insemination and the maintenance of male-dominated culture.' In Roberts, Helen, ed. *Women, Health and Reproduction*. Routledge & Kegan Paul, London and Boston: 163–90.

Harrison, Michael R. 1982. 'Unborn: Historical perspective of the fetus as patient.' *Pharos*, Winter: 19–24.

Harrison, Michael R., Mitchell S. Golbus and Roy A. Filly. 1981. 'Management of the Fetus With a Correctable Congenital Defect.' *Journal of the American Medical Association*, 246: 744–7.

Harrison, Michael R. et al. 1982a. 'Fetal Surgery for Congenital Hydronephrosis.' *New England Journal of Medicine*, 306: 591–3.

Harrison, Michael R. et al. 1982b. 'Fetal Treatment 1982.' *New England Journal of Medicine*, 307: 1651–2.

Henig, Robin Marantz. 1982. 'Saving Babies Before Birth.' *New York Times Magazine*, February 28.

Hollister, Anne. 1983. 'Treating the Unborn.' *Life*, April.

Holmes, Helen B., Betty B. Hoskins and Michael Gross, eds. 1981. *The Custom-Made Child?* Humana Press, Clifton, NJ.

Hubbard, Ruth. 1982a. 'Legal and Policy Implications of Recent Advances in Prenatal Diagnosis and Fetal Therapy.' *Women's Rights Law Reporter*, 7: 201–18.

Hubbard, Ruth. 1982b. 'Some Practical and Ethical Constraints on Genetic Decisions about Childbearing.' In Teichler-Zallen, Doris and Colleen D. Clements, eds. *Science and Morality*. Lexington Books, Lexington, MA.

Hubbard, Ruth and Mary Sue Henifin. 1984. 'Genetic Screening of Prospective Parents and of Workers: Some Scientific and Social Issues.' In Humber, James M. and Robert F. Almeder, eds. 1984. *Biomedical Ethics Reviews: 1984*. Humana Press, Clifton, NJ.

Hubbard, Ruth, Mary Sue Henifin and Barbara Fried, eds. 1982. *Biological Woman – The Convenient Myth*. Schenkman, Cambridge, MA.

Humber, James M. and Robert F. Almeder, eds. 1984. *Biomedical Ethics Reviews: 1984*. Humana Press, Clifton, NJ.

Kenen, Regina H. 1981. 'A Look at Prenatal Diagnosis within the Context of Changing Parental and Reproductive Norms.' In Holmes, Helen B., Betty B. Hoskins and Michael Gross, eds. *The Custom-Made Child?* Humana Press, Clifton, NJ: 67–73.

Kitzinger, Sheila. 1979. *Women as Mothers*. Random House, New York.

Labson, Lucy H. 1983. 'Today's view in maternal and fetal medicine.' *Patient Care*, January 15: 105–21.

Legal Advisors Committee, Concern for Dying. 1983. 'The Right to Refuse Treatment: A Model Act.' *American Journal of Public Health*, 73: 918–21.

McDonald, Marian, ed. 1981. *For Ourselves, Our Families, and Our Future*. Red Sun Press, Boston, MA.

Milunsky, Aubrey and George J. Annas, eds. 1980. *Genetics and the Law II*. Plenum Press, New York.

Neilsen, Caroline C. 1981. 'An Encounter with Modern Medical Technology: Women's Experiences with Amniocentesis.' *Women and Health*, 6: 109–24.

*Ob-Gyn News*. 1982. 'Intrauterine Dx Option Becoming Obligation.' September 1–14.

Perry, Ruth. 1979. 'The veil of chastity: Mary Astell's feminism.' *Studies in Eighteenth-Century Culture*, 9: 25–45.

Powledge, Tabitha. 1980. Letters to the Editor. *New England Journal of Medicine*, 302: 524.

Powledge, Tabitha. 1981. 'Unnatural Selection: On Choosing Children's Sex.' In Holmes, Helen B., Betty B. Hoskins and Michael Gross, eds. *The Custom-Made Child?* Humana Press, Clifton, NJ: 193–9.

Rich, Adrienne. 1976. *Of Woman Born*. W. W. Norton, New York.

Roberts, Helen, ed. 1981. *Women, Health and Reproduction.* Routledge & Kegan Paul, London and Boston.

Robertson, John A. 1983. 'Procreative Liberty and the Control of Conception, Pregnancy, and Childbirth.' *Virginia Law Review*, 69: 405–64.

Rodriguez-Trias, Helen. 1982. 'Sterilization Abuse.' In Hubbard, Ruth, Mary Sue Henifin and Barbara Fried, eds. *Biological Woman – The Convenient Myth.* Schenkman, Cambridge, MA: 147–60.

Rothman, Barbara Katz. 1982. *In Labor.* W. W. Norton, New York.

Rothman, Barbara Katz. 1984a. 'The Meanings of Choice in Reproductive Technology.' In Arditti, Rita, Renate Duelli Klein and Shelley Minden, eds. *Test-tube Women – What Future for Motherhood?* Pandora Press, London and Boston, pp. 23–33.

Rothman, Barbara Katz. 1984b. *The Products of Conception: The Genetic Tie.* (Working title) forthcoming. Viking, New York.

Royal College of Obstetricians and Gynaecologists. 1983. *Report of the RCOG Ethics Committee on In Vitro Fertilization and Embryo Replacement or Transfer.* Chameleon, London.

Rutenberg, Sharon. 1983. 'Chicago doctors tell of way to detect birth defects faster.' *Boston Globe*, August 18.

*Science News.* 1983. 'New test for birth defects.' August 20: 116.

Shaw, Margery W. 1980. 'The Potential Plaintiff: Preconception and Prenatal Torts.' In Milunsky, Aubrey and George J. Annas, eds. *Genetics and the Law II.* Plenum, New York: 225–32.

Stellman, Jeanne M. and Mary Sue Henifin. 1982. 'No Fertile Women Need Apply: Employment Discrimination and Reproductive Hazards in the Workplace.' In Hubbard, Ruth, Mary Sue Henifin and Barbara Fried, eds. *Biological Woman – The Convenient Myth.* Schenkman, Cambridge, MA: 117–45.

Stratmeyer, Melvin E. and Christopher L. Christman. 1982. 'Biological Effects of Ultrasound.' *Women and Health*, 7: 65–81.

Teichler-Zallen, Doris and Colleen D. Clements, eds. 1982. *Science and Morality.* Lexington Books, Lexington, MA.

Veitch, Andrew. 1983. 'Pre-natal tests urged to cut stillborn births.' *Guardian* (London and Manchester), May 11.

Wertz, Dorothy C. 1983. 'What Birth Has Done for Doctors: A Historical View.' *Women and Health*, 8: 7–24.

Wertz, Richard W. and Dorothy C. Wertz. 1979. *Lying-In.* Schocken, New York.

Williamson, Robert et al. 1981. 'Direct Gene Analysis of Chorionic Villi: A Possible Technique for First-Trimester Antenatal Diagnostics of Haemoglobinopathies.' *Lancet*, November 21: 1125–7.

# REPRODUCTIVE TECHNOLOGIES: THE FINAL SOLUTION TO THE WOMAN QUESTION?

Robyn Rowland

Feminists are now establishing our position with respect to the new reproductive technologies. Due to a resurgence of pro-motherhood attitudes within the women's movement, many feminists have welcomed technologies which give infertile women children. But we are not considering sufficiently who *controls*, markets, and gains financially by their use. The same people who gave women the Pill, DES, and the Dalkon Shield are now using our bodies once again as living laboratories. They develop technologies which increase the control men have over the actual conception and birth processes, among them sex-preselection and soon to come the artificial womb and placenta. These new technologies have the potential to take the reproduction away from women's bodies. If women do not act now, we may soon be marching for our *right* to bear children and give birth if we want to.

The advent of these new powers for human engineering means that some men may be destined to play God, to re-create other men in their own image.

Leon Kass

Kass is correct in his prediction: ultimately the new reproductive technology will be used for the benefit of men and to the detriment of women. Although technology itself is not always a negative development, the real question has always been — who controls it? Biological technology is in the hands of men.

Feminists have long ignored the movements forward in the reproductive area, being understandably confused and unsure about what position would be ideologically correct and which will be the safest. We have argued for many years that women should be freed from the drudgery and entrapment of enforced maternity. That freedom for some resulted in the imposition of two jobs with their encumbent workloads: home and the workplace. For others it meant the expansion of self and the fulfilment of their potential as human beings of worth.

The feminist position on maternity has often been misrepresented. Early platform statements can be quoted to indicate an anti-family position, and, indeed, the Western nuclear family came to be seen as the fortress of patriarchal dominance and chained, for the most part, to a financially dependent existence: married women worked for no wage, had little job security, could be sexually exploited or abused with the sanction of the law, and had the status of a minor. Within this context there was no *choice* for women – and this is what the women's movement has always fought for. We wanted women to choose to work in the workforce or at home, and to choose whether to have children or not. (These were, however, middle-class choices.)

At the basis of this claim for choice was a denial of an immutable 'maternal instinct'. Women re-evaluated the male 'experts' and found them wanting: 'expert' advice did not fit with women's experience. Bowlby's (1953) trauma-making statements on the fate of children left for an hour while their mother visited the dentist were rejected, though not without an enormous load of guilt for many women (and possibly the concomitant tooth decay!).

A variety of motives and causes were seen to guide women into motherhood. They had children because they were socialized to do so and convinced of the rewards of mothering; in order to gain a self-identity in a world which continually denied this to them; to have a power base from which to negotiate some terms in their lives; to prove their worth and their change of status to that of 'adult'. Feminists came also to validate the life of the childfree woman (childless by choice) and she ceased to be viewed as 'deviant'.

Books like Betty Friedan's *The Feminine Mystique* essentially changed the social attitudes of women to motherhood, freeing us from many of its myths. Effective contraception enabled us to separate sexuality from procreativity and was hailed as a release for women. 'The Pill' gave us greater control over the results of heterosexuality. We were yet to see the side-effects caused by this technology, used prematurely with insufficient research on a willing population of women with a need – the need to have choice.

The issue of choice is again with us, but this time it involves the very creation of human life as we know it. As usual, the technology enabling choice has direct consequences for the well-being and survival of women. Shulamith Firestone argued in 1970 in the *Dialectic of Sex* that 'pregnancy is barbaric . . . the temporary deformation of the body of the individual for the sake of the species' (1972: 188) and that women should be freed from 'the tyranny of reproduction by every means possible' (1972: 193). She envisaged *real* 'test-tube' babies as the answer for women, as long as what she called 'improper control' was not exercised by patriarchy. She had used the availability of contraception as an example of the wonders of modern technology! Indeed, Firestone's idea in its pure form does have its advantages for many women, the main one being that it would allow them to choose the manner in which their child is created and developed.

However, a groundswell of women within the movement has begun to reassess the value of biological maternity. Reacting against the feeling that the women's movement coerced them to give up having children, many feminists are striving to create the experience of maternity and family in a non-exploitative way. Adrienne Rich (1977) has pointed out that it is the patriarchal institutionalization of motherhood which is the problem, not motherhood itself. Betty Friedan, in her controversial book *The Second Stage* (1981), made a desperate attempt to reclaim the family as of value, writing that 'our failure was a blind spot about the family' (1981: 203), and that the women's movement has had an extreme reaction against motherhood. Right-wing antifeminist women have used this book as a stick with which to beat feminism, claiming that the only true role for women is motherhood – also an extreme reaction. In a book I recently edited, *Women Who Do and Women Who Don't, join the women's movement*, this issue clearly arose as a major division among women. Antifeminists in fact experience motherhood and the family as their primary power base while many feminists have argued that, for many, motherhood is experienced as inferior. The social class of the woman has a great bearing on this of course: motherhood is more enjoyable the richer you are.

In *Women Who Do and Women Who Don't* Anne Curthoys as a feminist has written a provocative view of the family, claiming that for all its disadvantages, the family does fulfill the real needs of people for 'security, commitment and continuity'. Barbara Wishart (1982), an Australian lesbian mother who conceived her daughter through artificial insemination, has also stressed that it is not motherhood itself that oppresses women but the structures within which motherhood is experienced. There is still 'something *positive* or *worthwhile* or even *wonderful* about being a mother' (1982: 27). In fact then, the dilemma over motherhood and the family remains strong within the women's movement.

The advent of the Pill is now viewed with some scepticism by feminists. We found that there was a price to pay in terms of women's health, and in the fact that we could be even more readily exploited as sexual objects for male gratification when there was no fear of pregnancy, and therefore no responsibility for their actions on the part of men should a pregnancy result. Many feminists suspect that the 'sexual revolution' was a new form of enslavement for women. We have to ask did we learn anything from the invention and use of the Pill. As Roberta Steinbacher says: 'Who invented it, who manufactured it, who licensed it, who dispenses it? But who dies from it?' (1981: 189).

Today we are about to see the separation of reproduction from women's bodies and it is time *now* to consider the possibilities this opens up for women and the dangers to us which lie ahead. We should not wait, as we did with the Pill, until we are twenty years too late.

I have been conducting research into the social and psychological consequences of artificial insemination using unknown male donors and have had contact with many infertile couples. The need for a child and the desire towards that end is so strong that initially it shocked me. Over a period of two years I have developed an overwhelming sympathy and empathy for the plight of the infertile. But I cannot divorce this from the feeling that they are being used by the medical profession in order to gain funding for research which is not necessarily intended to help the infertile person. We have all heard, and at times been swayed by, the argument that medical advances which help people are often off-shoots of seemingly distant or unrelated research. These studies help to keep funding available for the seemingly unrelated research – because you just never know what might turn up!

There are so many issues involved in this area of technology that we are just beginning to formulate the questions. Trust in the medical profession on the part of clients and of the community is incredibly strong. Time and again women have taken the brunt of the mistakes and exploitation of medicine (see Ehrenreich and English, 1978) and yet we continue to allow the 'profession' to use our bodies as laboratories. The trust is so often misplaced. I came across an incidence in my research on artificial insemination where a physician, Schoysman, in two separate incidences, used a brother's sperm to inseminate a wife without her knowledge or consent. He writes:

> In order to limit as much as possible future
> indiscretions the wives both of the donor and of the
> receiving couple were not made aware of this decision.
> Considering that the result of these two particular cases is
> the creation of happy family relationships, we have no
> regrets. (1975: 35)

Schoysman, in fact, could not judge the happiness or otherwise of the relationships involved, but in the name of 'happy families' unethical situations can be easily reconciled to conscience.

From the same medocrats who gave us the Pill, DES and the Dalkon Shield, now comes a new adventure which may end with the artificial baby – sex of choice – and synthetic birth. Is this the beginning of 'previctimization,' as Janice

Raymond calls it – the destruction of women before they are even born? Two areas of research which are speeding ahead and warrant a close look are sex preselection and the development of the artificial womb and placenta.

There are two ways of ensuring the sex of a child. The first is to use amniocentesis to assess the sex of the foetus and abort if the sex is undesirable. This allows the couple to avoid actually killing a *baby* if it is a girl – it's tidier femicide. The other more subtle method is to determine the sex of the child *before* conception – preconception sexism. Researchers are currently working on a number of methods of conducting this preselection but most involve artificial insemination at the moment (see Betty Hoskins and Helen B. Holmes in this collection for details on sex-selection technologies).

Studies by a variety of social scientists have shown that a majority of all societies have a strong preference for male offspring. Social values in most societies mean that males have greater prestige and power, and male children are therefore more status-generating for the parents. Women who bear sons are still rewarded by social approval in a variety of forms and the line of inheritance is assured within patriarchy. Nancy Williamson (1976) has conducted studies in a variety of countries and finds this predominance of male-preference. Those 'very few' societies which desire female offspring were classified as indicating a 'deviant preference'. These communities are not female-dominant and do not value women because they signify power and status, but because they are valuable chattels or commodities within the marriage or work markets. Colin Campbell (1976) has indicated, furthermore, that in China where abortion is available and people are encouraged to have only one child, most aborted foetuses are girls.

In societies where people could still have two children, the rate of first-born males would dramatically increase. Roberta Steinbacher (1981) has indicated the strong documentation in support of this. The frightening aspect is that first-borns have been shown to be generally more intelligent and achievement-oriented, more successful, independent and higher in self-esteem than their brothers and sisters. We would therefore be building the traditional sex-role stereotypes *into* a biological determinism. Males would be more stereotypically male; and second-born females more stereotypically feminine. Second-class status would be assured; pre-determined.

And the class situation is even more invidious. Abortion is more difficult for poor women to obtain; so too would access to sex preselection be class-regulated. These women would be trapped into normal birth/sex ratios. Already the issue has arisen with surrogate mothers. Those seeking surrogates have been found to be 'highly intelligent professionals in the thirty to forty age group . . . they know a lot about surrogacy; they know what they want and they know how to bend the rules their way'.[1] And who are the surrogates whose bodies are used as incubators? Could they be working-class women who need the money? Remember the wet-nurse system of the nineteenth century when working-class women were exploited by those who could afford them. If surrogate-users decide to sex preselect as well we will have an interesting situation: working-class women's bodies used to produce the next generation of male power-holders. Non-surrogate women in the working class will still produce girls, sex preselection being costly, while the powerful will select male offspring. The majority of women will still therefore be locked into poverty and locked out of access to financial power. The basic racism of whites will also ensure that non-white women have limited access to the new technology.

The scenario to this is very unpleasant. With an increase in males, particularly first-born males, Campbell predicts a concomitant rise in male values: aggression, sexual pressure on women, alcoholism. 'More of everything, in short, that men do, make, suffer, inflict and consume' (1976: 88). In addition, as males are physically the weaker sex, more ill-health and early death will result. Women will be run off their feet supporting the sick and dying, as well as the wounded and battered, results of male violence and war. Already women are the less powerful, more exploited, raped and poor social group – and we have the numbers! Imagine how tenuous will be our hold on life and security if our numbers are severely depleted. Women's culture, which is already systematically discarded, will be crushed, and without a sense of community of culture, our sex would lose the bonds of strength we now grapple to share. Without women we face a future without hope.

It is that life-force in women which men have always sought to control. How powerful we have always seemed; we who can bleed regularly and not die; we who can grow another human being inside our own bodies. Dubious though it has been in real terms, this has since 'primitive' times been a source of mythical power for women when all else was kept from them. For many women it is the *only* experience of power they will ever have. And men have coveted that last of powers. Men's myths have continuously expressed their fear, awe, and envy of it, and they have repeatedly tried to control it. They renounced the midwives and made a profession out of studying women's bodies; they frequently express their anger, resentment, and hatred of women through violence against our bodies; they have controlled and regulated our choice with respect to our bodies, controlling contraception, controlling abortion. Now, with the possibilities offered by technology they are storming the last bastion and taking control of conception, foetal development, and birth. There is nothing 'rational' in this, as Campbell warns, 'there are also dreams at work, and ancient aspirations'. (1976: 91)

A second development of immediate concern is that of the artificial placenta and womb. Babies born prematurely can now be adequately cared for in an incubator. Research into perfecting these incubators can thus be justified so that younger and younger premature babies can be kept alive. If we look at it now from the conception end, after in vitro fertilization, embryos are being kept alive no longer than seven days. Imagine the potential of the perfected artificial womb. An egg could be fertilized and grown to maturity within an incubator. What would it be like to be an adult who had never been borne or experienced birth; who had never grown to life within a woman's womb?

R. John Buuck (1977) has pointed out that the greatest challenge still in this area is the perfection of the placenta. An incubator can supply heat and oxygen and force the foetus to breathe, but the exchange of waste material for nutrients, which the placenta carries out, has not yet been imitated.

Buuck then concluded that the only obstacle at that time was a lack of national commitment to such a development. He pointed out that after the artificial womb is perfected the relationship 'of women to children and women to men will be affected' (1977: 546). But he did not suggest *how* they will be affected!

Edward Grossman (1971) does attempt predictions. He discusses the new branch of medicine called 'fetology'. The advantages to the nation of the artificial womb are as follows: foetal medicine would be much improved (!); the child could be immunized while still inside the 'womb'; the environment would be *safer* for the foetus than a woman's womb, and geneticists could programme in some superior trait 'on which society could agree'; sex preselection would be simple: women would be 'spared the discomfort' of childbirth and the danger of miscarriage; men would be able to prove for the first time who is the father of the child; and women could be permanently sterilized. He sees these advances as a great advantage for women who would 'gain the most'. Day care would be no problem as children could be kept in communal centres after their laboratory births.

Grossman writes that 'natural pregnancy may become an anachronism . . . the uterus will become appendixlike' (1971: 49). Do you get the feeling that Firestone's vision has been manipulated? Isn't it true that feminists have wanted relief from pregnancy and child-rearing; isn't it true that we wanted technology to help the infertile and save premature babies? As Dr Robert Edwards, the medical 'father' of the first 'test-tube' baby in Britain, said: 'We tell these women, "Your only hope is to help us" ' (Grossman, 1971: 45). And women have been helping, colluding in the development of new technology by offering our bodies once again as living laboratories. Grossman points out that it was women who first saw the 'greatness' of their 'benefactor' who introduced anaesthetics in childbirth, and 'displayed uncomplicated enthusiasm, which finally proves more effective than anything else in overcoming tradition' (40). So our enthusiasm certainly helps. But Grossman also points out the inevitability of these advances, even if no support is forthcoming, concluding: 'Certainly it would take more exertion over the long term to prevent it, than to achieve it, and why prevent it.' (50) This is resonant of Buuck's comments that little is being said about cloning because the reaction of the public might reduce the limited money available for research. We have fought so hard against women being *impelled* to have children. Will we soon be fighting for the *right* to have them, and to have them naturally?

Well, why prevent it? And *can* we prevent it? Women are grossly underrepresented in the medical and biological research fields, as well as in the areas where policy decisions are made. As man gets closer to reproducing himself, what forces can possibly stop him? One way is to stop colluding, but we need first to convince people of the dangers ahead. These are for the most part unknown, which stops us from even attempting to imagine them. The attitudes of the researchers are evident. Grossman comments that 'it will mean that the awefulness associated with pregnancy and childbirth will have nothing to feed on, and motherhood, if it continues to excite any awe at all, will not do so more than fatherhood.' (48) Here is man's control of the awesome power of women; the last stronghold of nature which he can finally dominate. Will this last act of power make woman obsolete; permanently unemployed; disposable? Will it allow the bodily mutilation which has been so much a part of our herstory to be concluded, manifesting the inevitable culmination of misogyny? In discussing hysterectomy, Richard Taylor quotes one gynaecologist thus: 'After the last planned pregnancy the uterus becomes a useless, bleeding, symptom-producing, potentially cancer-bearing organ and therefore should be removed' (1979: 162). Is this woman hating, womb envy? What would be the scenario if there were *never* a need for planned pregnancies in the first place? Surely it would seem logical to eliminate this so-dreadful a part of women's bodies at puberty to avoid all this potential harm, and the possibility of an unplanned natural pregnancy.

Two notable men have already presented their misogynistic visions of the way ahead. John Postgate, professor of microbiology in Great Britain, has given a horrendous picture of the future, which Campbell warns is not intended as satire. Arguing that the world population is out of control,

Postgate suggests the need for a pill which would ensure
male offspring – the Manchild Pill. He points out that, after
all, in the great majority of countries people primarily *want*
male children. And a pill for selecting female offspring 'would
not work' because women will not or cannot stop breeding!
The transition stage of this new world would be a little
difficult to adjust to at first. A form of 'purdah' would be
necessary; 'women's right to work, even to travel alone freely,
would possibly be forgotten transiently' (1973: 16). (Does
anyone remember that mythical period?) Polyandry would be
necessary and some societies 'might treat their women as
queen ants, others as rewards for the most outstanding (or
most determined) males' (16). Homosexuality among men
would be supplemented with artificial forms of sex. Postgate
is uncertain about whether the world would resemble a huge
male prison or a boy's public school – we can wonder at the
difference he imagines between the two – but he does imagine
that the difficulties would be mainly a matter of 'taste'.

Postgate's article is resonant with its lack of understanding of the complexity of social relationships and its failure to
consider even momentarily the experience of women in such
a sexual imbalance. A scarcity of women has never led to
their rise in status, as evidenced in the brutality of the early
west of America and the foundations of Australian society. In
these instances women are forced to be extremely moralistic
in order to protect themselves, or to prostitute themselves for
a different kind of protection. In Australia, where men
initially outnumbered women five to one, this led to the
division of women into *Damned Whores and God's Police*
(Summers, 1975). In Postgate's world the abuse of women
would be on a massive scale, as men demanded sexual satisfaction and breeding rights from the diminishing numbers.
In all probability, suicide rates for women would escalate
dramatically. Another male expert's viewpoint – William
Shockley's – is much 'tidier' than Postgate's, possibly
reflective of his standing as a Nobel Laureate for his work
with transistors! It does still rely on 'natural' childbirth, but
gives us an idea of the controls envisaged by some of our
scientists. He suggests that all girls be sterilized on entering
puberty by an injection of a contraceptive time capsule which

seeps contraceptives into the girl until it is time for her to conceive. At marriage she is issued with deci-child certificates, payment of which will enable her to have a doctor remove the capsule. It is replaced when the child is born. If the state deems it desirable that a couple have two children, the appropriate number of certificates would belong to the couple. If they decided to remain childfree or have only one child, they could sell their surplus certificates on the open market. Thus the child as property concept reaches its logical conclusion in the child as commodity concept.

And who would control this dystopian bleak future? The state would ultimately have to organize and run things, with particular expertise from medical researchers. As Kass, himself a doctor, has said, power 'rests only metaphorically with human kind, it rests in fact with particular men geneticists, embryologists, obstetricians' (1972: 45). Males run the governments, train the doctors, make birth control devices, decide on the availability of abortion, own the companies who will market the products and make the money. And man *will* reproduce himself in his own image as he has managed to produce God in his own image.

The fact is that *all* women are guinea pigs in this exercise. We have not been included in decisions about the technology, not asked if we want it. Are we again to collude with patriarchy because our own momentary needs or desires blind us to the social responsibilities we must have to our daughters; to those who come after us and want the experience of natural conception and childbirth? Jalna Hanmer and Pat Allen have commented that 'women have acted, and do act, as agents of male individual and social power' (1982: 69). Often this compliance is through ignorance. We must not turn from this difficult area of technology as if it is only relevant to infertile couples seeking children, and that any statements of hesitation on our part strikes at their 'rights' to have a child if they can. What may be happening is the last battle in the long war of men against women. Women's position is most precarious. The medical profession continues to work in many areas unknown to the general community, and does so in the guise of helping women. We need to draw a distinction between helping the infertile and experimenting further with the most basic aspect of human life – its creation. In terms of the marketplace, if we do not educate ourselves on these issues, and develop a viewpoint on which we can act, we may find ourselves without a product of any kind with which to bargain. For the history of 'mankind' women have been seen in terms of their value as child-bearers. We have to ask, if that last power is taken and controlled by men, what role is envisaged for women in the new world? Will women become obsolete? Will we be fighting to retain or reclaim the right to bear children – has patriarchy conned us once again? I exhort you sisters to be vigilant.

In her moving poem 'The Right to Life' Marge Piercy writes: 'Without choice, no politics, no ethics lives'. (1980: 97) This choice includes the choice to create children the way we want to create them.

## NOTE

1 Newspaper article by Lucy Twomey. 1983. 'Surrogate motherhood: A blessing or exploitation?' *Australian*, May 2.

## REFERENCES

Bowlby, John. 1953. *Child Care and the Growth of Love*. Penguin, Harmondsworth.

Buuck, R. John. 1977. 'Ethics of reproductive engineering.' *Perspectives*, **39**, (9): 545–7.

Campbell, Colin. 1976. 'The Manchild Pill.' *Psychology Today*, August: 86–91.

Curthoys, Ann. 1984. In Rowland, R., ed. *Women Who Do and Women Who Don't, join the women's movement*. Routledge & Kegan Paul, London.

Ehrenreich, Barbara and Deirdre English. 1978. *For Her Own Good: 150 Years of the Expert's Advice to Women*. Doubleday, Garden City.

Firestone, Shulamith. 1972. *The Dialectic of Sex*. Paladin, London. First published in 1970 by Morrow, New York.

Friedan, Betty. 1963. *The Feminine Mystique*. Penguin, Harmondsworth.

Friedan, Betty. 1981. *The Second Stage*. Summit Books, New York.

Grossman, Edward. 1971. 'The Obsolescent Mother. A Scenario.' *Atlantic*, 227: 39–50.

Hanmer, Jalna and Allen, Pat. 1982. 'Reproductive engineering: The final solution?' *Feminist Issues*, 2 (1): 53–75.

Kass, Leon. 1972. 'Making babies – the new biology and the "old" morality.' *Public Interest*, Whiter: 13–56.

Piercy, Marge. 1980. 'The Right to Life'. In *The Moon is Always Female*, Alfred Knopf, New York.

Postgate, John. 1973. 'Bat's chance in hell.' *New Scientist*, 5: 11–16.

Raymond, Janice. 1981. In Holmes, Helen, Betty Hoskins and Michael Gross, eds. *The custom-made child? Women-centered perspectives*. Humana Press, New Jersey.

Rich, Adrienne. 1977. *Of Woman Born. Motherhood as Experience and Institution*. Virago, London.

Rowland, R., ed. 1984. *Women Who Do and Women Who Don't, join the women's movement*. Routledge & Kegan Paul, London.

Schoysman, R. 1975. 'Problems of selecting donors for artificial insemination.' *Journal of Medical Ethics*, 1 (1): 34–5.

Steinbacher, Roberta. 1981. 'Futuristic implications of sex preselection.' In Holmes, H., B. Hoskins and M. Gross. eds. *The custom-made child? Women-centered perspectives*. Humana Press, New Jersey.

Summers, Anne. 1975. *Damned Whores and God's Police. The Colonization of Women in Australia*. Penguin, Melbourne.

Taylor, Richard. 1979. *Medicine out of Control*. Sun Books, Melbourne.

Williamson, Nancy, 1976. *Sons or daughters. A cross-cultural survey of parental preferences*. Sage, London.

Wishart, Barbara. 1982. 'Motherhood within patriarchy: A radical feminist perspective.' *Third Women and Labour Conference Papers*, 1: 23–31.

# WOMEN TAKING CONTROL: A WOMB OF ONE'S OWN

# CHILDREN BY DONOR INSEMINATION: A NEW CHOICE FOR LESBIANS

Francie Hornstein

In spite of the many difficulties involved in making any kind of far-reaching change, donor insemination has been an enormously exciting step in breaking through the constraints placed on women by sexist prohibitions. It has opened the door for allowing women to arrange their lives in a way that best suits their needs. For lesbians and some heterosexual women, donor insemination represents a new reproductive choice — and one which can remain in our control.

My decision to conceive a child by donor insemination was a long time coming. It was nearly seven years between the time I first considered the possibility and when I began trying to get pregnant. The one recurring reservation in what had become a passionate desire to have children was my fear for how the children would cope with being from a different kind of family.

I knew I would be sorry if I never had children; sorry not only for giving up a part of life I really wanted, but for not making a decision that I believed was right. I felt I was as worthy of having children as any other person. To not have children simply because I was a lesbian would have been giving up on a goal that was very dear to me.

I had always wanted to have children. I can remember when I was very young, as far back as elementary school, being afraid that I would never have children because I didn't think I would ever get married. Of course when I was eight years old I didn't realize that I was lesbian — I just could never imagine myself married to a man. Marrying a woman might have been more appealing, but that option was never presented to me.

No one has yet written a chronicle of feminist-controlled donor insemination, though some of us are beginning to collect information. It seems that small groups of women in different parts of the country began discussing and actually doing donor insemination beginning in the middle to late 1970s. For the most part, we were unaware of one another's existence. It wasn't until after several of us had children and either heard about each other through the grapevine or met at conferences that we began comparing notes.

I first tried donor insemination in 1973, while I was working at the Feminist Women's Health Center in Los Angeles. I was unable to use the services of the sperm bank because they would only accept married women as candidates for insemination. It was difficult finding donors and I was absorbed in long hours of work in the women's health movement, so the work involved in my getting pregnant was shelved for a few years. With the help of my co-workers and the encouragement of my lover, I finally began trying to get pregnant in 1977.

I think it was significant that I was working at the Feminist Women's Health Center at the time I got pregnant. It seemed particularly fitting that the same women who developed the practice of menstrual extraction, a procedure which could be used for early abortion, also were among the pioneers in the practice of self-help donor insemination. We figured if we could safely help a woman end her pregnancy without the help of physicians and patriarchal laws, we could certainly help women get pregnant.

My co-workers at the FWHC and I learned how to do the insemination in the same self-help way we learned about other aspects of women's health. We read medical journals and textbook articles, talked with physicians who did the procedure and combined that information with plain, down-to-earth common sense.

Finding donors was the most difficult part of the whole process for me. At the time I got pregnant, there was only one sperm bank in the city. It was owned and operated by a physician who had a private infertility practice and who was very conservative in selecting his clientele. He declined to make his services available to women who were not married, not to mention lesbians.

The only option open to us at the time was to find donors through our friends. I wanted to be able to give the children the option of knowing their father, so we preferred a situation in which the donor was known either to us or to a friend. Eventually, we were able to find donors.

The insemination itself was simple. All we had to do was have the donor ejaculate into a clean container, draw up the semen into a clean syringe (with the needle removed) and inject it into the vagina. We already knew how to do vaginal self-examination with a speculum, so we were familiar with the anatomy of the cervix, the opening of the uterus where the sperm needs to be put. Other women we later spoke with who didn't have access to medical supplies, such as syringes, improvised with common household items. A turkey baster, now synonymous with self-help insemination, works just fine. One innovative woman had her donor ejaculate into a condom, then she simply turned the condom inside-out in her vagina. Some women either insert a diaphragm or cervical cap to hold the semen near the cervix or they lie down for a half-hour or so after inserting the semen.

After our son was born, in the fall of 1978, my lover and I were asked to talk about our experiences at a variety of feminist conferences and programs. It was then that we began meeting other women who either had children or wanted to have children by donor insemination. Since that time, we have personally met women from several states and Canada and have heard about women from England and throughout Europe who are also having children by donor insemination, without the assistance of physicians. We have met two women who had children before 1978, but are sure there must be others. We had also heard that women in England had been using donor insemination for a number of years before women in the US. A friend visited a woman in England who has a 12-year-old son conceived by donor insemination.

The majority of women we have met who have had children by donor insemination are lesbians, though there is now a growing number of single, heterosexual women who are choosing donor insemination as a way of getting pregnant. Some of these women prefer being single, but want to have children; others haven't yet met men they want to live with or have children with, but because of their age or other reasons, don't want to wait for marriage before having children.

Several feminist health groups have begun making donor insemination available to women who ordinarily would not be able to use the services of sperm banks. In 1978, the Feminist Women's Health Center in Los Angeles began a donor insemination program. A commercial sperm bank had just opened up in the city and the only requirement for obtaining sperm from them was a physician's order. The FWHC used their staff physicians to order sperm for women requesting insemination. The Vermont Women's Health Center and the Chelsea Health Center in New York City also assisted women in getting pregnant by donor insemination. In 1982, the Oakland Feminist Women's Health Center began their own sperm bank, the Sperm Bank of Northern California, tailor-making the health services to conform to their own feminist values and expectations rather than the medical model of the traditional sperm banks.[1]

The Oakland FWHC program varies from other sperm banks in a number of important ways. The aspects that distinguish their services are their willingness to provide sperm to any woman, regardless of her marital status, sexual preference, or physical disability; their provision of extensive, but non-identifying social and health background information of donors; a policy which permits women to examine a catalogue of donor information and to select their own donor; and possibly most important, a donor 'release-of-information contract' which donors have the option of signing which gives their consent to provide their name to any children conceived from their sperm, when the child reaches the age of majority.

One thing the feminist health services have in common with one another is their attempt to demedicalize the procedure of donor insemination. In most instances, physicians do not perform the insemination. Although the feminist health workers are willing to assist their clients who ask for their help, they prefer to provide the information so that women can do the insemination themselves, most often with the help of lovers or friends.

The intention on the part of feminist health services who provide donor insemination is less a desire to branch out into additional services but rather a strong political statement in support of a woman's right to make her own reproductive decisions. The feminist clinics find themselves in the unique position of having physicians on staff who have access to commercial sperm banks and want to make the resource available to the community. But they are adamant about their belief that physicians should not make decisions for women about whether or not they will have children. Because of the services provided by the Oakland Feminist Women's Health Center and the other clinics, and the work of women who have done self-help donor insemination and who are talking publicly about their experiences, a great many women, particularly lesbians, are now able to have children by donor insemination.

In discussing women's rights to make reproductive decisions, the positive impact of self-help donor insemination cannot be underestimated. But the practice does not exist in isolation and carries its fair share of potential problems and unanswered questions.

A woman deciding to have children on her own terms and without the inclusion of an on-site father is seen as attacking the traditional notion of a proper family. In spite of the fact that a large proportion of children end up living with their mothers only, it remains more threatening to patriarchy for a woman to *choose* to set up such an arrangement than to merely end up that way as a result of divorce, desertion or death.

While feminists are trying to make room for a variety of acceptable models for families, a number of patriarchal institutions are objecting to donor insemination as a means for creating a different kind of social unit. One incident is particularly illustrative of the reaction of the medical establishment and the state and local government to a woman's choosing to become pregnant by donor insemination.

In 1981, a woman in Milwaukee, Wisconsin, was inseminated by a physician and became pregnant. The woman was single and employed in a part-time job which did not provide health insurance coverage. She subsequently applied for medical assistance from the county social service agency for help in paying her maternity care bills. She was told that she would also qualify for Aid to Families with Dependent Children (AFDC) after her baby was born. The incident began the first public skirmish in the country about the rights of a single woman to have children by donor insemination.

The medical community was divided on the issue, with a number of outspoken physicians calling for a ban on the insemination of single women who could not prove financial stability. Although the physician who inseminated the woman held firm to his belief that a woman has the right to decide to bear children, the situation incensed other physicians and politicians who thought a single woman, especially a low-income single woman, had no right to intentionally have children.

Conservative politicians in the city and state governments called for actions ranging from a resolution for the county to file a paternity suit against the woman's physician to an amendment to a bill introduced into the state legislature which would have considered it unprofessional conduct for a physician to inseminate a woman under similar circumstances. The bill was vetoed by the governor.[2]

For the most part, women who are having children by donor insemination are not in such a public spotlight. Yet there are still a number of difficult issues we must face – even under the best of circumstances. We must all decide what to tell our children about their fathers. Our families, who may not share our feminist perspectives yet whose attachments we don't want to lose, often find it difficult to accept our lesbian families and our decisions to have children. Our children may well want to have contact or relationships with their fathers (in the event that they are known and can be located). We need to establish and protect the rights of partners of lesbians who may not be biological parents of the child, but who may be parents in every other sense of the word. And what do we do when a known donor who, after the baby is born, has a change of heart and wants more of a relationship with the child than was his original intention? These are all real issues that have and will continue to come up.

In addition to creating a new option for lesbians and other women who find that donor insemination is, for them, the best way to have children, it has been reassuring and exciting that a variety of support systems have grown right along with the numbers of women who have children by this method. Several feminist attorneys around the country have acquired considerable information about legal implications of donor insemination and have provided invaluable assistance to those of us having children. In many cities, women who have children or want to have children by donor insemination have started information and support groups. The groups provide as much benefit for the children as for the mothers. Even though the children are all still fairly young, they are growing up knowing that there are other children whose families are like theirs.

I think it is unwise and dishonest to gloss over many of the complex issues involved in donor insemination. Serious consideration and care must be taken for our children as they grow. Our children are not subjects in a social experiment but human beings with feelings whom we deeply love. There needs to be continuous support for mothers and for the rights of non-biological mothers who are part of the children's lives. We need to recognize the interests of the donors. But in the midst of trying to carve out new ways of doing things in an ethical way, we should also take joy in the fact that we have broken new ground. We have created new and important life choices for many people. We have taken back a little more of what is rightly ours – the chance to make decisions about how we will live our lives.

## NOTES

1 Information about the Sperm Bank of Northern California was obtained in a personal communication with Laura Brown,

Director of the Oakland Feminist Women's Health Center. The services of the Sperm Bank can be made available to interested people living outside the Northern California area. For more information write: Sperm Bank of Northern California, 2930 McClure Street, Oakland, CA. 94609.

2  Facts about the Milwaukee, Wisconsin, donor insemination case were provided in a personal communication with Dan Wikler, Program in Medical Ethics, Center for Health Sciences, University of Wisconsin.

## BIBLIOGRAPHY OF RELATED ARTICLES

Annas, George J. 1978. 'Artificial Insemination: Beyond the Best Interests of the Donor.' Hastings Center Report, August. A look at the legal aspects of donor insemination with emphasis on unanswered questions for the recipient of the sperm and for the child born as a result of the insemination.

'Artificial Insemination Packet.' 1981. Available from Lesbian Mother National Defense Fund, P.O. Box 21567, Seattle, Washington, 98111; $3. A collection of articles that cover the 'how to' medical and legal aspects of donor insemination.

Federation of Feminist Women's Health Centers. 1981. A New View of A Woman's Body. Simon & Schuster, New York.

Federation of Feminist Women's Health Centers. 1981. How to Stay Out Of the Gynecologists Office. Peace Press, Culver City, CA. Both of the above books include short sections on donor insemination.

Hitchens, Donna J. 1981. 'Lesbians Choosing Motherhood: Legal Implications of Donor Insemination.' Available from Lesbian Rights Project, 1370 Mission Street, San Francisco, CA. 94103; $1.50 incl. postage. An article describing the legal implications of donor insemination (custody, child support, visitation, and nomination of a guardian) with a focus on the special problems encountered by lesbians. The article discusses the benefits and risks of doing one's own insemination, using a known donor and entering into a contract with the donor. Also included are sample (1) donor-mother agreement; (2) nomination of a guardian for the child; (3) agreement for co-mothers; and (4) will provision for nominating a guardian.

Hornstein, Francie. 1974. 'Lesbian Health Care.' Available from the Feminist Women's Health Center, 6411 Hollywood Boulevard, L.A., CA. 90028. A first-person narrative outlining the issues of lesbian health care in the context of the feminist movement. Includes a section on options for lesbians who want children. Since this article was written in 1974, it is now more an interesting piece of history rather than an up-to-date monograph.

Kritchevsky, Barbara. 1981. 'The Unmarried Woman's Right to Artificial Insemination: A Call for an Expanded Definition of Family.' *Harvard Women's Law Journal*, 1. An excellent and comprehensive article on the legal implications of donor insemination. The only resource that pulls together cases and statutes on artificial insemination.

Moira, Fran. 1982. 'Lesbian Self-Insemination: Life Without Father.' *Off Our Backs*, XII, January 1982. Interviews with women considering donor insemination; an overview of what's happening and the concerns of lesbians.

'Self-Insemination.' 1980. Available from the Feminist Self-Insemination Group, P.O. Box No. 3, 190 Upper Street, London, N1, United Kingdom; £2.00. (See article in this publication by Renate Duelli Klein.)

Stern, Susan. 1980. 'Lesbian Insemination.' *Co-Evolution Quarterly*, Summer. Accounts of several lesbians conceiving by donor insemination and the gay men donating sperm to them.

Sutton, B. 1980. 'The Lesbian Family: Rights in Conflict Under the CH Uniform Parentage Act.' 10 *Golden Gate Law Review*, 1007. How the rights of a lesbian mother might be limited where there is a known donor. The first article that discusses the legal implications of artificial insemination for lesbians.

# DOING IT OURSELVES: SELF INSEMINATION

Renate Duelli Klein

The following report introduces the concept of women-controlled artificial insemination. Self insemination, as defined by a London-based group of lesbian feminists, is much more than the actual process of getting pregnant without the interference of a man as sexual partner or medical adviser. They see it as a liberating new approach to the concept of parenting in which the conventional 'one child-one mother' relationship is exchanged for a close interrelationship of a group of mothers and their children.

> In October 1978 a small group of lesbian feminists met together through an 'ad' in the London Women's Liberation Newsletter to talk about artificial insemination and to work out ways of getting pregnant through insemination by organising it ourselves. We called our process Self Insemination. (Feminist Self Insemination Group, 1980: 3)[1]

By 1980, 6 women had organised themselves as The Feminist Self Insemination Group and had produced a fifty-page pamphlet which explained the practicalities as well as the personal processes and decisions of their involvement with Self Insemination (SI). The women describe themselves:

> We are all white, middle class lesbian-feminists (and later inserted 'able bodied'). We all have to work full or part time to support ourselves, or claim Social Security. Jobs we have had include teacher, social/community workers, advice worker. Housing is a problem, but we all have a roof over our heads. We live in multi-ethnic areas of London. Some of these factors helped us in following the SI process, and help

us now we have children. (Feminist Self Insemination
Group, 1980: 6)

By 1983, more than 1,000 copies of their self-published
pamphlets had been sold, and, importantly, several children
have been born.

Five of the women continue to meet as friends, and as
*joint mothers* to their children. They also function as a
support group and continue to distribute their pamphlet and
to empty their P.O. Box with its innumerable letters from
readers world-wide: there is a constant flow of international
queries and comments which began with the publication of
their pamphlet in 1980, and puts considerable strain on the
small group of women who give advice – all unpaid and in
their spare time.[2] Although no official figures are known, it
appears as if some other SI groups exist in the UK (and in
other European countries, notably Holland), one of which is
known as the Girl Babies Group (London).[3]

That there must be a self-organised, autonomous way for
women who want to get pregnant by artificial insemination
by donor (AID), without the restrictions of 'expert' help by a
doctor, was the starting point of the group's research into IS
in 1978. Intrigued by a piece on AID published in 1978 in the
*Evening News*[4] which made artificial insemination the prerogative of the (male) medical establishment and was critical
of lesbian motherhood, the women set out to challenge such
patriarchal wisdom. As they say in their SI pamphlet
(Feminist SI Group, 1980: 3):

> In writing and publishing it we recognise, validate and
> make public our effort to find a woman-controlled method
> of conception. We wish to make our information and
> feelings available as widely as possible to combat incorrect
> information and mystification, and make self insemination
> something which can be openly discussed, as well as giving
> other women information on which to act.

Indeed, the 'mechanics' of SI are incredibly easy (ibid.: 11):

> Self insemination is very straightforward. The semen is
> placed inside the vagina near the mouth of the cervix, (or
> not even that far up (see section on Girl/Boy choice), where

it would usually be deposited during intercourse. It is as simple as putting a tampon or a finger inside your vagina. We used a needless syringe, which can be obtained at a chemist, but on occasions one woman just tipped the sperm into her vagina. One woman in our group told a friend of her plans – 'But it's supposed to be painful, isn't it?' her friend said. This is completely untrue.

It was so easy, in fact, that many women who wrote to the SI Group in response to their pamphlet asked for 'more information', as if to say 'surely, it can't be *that* easy' – why otherwise all the fuss about medically controlled AID with sperm banks, complicated donor/receptor screenings and clinical supervision of the women's insemination?

While the insertion of the sperm is simplicity itself, what is difficult to know is the time when a woman can conceive, that is to determine one's ovulation (which occurs usually twelve to sixteen days before the onset of menstruation). Especially, as the SI group states, because women know so little about our bodies and reproductive cycles (ibid.: 14).

The SI booklet does provide practical help for self-help: examples of making temperature charts and of recognising changes in the amount of mucus at the entrance of the vagina to determine ovulation. A further component is the longevity of the sperm: one to two hours outside and two to three days inside the body seems to be the average life-time of sperm with female x-sperm living longer than male y-sperm.

SI, in the way the Feminist SI Group defines it, however, is much more than the mere act of a woman getting pregnant without heterosexual intercourse and without help of the medical establishment.[5] It is more than the woman giving birth to her baby. It is nothing less than a radically different approach to the concept of parenting as well as to the question of 'what *kind* of children do I want?'. SI has decisive implications on the concept of biological parenting – of who the sperm donors are and who will be the future 'family' of the child, including the biological and non-biological mother(s) and friends of both sexes. It questions the values which, in western patriarchal society, define what a 'desirable' child is: white and able-bodied, preferably male (at least when it is a first child), preferably blond and blue-eyed (when born into a Germanic or Anglo-Saxon culture), and preferably within the legitimacy of marriage. SI, as perceived within a lesbian feminist politics that sees women as self-determined human beings, challenges all these norms and assumptions. It aims at creating a different value system for the women, for the children – and for the fathers.

'Setting up the Donors Group' as the SI pamphlet explains (p.12) implies finding men who are prepared to view biological fathering from a different perspective: 'We wanted to be sure that all the men who might become donors were clear that they would be biological fathers only and have no contact (or right to a relationship) with the child(ren).' A group of homosexual men was contacted and they met with some of the members of the SI Group (ibid.: 12–13):

> After this meeting a group of men emerged who felt they could fulfil the requirements. Their contribution to our self-insemination group came from a strong political motivation, they never wanted to be fathers, but felt that lesbians who wanted to should be able to be parents. On this basis they were contributing to the disempowering of one of the basic rights claimed by patriarchy – that biological fathering gives men power over women and children.
>
> There was no model that we knew of for our relationship to our donors. Most of us at the beginning had contact with them based only upon a shared understanding of what part each of us played in the process towards conception, and some shared analysis of the political significance of the link.

The communal household of some of the donor men was used to facilitate the transfer of the sperm between the donor and the woman. She would thus be able to inseminate herself as quickly as possible. But as pregnancy in no case happened during the first attempt it turned out to be a somewhat draining experience for donors as well as the woman who had to go to the men's house and repeat the process for two to five days each month. It was easier on the men who, in order to protect the anonymity of the donors as requested by the women and themselves, made sure that different men provided the sperm on each day the woman inseminated herself during one month. The men had also agreed to have regular VD and AIDS check-ups, and to be honest about their medical (family) history.

When the London women got together in 1978, as they say:

> Our group of donors were all white. We do not know if any of their black friends considered being donors. We did not at that time think through the implications of having black donors, as we were not presented with the possibility. We acknowledge that this lack of thought is in itself a covert form of racism. (ibid.: 6)

Today, one of the women says if she considered having a second child by SI she would plan a racially mixed group of donors. This would be another step out of narrow cultural boundaries: trying to expand one's horizons, to unlearn one's own racism while at the same time exploring other cultural heritages.

Such thinking, again, goes totally against the conventional concept of 'motherhood' and parenting. And so does the issue of disabled children. Two members of the SI Group have children with disabilities.[6] This has given them yet another view of parenting, and contributed, in their view, to a significant learning experience for all people involved: 'what are our expectations, what kind of child do we call "normal"?' In a leaflet now inserted in the pamphlet they say

> we are conscious of the very deep seated nature of our (ablebodied) assumptions about the 'normality' and 'preference' of being able-bodied. (It is better and more 'normal' to be heterosexual too!) And . . . we think women's attitudes to disability must be challenged.

They feel this includes potential parents' attitudes to the 'ability' of their future children.

The inseminated woman – the biological mother-to-be – within the SI Group's concept is *not* the only woman concerned with having the child. In fact, in addition to their own mothers, sisters and friends who usually (after an initial period of shock and confusion) accept SI and the resulting child, in lesbian relationships there is often 'the other woman' who may make a conscious decision to be just as much involved with (and responsible for) the child as its biological mother. One of the women who has been a member of the Feminist SI Group from its start speaks openly about the unresolved problems in being the non-biological mother: 'I feel just as "real" as the child's "real" mother, but some people tell me that I'm not in control, that I'm being ripped off – she'll go away with the child and I'll be had.' The 'real' mother, in turn, has to cope with her conditioned responsibility to opt out of prescribed motherhood, that is, for example, to consider leaving her small child with the non-biological mother – or mothers – or other friends, while she pursues some other interest in her life which may be difficult to combine with mothering (e.g. studying abroad).

The SI pamphlet and the women I talked with about SI make it very clear that the decision – and later the process – of having children by SI is not an easy one.[7] Firstly, there is the question of guilt – this was especially striking in many letters the SI Group got from women who were justifying at length why as lesbians they felt they had a 'right' to a child (for instance because of a long and stable relationship with their lovers). Secondly, there is the long – and often desperate – struggle to become pregnant. Of rushing through London's traffic in order to arrive in time for the sperm survival. Of waiting and hoping . . . and then (ibid.: 23):

> A few days more. Those pains, cramps. The slightest brown stain on a piece of toilet paper. Hope you're mistaken. Know I'm not. Pains go. For a day or two maybe. Maybe they won't return. Know they will. A period starts between 12 and 14 days after ovulation – just like the books say. Resignation. That's the way it goes. Just have to try again next month. Despair. I won't ever get pregnant.

The SI pamphlet – and the women who produced it and *are* the Feminist SI Group – do not shy away from such pains and difficulties. The process of becoming pregnant – of repeatedly disappointed hopes, of finally being pregnant, places considerable strain on the future biological mother as well as on those women who have chosen to be non-biological mothers, in particular the woman's closest friend(s) and lover(s).

And then there is the problem of once the child is born and then grows up – what should s/he be told about her or his 'origins'? How does one deal with people's questions about 'but who's the father?' or worse 'don't you think the child will *miss* a father?' Again, as one SI-mother put it: in a patriarchal world having children is not easy. In a way, not even the myth of the happy heterosexual tandem – husband and wife – is sufficient to fulfil the child's needs: what is required, it seems, is *more* than two parents – maybe three or four. . . .

Ideally, an SI Group as close as the one described in this paper, can satisfy these needs. Little Catherine says that she has three mothers – mum Pauline, mum Claire and mum Ann. It appears as if she isn't going to be upset that she has no father, but, rather, is pleased that she has multiple mothers and such a loving environment!

The Group's oldest children are four years old, but, as the following remark indicates, they seem to be going in the footsteps of their independent mother(s): 'When I'm grown up I'll get a sperm and grow a baby in my tummy.' And, one of the boys, listening to a discussion on the question of racially mixed donors for another SI pregnancy, offered his advice: 'The black workman fixing the windows outside could give you a seed.' Yes, it is going to be tough for them as they grow up; in a similar way as it is tough for their mothers to be lesbian, thus 'different'. But then, as one of the women from the feminist self insemination group summarised it: 'Women who decide to do SI will go through a fundamental reconceptualisation of their lives: they will question the patriarchal concept of biological parenthood, able-bodiedness, racial and cultural barriers. They will draw strength from non-biological but instead consciously chosen families.' The links among the five members of the SI Group and their children are strong. Maybe they will be able to transmit this strength to their children, especially their daughters[8] to become autonomous strong women. For as they put it: 'SI deals a blow to the power of the fathers' (Ibid.: 7). 'Doing it ourselves' seems one of the roads to getting in charge of our reproductive capacities.

## NOTES

1 *Self Insemination*, 1980, is available from the Feminist Self Insemination Group, P.O. Box 3, 190 Upper Street, London N1, UK at £2.00

2 This article is made up of information extracted from the SI leaflet and from a conversation with three members of the Feminist SI Group. I am most grateful to them for taking the time for our talk as well as for revising and commenting on the manuscript. This piece is as much theirs as it is mine.

3 The Girl Babies Group describes itself as lesbian feminists interested in maximising chances of having girl children by SI, but also by heterosexual intercourse AID and (artificial insemination by donor using the services of an official sperm bank). The group is gathering accounts on women's experiences and can be contacted c/o *A Woman's Place*, Hungerford House, Victoria Embankment, London WC2, UK.

4 *Evening News*, January 1978.

5 Although the majority of women interested in SI are lesbians, some celibate and heterosexual women have contacted the Feminist SI Group. The SI pamphlet points out that (in 1979)

> The British Pregnancy Advisory Service is prepared to consider arranging AID for single women, including lesbians. BPAS charges £20 for the initial counselling and £30 for the first three months 'treatment', but we don't know how many inseminations you get. Some doctors will arrange it privately. They work out expensive – in 1978 Dr. D charged £12 for the initial consultation and £12 *per specimen.*' (20)

6 Both cases are explicable with virus infections which the women had while pregnant. There is no proven connection at all between the disabilities and SI. Up to date, research into the question of heightened disability risks for SI (or AID) children indicates that it is unsubstantiated to assume that SI increases the chance of having a child with a disability. (For more information see the SI pamphlet: 19.)

7 The SI pamphlet does not deal with the question of 'child or child-free?' It assumes that the woman who goes in for SI has made up her mind to become a mother.

8 'Although', as one member of the Feminist SI Group puts it, 'we would all prefer to have girls, the decision to have a *child* seems more important to us than the decision of whether it's going to be a boy or a girl' (The SI pamphlet does list some recommendations of how to maximise chances to conceive a girl or a boy.)

# REFERENCES

Feminist Self Insemination Group. 1980. *Self Insemination*. P.O. Box 3, 190 Upper Street, London N1, UK at £2.00.

# EQUAL OPPORTUNITY FOR BABIES? NOT IN OAKLAND!

## The Coalition to Fight Infant Mortality

This article describes how, in 1978, the Coalition to Fight Infant Mortality, a community-based group in East Oakland, California, organized the community to demand early and comprehensive prenatal care for low income women and women of color. The Coalition has become a model for other groups in the country trying to lower infant mortality rates in their communities.

In the spring of 1978, several Bay Area newspapers carried headlines revealing that East Oakland had one of the nation's highest infant mortality rates. In a country that spends more on health care than any other nation in the world, East Oakland had a higher rate of infant deaths than such Third World countries as Jamaica, Thailand, and Jordan.

The infant mortality rate is defined as the number of infants who die within the first year of life per 1,000 live births. Infant mortality rates are commonly used as indicators of both access to health services and quality of life. In the US, the infant mortality rate for Blacks is almost twice the rate for Whites. In 1978, it was discovered that, during the years 1974 to 1976, twenty-six out of every 1,000 pregnant women in East Oakland, a primarily low-income and Black neighborhood, lost their infants within the first year of life. By way of contrast, only blocks away in the affluent White suburb of Piedmont, the infant mortality rate was 3.5 deaths per 1,000 live births. The line dividing the privileged class from the economically powerless in our society could not have been drawn more clearly.

The public outcry that accompanied these revelations

prompted the formation of the Coalition to Fight Infant Mortality, a local organization made up of concerned citizens, including health workers, educators, and representatives of other community groups.

The main purpose of the Coalition to Fight Infant Mortality (CFIM) is to catalyze community pressure and involvement in demanding improved health services from various levels of government. The Coalition believes that health care is a right of all people, and that all people have a right to have healthy babies. It is the responsibility of the government to assure that these rights are a reality for all people. The Coalition also believes that the community has both the right and the responsibility to participate in and give direction to the health care system. CFIM sees infant mortality as a reflection of racism and discrimination against women, poor and working people, and as a result of the profit orientation of our health-care system.

From December 1978 to September 1979, the Coalition's work focused on researching the problem of infant mortality and assessing the key factors that caused this problem. Through this work, the Coalition came to realize that the most important factor causing infant mortality was the lack of early, comprehensive prenatal care.

Because the county hospital was the only public hospital offering obstetrical services accessible to low-income women, the Coalition decided that this hospital should be the target of its activities and began investigating its quality of care for perinatal services. Since the county Board of Supervisors are the trustees of the hospital, CFIM mobilized the community to demand from the Board a 'community-based investigation' of the problem of infant mortality, and, in particular, the quality of care at the county hospital. Over 5,000 signatures were obtained on a petition demanding a community-based investigation. The purpose of this strategy was to stress the importance of community participation by obtaining community input on the problems and possible solutions. Through the community investigation, outreach and education could be carried out and serve as a means of developing a network of support.

The Board of Supervisors rejected the Coalition's

proposed inquiry on the grounds that a grass-roots investigating team would be biased and would not have enough expertise. Instead, a Grand Jury was assigned to evaluate the county hospital's performance. The Coalition went on to form its own community-based Investigating Team, known as the I-Team.

The central focus of the I-Team was to obtain community participation during the investigation through a process of educational meetings with low-income and women of color and surveying them about their experiences in getting prenatal care. CFIM recognized that there were many barriers to the community in going to meetings, or becoming immediately involved. Therefore, the Coalition not only organized two community meetings, but also set up meetings through various social service agencies, child care centers, etc., to conduct presentations and have people participate in the survey. The results were then taken back to the community for input and discussion on how to get the I-Team's recommendations implemented.

The I-Team found that the community identified four primary barriers to women seeking prenatal care:

1 *The high cost of prenatal care.* Women again and again cited the high cost of medical services as the single most important barrier discouraging them from obtaining prenatal care. Working-class women with incomes too high for Medi-Cal, but too low to afford private insurance, frequently could not afford expensive prenatal care. Women on Medi-Cal talked about problems finding obstetricians that would accept it and bureaucratic delays in getting coverage.

2 *Inaccessible services.* The I-Team found that perinatal services are currently most concentrated in areas of Oakland far removed from where there is the greatest need for those services. Working-class and poor women thus frequently have to travel long distances to obtain medical services related to their pregnancies. The access problem is compounded by slow and expensive public transportation, a major problem for women without care.

3 *Provider attitudes about women.*

4 *Provider attitudes about racial minorities in the United States.* Community members frequently told the I-Team how the hurried, unconcerned attitudes of health-care workers discouraged them from continuing to seek prenatal care. Women visiting doctors often find the doctor only spending a very brief amount of time with them, with little explanation of what is happening to them. They felt their treatment was a result of racism and discrimination against them as women on the part of the medical professionals.

A great deal of effort was also put into setting up a press conference and hearings with the Board of Supervisors, once the results were developed from the investigation. Newsletters, leaflets, and other handouts were developed, concentrating on what happened at the board meeting in order to expose the racist comments and attitudes of the Board of Supervisors.

It is important to note one of the main intentions of these activities was to expose the community to how decisions are made regarding the community's needs and what the priorities are with the county government in addition to lobbying the board to win concessions. It was important to develop a strong political analysis in order to draw out the real causes of infant mortality.

Although the Board shifted from not recognizing the infant mortality problem to now acknowledging it, a substantial commitment could not be obtained from them. However, positive changes did take place through the support of the Alameda County Health Care Services Agency. One result was the Board's willingness to contract a more community-based obstetrical staff at the county hospital which implemented many of the recommendations made by the community investigation. A community relations department was developed to address the need for translation services for non-English-speaking patients at the hospital. The midwifery service was expanded as a result of continual community support. Thus, important changes were achieved. Through the Coalition's work, the awareness of infant mortality was and continues to be raised. The presence of the CFIM has grown, upon which a base in the community can be developed for on-going organizing efforts.

The Coalition to Fight Infant Mortality has been able to share its experience and political perspectives with others through the participation in two hearings on infant mortality: one sponsored by the California Department of Consumer Affairs, and a national hearing sponsored by Congressman Dellums. CFIM has also assisted in supporting the continuation of the Oakland Perinatal Health Project, a special program offering comprehensive, perinatal care through a network of community clinics.

The Coalition has spent most of the last year analyzing the most recent statistics on infant mortality in Alameda County. After declining for several years (1977 through 1979), the infant mortality rate in East Oakland increased in 1980 and 1981. Infant mortality in East and West Oakland is still approximately 50 percent higher than the county average and, county-wide, Black infants continue to die at a rate 40 percent higher than the rate for White infants. In addition, the percentage of low birthweight infants, a good predictor of infant mortality, morbidity, and disability, is over 60 percent higher in East and West Oakland than the county average. Alameda County ranks third highest out of California's fifty-eight counties in the percentage of low birthweight infants.

The Coalition completed an investigation of changes that have been made in perinatal services in the county in the last year. Based on this information, CFIM developed three recommendations for improving the quality and accessibility of perinatal services for low-income women and women of color in the community. The Coalition held a press conference to announce its recommendations and then a hearing in front of the Board of Supervisors. The three recommendations were:

1 The County Health Care Services Agency should take the lead in organizing a comprehensive, county-wide perinatal services system; this system should include the county hospital, county and community clinics, and private providers of perinatal services.

2 The county should improve perinatal services at the county hospital by having a pediatrician in the hospital twenty-four hours a day.

3 The county should expand community outreach and education about the importance and availability of prenatal care.

The Board directed the Director of the County Health Care Services Agency to review the Coalition's recommendations, to estimate the cost of implementation, and report back to the Board. The Coalition will monitor closely the report of the Director and the Board's response.

The Coalition to Fight Infant Mortality is currently involved in several other activities as well. They publish a quarterly newsletter[1] and have been active in organizing assistance to monitor cuts in state and local funding for health care. The Coalition also is participating in support work on two legal cases in which women are suing the county government and a private hospital because their infants died due to inadequate health care. These lawsuits advance the idea that people have the right to decent health care, and that both the government and private hospitals have a legal obligation to provide care for all who need it. Publicity about the lawsuits also helps maintain political pressure on the county government to improve perinatal services for low-income women and women of color.

The Coalition to Fight Infant Mortality has been successful at the local level by showing how high infant mortality in low-income and minority communities reflects racism, discrimination against women, and the profit motive of the health-care system. Based on the experiences of the Coalition, groups in other parts of the country have begun organizing to lower infant mortality in their communities.

## NOTE

1 To order copies of the Report of the Community-based Investigating Team ($10.00) or to subscribe to the newsletter ($10.00/year) write to: Coalition to Fight Infant Mortality, P.O. Box 10436, Oakland, California, 94610.

# WHO IS GOING TO ROCK THE PETRI DISH? FOR FEMINISTS WHO HAVE CONSIDERED PARTHENOGENESIS WHEN THE MOVEMENT IS NOT ENOUGH

## Nancy Breeze

Intimately acquainted with the realities of mothering, 1950s style, Nancy Breeze has integrated her personal experience with her observations of motherhood today. She believes that new reproductive technologies may be the key to more positive, functional ways of raising children.

It is quiet. Lesbians are sitting in a full-moon circle. One breaks the silence. 'I'm going into the ocean at midnight. I am ovulating and I want to see if I can start parthenogenesis. I'd like to have a child.' Across the room, the only woman in the group who now HAS a child, struggles guiltily with her wish to give up custody of her five-year-old daughter.

I gasp, not only because I think that going swimming in December is extreme, for any reason. I, who was subjected to the efficient reproductive technology of the 1950s, know only too well what it means to HAVE a child; the dailiness (and nightliness) of it all. Pregnant at nineteen, a mother at twenty, I, unlike the mother of the five-year-old, had not yet developed a 'self' which would inevitably be suppressed when its needs collided with those of a baby. I, who chose to study shorthand rather than teaching, because I 'didn't like children,' never considered not having any. Motherhood was the unexamined, 'chosen,' future for most of us who grew up back then. Once I had a baby, I went about my boring, exhausting, tasks dutifully. I gave birth to four children in seven years and was praised for being a drudge. When others said, 'I just don't know how you DO it,' I beamed. Still, I often wished I could be more patient with the children, and sometimes I wondered why my life seemed so unsatisfying.

At the close of the moon circle, the other mother, Carey,

and I talk. 'It's just so hard to get help,' she says in exasperation. 'Back in Connecticut, where I live, the women's community is strong and active. Some women are thinking about having babies themselves. They say it's awful for me to even consider letting my ex-husband raise Susie.' She pauses, shrugging. 'Sometimes women offer to help me out by taking care of her for a while. But they're all so busy, I can't count on it. You know how it is, they can never tell when something else might come up.' She laughs, but she doesn't look amused. Our eyes have locked together in stereo, every time she uses the word, 'help.'

The next day I take my lunch break on a bench in the park. A fat-cheeked boy toddles over to inspect the aerial on my transistor. He smiles up at me. I notice a woman hovering, unobtrusively nearby, ready to intervene if he should start toward the road, pick up a piece of broken glass or a cigarette butt. Suddenly I realize that I must have spent at least eight years of such hovering. Watching a small child has its delightful moments, of course, as we discover with them many hidden treasures. But it is also a job which is largely unstimulating, while requiring our full attention.

My mind travels back to our first house, on road M-59 in Michigan. I was always afraid that the two-year-old would wander onto the highway. We didn't have enough money for a fenced-in yard, and he loved to be outdoors. When I ran inside to catch a phonecall, or stir the spaghetti sauce, I always made sure he was in his sandbox near the door. But he was so quick I never knew if he would stay there. Later, when we lived on a quieter street, I remember furtively taking a bath in the afternoon, continually running to the window to see if he was still in the backyard.

I wondered what eight years of that kind of fragmentation did to my brain cells. Would it be like a lobotomy?

In the early 1970s, when I backed out of marriage and into the women's movement, I was startled by all the new ways of looking at my past. I wanted to analyze everything. It was especially shocking to realize how subtly my youthful energy had been channelled into motherhood. I naively imagined that everyone was, like myself, turning their backs on all that. However, after years of working as an abortion counsellor, I admit it isn't all that simple. Women often are pulled equally in opposite directions, feeling the need to 'mother' like their mothers did, simultaneously with demands to be successful in careers. I agonized with these women over their decisions about the unintentional pregnancies.

Still, I expected that the women's community would be dealing largely with children who were born before their mothers 'found feminism.' I was completely unprepared to pick up an issue of *Off Our Backs* last year (1982) and read interviews with lesbians who were trying to get pregnant, especially in couple relationships.

Presently, many of my closest friends are practicing mothers. And they've heard enough feminist criticism of traditional motherhood that they're genuinely trying to create better ways of raising children. But it is difficult. I signed up for an assertiveness training class at the Women's Center. Our teacher, a married mother of an infant, had planned some role-playing exercises for us. First we all relaxed by sharing events from the past week. About halfway through the class, there was a knock at the door. The instructor's husband came in carrying the baby. 'She's fussy,' he explained. 'I guess she wants to nurse.' In a moment he was gone. I watched from the window, as he stepped lightly down the street, swinging his arms.

My best friend has a three-year-old daughter, Jane. One afternoon a group of us were at her house, drinking coffee and arguing over the details of a planned Take Back The Night march. Another friend dropped Jane off from daycare. As soon as she was in the house, she was determined to get her mother's undivided attention. Although several of us offered to get her the drink she wanted, she was not satisfied until her mother gave up trying to carry on a conversation and took her for a walk. Even though Jane has been raised more collectively than any of my children were, she and her mother are still captives of the belief that she has the right and an emotional need to demand the full attention of one particular person. I wondered what it would be like for five women, none identified as THE MOTHER, to raise a child together. No one would have a special 'guilt string' to be pulled when the child came home from school.

I remember seeing a play in Washington, DC in the late 1970s. The female characters were trying to sabotage a test-tube baby project. They had discovered that, once the 'mad scientists' had created babies, they would exterminate the no-longer-needed women. Then I remember Shulamith Firestone's assertion, in *The Dialectic of Sex* (Firestone, 1970), that artificial reproduction and other scientific discoveries, are 'liberating unless they are improperly used.' She advocated 'concentrating full energy on demands for control of scientific discoveries,' rather than opposing them because they could be misused.

Recently I read Marge Piercy's *Woman on the Edge of Time*. Piercy has created a loving, child-centered environment for the babies of non-womb procreation. Each child is nurtured by three co-parents, all adults are equipped with fully-operating mammary glands, and teenagers choose their own significant adults. I felt encouraged by what seemed a visionary movement away from isolated, biologically-assigned, childcare.

But recently I walked out of the hospital just in time to overhear a woman say to a young girl: 'Other people's babies are boring, but when you get your own. . . .' In the parking lot, car bumper stickers quiz, 'Have you hugged YOUR Kid today?' My son and his wife agree that she should stay home with my grandchildren while they are young!

I am impatient for change. One of the many friends who have been subjected to the passion of my ideas asserts, 'Let's not change the way babies are made. Let's just change what happens when they get here.'

However, the good-faith efforts I've observed seem unable to substantially change 'what happens after they get here.' It seems that society-wide involvement in the process of creating babies could structure a society-wide sense of responsibility for their care.

Two thousand years of morning sickness and stretch marks have not resulted in liberation for women or children. If you should run into a Petri dish, it could turn out to be your best friend. So, rock it; don't knock it!

## REFERENCES

Firestone, Shulamith. 1970. *The Dialectic of Sex*. William Morrow, New York.
*Off Our Backs*. 1982. 'Creating Sappho's family. Interview with Jackie Forster,' XII, 10 November. Washington DC.
Piercy, Marge. 1980. *Woman on the Edge of Time*. Alfred A. Knopf, New York.

A version of this chapter first appeared in *Trivia, A Journal of Ideas*, April 1984.

# TAKING THE INITIATIVE: INFORMATION VERSUS TECHNOLOGY IN PREGNANCY

## Maureen Ritchie

This article is an attempt to set my personal quest for a good birth in the context both of my own birth forty years earlier, and of the current childbirth scene in the UK. There is a brief account of the development of the 'natural childbirth' lobby, and organisations and publications are described and listed. This growing support and information available to women makes it more possible for us to take decisions back into our own hands, and I describe some of the decisions I managed to 'take back' and why. Whatever the shape of the eventual birth, if we control it our integrity is not so threatened.

A decision to have a child, and certainly a successful conception, immediately raises the question of what sort of pregnancy and birth we expect and need, and of whether these needs will be met in the present medical environment of western childbirth. Many of us, some from bitter experience, now know that we will not 'be given' a good birth, we have to 'take' it. In other words, to retain control over our bodies and our babies in pregnancy and childbirth we have to resume much more responsibility for ourselves than we are usually expected to. For many of us it's difficult to find enough confidence to do this successfully; partly because we have been taught to ignore the information about her own body available to a pregnant or labouring woman, and partly because access to codified 'scientific' information is made difficult by the paternalistic attitudes of the medical profession,[1] and by the complexities and expense of medical literature itself.

In this essay I want to show how I gave my smallest

daughter as nice a birth as I had had myself. Knowing of the change in control over pregnancies and births since I was born, I did this by searching for the information needed to give me the knowledge and confidence to turn down some of the offerings of modern obstetrics; and I also chose the expert help as carefully as possible.

In the last thirty years in western industrialised countries, childbirth and, to some extent, pregnancy too, has been almost totally separated from the traditionally woman-controlled sphere of child and home, with disastrously alienating results. Done explicitly in the name of safety, and implicitly for the juggernaut of male-dominated obstetric technology. This process has resulted in some really dreadful experiences for many women and their babies (e.g. Thorne, 1983). But it wasn't always like this. When I and my brother and sister were born, in the 1940s, my mother found pregnancy normal, and childbirth positive and enjoyable. This is her account:

> When I became pregnant in 1941 it was not difficult to arrange a home confinement. My doctor recommended a midwife, and she visited me several times – as a friend rather than in her role as midwife. A friend had suggested that I read *Natural Childbirth* (Read, 1933). She had been to his clinic when she was pregnant, and I thought his approach was right for me. I think his routine was probably responsible for a very quick and easy labour – the midwife was only in the house for ½ hour before the baby was born. I think if I had gone to hospital when I first had some 'pains' it would have taken much longer. I remember it as a very happy relaxed experience (no stitches or drugs needed).
>
> My second confinement was in a nursing home because the midwife I had before now ran this home which had been opened by my doctor. I had confidence in them, and thought I would do better there than at home with strangers. This was a longer labour, about 4 hours, partly because the baby was bigger, but also I think because I had to go to the home earlier as we had no petrol for private transport and the roads were dangerous with snow and ice (Dec '44). My doctor was present and suggested I had some 'help' but I

refused and he said he wouldn't ask again, *I* would have to ask *him* – at least we understood each other. I was happy in the home, but the babies were kept in a day nursery (where we could go if we liked), and also my small daughter couldn't come to see the baby (I didn't think anything of this at the time; it was normal practice in hospitals; there is a great improvement now). My parents lived about ten minutes walk away, and as soon as possible I went there each day to see my daughter. There was no question of me going home for a fortnight after the baby was born (again normal at the time).

A third confinement was in a nursing home, though not by choice; we had booked a midwife and I was looking forward to a home confinement when I could see my daughters and be relaxed in my own surroundings, but sadly she broke her leg a week before the baby was due and we had to find a nursing home quickly. I hadn't met the midwife till I went into labour, and this time I delayed as long as I dare. Here for the first time I was left alone for about 20 minutes. I was shown how to use the gas and air apparatus if I wanted it but instead I had to call the nurse and the baby was born in ten minutes. Perhaps because it was Christmas and I had expected to be at home, I think this was the least satisfying confinement. I did have the baby with me except at night, but I was anxious to go home. It was a difficult time with rationing and no petrol for visiting, although I have nothing but praise for the midwives (my doctor didn't arrive in time for this birth either!). I never needed stitches, and had no problems, but if I had had any, I'm sure I would have been cared for equally well each time. I think women were often torn and had stitches. Some had quite a lot if the babies were big, but it doesn't seem a good idea to cut if it's not necessary.

I'm sure I enjoyed your birth the most, partly because I knew and liked Sister Allison, partly I think because I could stay in my own environment without worrying about when to go to hospital, and what would it be like. It was all so quick that there was no time to feel apprehensive. I was lucky, having read Dick Read and decided I wanted my baby completely naturally so that I was aware of what was going on, it happened that way without any effort on my part.

Since my mother's time, with the establishment of the National Health Service, no one in the UK has to pay for the services of midwife, doctor or obstetrician, but pregnancy and birth have become more and more hospital-centred and (male) doctor-dominated. Hospital midwives deliver fewer babies and community midwives fewer still. In the course of the 1970s hospital birth became more technological, with the widespread use of scans, induction, monitors and, of course, drugs, one intervention frequently leading to another. With 'normal' births becoming a rarity, and over-reliance on machines, skills and experience built up over decades began to be lost. Now it is common for obstetricians to refuse to deliver a breech baby vaginally, so the Caesarian section rate is climbing as well. This could only happen in a society where not only are women powerless, but those with power have utter disregard for women's integrity, and scant respect for their bodies; often coupled with considerable ignorance, despite their official expertise, of pregnancy, birth and babies. We have to take back that power and control, and reassert our own knowledge.

My first child was born in 1976, just about the heyday of unquestioned man-management of labour and birth; not a good time to wage a rather uninformed and isolated battle for power. Nevertheless I tried, and I found my mother's positive views enormously encouraging. Although I am a natural pessimist where health and medicine are concerned, her influence helped me regard pregnancy, birth and lactation as normal, almost everyday happenings. Without that confidence I'm sure my firstborn would have had a rotten time. Even so it was far from perfect – I had two scans, because I wasn't clued up enough to refuse them, accepted pethidine when I and the hospital sister should have known better (half an hour before the birth) and had an episiotomy I could have done without. But I did manage to refuse an epidural and to avoid (just) a forceps delivery. Compared with many women's experiences I was amazingly lucky.

By the time I was pregnant again, in 1978–9, the climate

was changing; women's assertions were being heard if not heeded. The National Childbirth Trust (NCT) and the Association for Improvements in the Maternity Services (AIMS) were becoming more visible and articulate. The La Leche League still has rather a low profile in the UK; in part the need is filled by the breastfeeding counselling service of the NCT. In 1980 the Association of Breastfeeding Mothers was set up as well. The London Birth Centre started in 1977, to be followed by others; the Association of Radical Midwives began in 1976 (Spinks, 1978; Jennings, 1982). Foresight, the organisation for pre-conceptual care followed, and later, in 1980, the Maternity Alliance was set up.

Most of these organisations publish newsletters or journals; all are to some extent influenced by feminism, in some cases feminist principles inform their policy and attitudes; the *AIMS Quarterly Journal* is a uniquely informative and supportive publication. Two important 'how to' books were published in 1978; these were the path-breaking, woman-centred *Childbirth Book* (Beels, 1978) and *Breast is Best* (Stanway, 1978), which, though not explicitly feminist, certainly reaffirms our ability to feed our babies. I wished they had been around three years earlier. In the US *Spiritual Midwifery* (Gaskin, 1978) came out, and its accounts of the childbirth customs and achievements at The Farm in Tennessee began to be wider known in the UK too. On a more academic level a study was published (Wynn, 1979), relating the health of mothers and their babies, using statistics from several countries, and paying particular attention to nutrition. The picture that emerged was a gloomy one of low birthweights related to class, partly a direct result of poverty, partly due to the poor nutritional standards of the British in particular, and to the total absence of good dietary advice or support to pregnant (or any other) women. In my experience this is still true. The influence of food on the outcome of pregnancy is also the theme of an American book (Brewer, 1977) by a doctor who has reduced the incidence of toxaemia by improving the diets of pregnant women.

With the confidence provided by experience and this climate of increasing demands, my second birth was not too bad. My son was born with no scans, no drugs and no monitors; but I still had an episiotomy, and was delivered by strange hospital midwives, who had no interest in my wishes, and perhaps not enough skill or confidence themselves either. The atmosphere was altogether wrong.

My third child was born in 1982, at a time of considerable media interest in childbirth, which stemmed from the visit to Michel Odent's maternity ward in Pithiviers in France by television personality Esther Rantzen, and the television film and programmes which resulted (Paul, 1982). Odent, who has been almost lionised by the natural childbirth movement, runs a labour ward where intervention is a rarity. He and his midwives spend most of the time simply waiting and watching for a baby to be born. He believes that most women will give birth successfully on their own, if their access to their instincts or powers is not blocked by outside demands such as lying down, being strapped to monitors, etc. For him, the labouring and parturient woman is not a threat but a goddess; albeit still a goddess owing her position to one man's vision and power, not to her own. Nevertheless, the calm atmosphere, respect, and the peaceful births – so far from what is attained here – were moving and thought-provoking in the films. (For an account of a Pithiviers birth, see Grierson, 1983.) This was followed by the public eruption of a conflict between two obstetricians at the Royal Free Hospital in London on how birth should or shouldn't be managed; the 'natural childbirth lobby', as it was dubbed, held a well-publicised demonstration outside the hospital. Another television programme, again by Esther Rantzen, led to the publication of *The British Way of Birth* (Boyd and Sellers, 1982), a depressing survey of birth experiences. 'Active birth' became the buzzword, and at least one private (i.e. fee-paying) clinic was set up. An excellent digest of research on various aspects of birth (Inch, 1982) cast further doubt on many modern practices, and pleaded for an end to the erosion of the British midwife's role.

The 'ideal' births of Pithiviers, and the apparent success of Odent in functioning within state-run medicine raised the morale of the childbirth movement, and heightened the awareness for individual women of what was possible.

Although after a few heady days I realised I probably was not going to go to France for this baby, I was really determined to organise a good birth if I possibly could. I decided not to fight for a home birth but to have the baby delivered by my own midwife, who would also do most of the antenatal care. I wanted no intervention at all, and I would come home a few hours after the baby was born. In the UK this system of delivery by the community midwife is called a domino (i.e. *dom*iciliary *in – o*ut). I did eventually get more or less exactly the birth I wanted; however, the pregnancy was marred in the early stages by having to make decisions about procedures offered us, mainly because there was *never* enough accompanying information; nor was our desire to find out necessarily sympathetically received.

The first major issue that arose was amniocentesis. Because I was forty, I could easily have had this test, which involves the insertion of a needle into the amniotic sac to withdraw some fluid. This is then cultured, and is a fairly reliable way of detecting a baby with Down syndrome or spina bifida and other irregularities. Because some types of Down syndrome babies are more often born to older parents, this test is now fairly common in large hospitals. There are two main problems: one is that the test cannot be reliably performed until the foetus is fourteen–sixteen weeks old. Add three–four weeks for the laboratory procedures and you have to face the possibility of a second-trimester abortion, after the baby has been felt moving. Even with an unwanted baby this is a painful and traumatic experience. The other problem centres on the invasive nature of the test and the risk involved. Firstly, in order to minimise the risks of sticking the needle in the baby, it is normally done in conjunction with an ultrasound scan (of which more later). There is a well-established 1–1.5 per cent risk of a miscarriage shortly afterwards; there is a small increased risk of ante partum bleeding, of abnormalities like club foot and dislocated hip, of breathing difficulties at birth and of rhesus sensitisation in the mother. There is also an increase in the miscarriage rate of future pregnancies (Medical Research Council Working Party on Amniocentesis, 1978) reported in the *British Medical Journal* (1978). The only one of these drawbacks which is openly mentioned is the risk of immediate miscarriage. To find out about the rest you have to dig. My General Practitioner (GP) didn't know, but he did refer us to a genetic counsellor who was really good – she told us what she knew *and* what she didn't know, and did not try to push us around.

Apart from the mechanistic aspects of amniocentesis, the other information we needed to make a decision was statistical. Needless to say this was not easily available either. The most we were usually offered was a simple graph, showing Down syndrome babies born by maternal age. Since then some other figures have been published relating Down syndrome babies to parental (i.e. father's) occupation (OPCS, 1982). We decided in the end that our risk of bearing a Down syndrome child was not high enough to justify exposing a normal baby to the risks of the test. But it is a very tricky decision to make. For some women, amniocentesis offers hope of a 'normal' child, without which they might not risk pregnancy, and for others it provides a relatively worry-free second half of pregnancy. But whatever decision is made, it should be with the benefit of full information, not just whatever scraps have stuck in the obstetrician's mind.

Issue number two, of course, was ultrasound. Scans have become standard in many or most hospitals in the UK: at least two per pregnancy and very often many more. Although they can provide information, particularly early in pregnancy, which is harder to detect otherwise (e.g. twins), they tend to be used just as a substitute for experienced judgment. They are open to misinterpretation – erroneous diagnoses of placenta praevia based on scans are not uncommon – though presented by hospital staff as if they are an oracle. But the worst aspect of ultrasound is that it has not been tested properly, and nobody knows for sure that it is not harmful. Studies are now underway, but not before many thousands of women and babies have been exposed, both to antenatal scans, and to ultrasonic foetal monitors used in labour. Moreover, because people are looking for long-term effects, by the time they report countless more scans will have been done. A recent report of a symposium on ultrasound and its effects on the foetus ended thus: 'Don't assume diagnostic ultrasound is innocuous, keep up with research developments on bioeffects, and use the procedure only when clinically indicated.' (*Journal of the American Medical Association*, 1982.) This advice is ignored many times a day in most British hospitals, and, because of this enthusiasm, it is very difficult to get a sympathetic response to a suggestion that you do not want a scan. The standard, and in the light of the above, scandalously insulting reply is that they are perfectly safe. In the interests of low blood pressure, I chose to approach the problem circuitously; namely to cancel, or not make, appointments for scans, and wait and see. Throughout two pregnancies, involving about twenty antenatal visits, only one hospital doctor ever noticed.

Amniocentesis and scans are technological procedures affecting pregnancy rather than birth. By having the domino type of delivery described earlier, I hoped to avoid, rather than refuse, the procedures usually applied to labour and birth, so I didn't search out the arguments against them. They are well presented in Inch (1982) for anyone who needs them. More on technology and pregnancy can be found in Rakusen and Davidson (1982). During the pregnancy my two main sources of information were the midwife (and to some extent the GP), and AIMS (Association for Improvements in the Maternity Services). The women who run AIMS are amazingly well informed and helpful. I corresponded with them a lot, and found their support absolutely invaluable. They are practically an alternative information service on birth, which for a voluntary organisation is quite an achievement.

I saw the midwife at most of the antenatal visits, and she eventually delivered the baby. In this part of England the midwives are keen to do dominos and do get involved with 'their' mothers. Although I don't think my midwife and I actually had much in common save giving birth, we did both get to know enough about each other's expectations to make the relationship successful. She was worried about delivering a baby from a standing or squatting woman as she feared she could not control any tearing; on the other hand she was no advocate of supine labours, and was understanding of my need not to have an episiotomy. (Shaving and enemas were never mentioned by either of us!) In the event the birth was fantastic; the baby surged out effortlessly, sucked straight away, and the whole thing was lovely. Somehow this time, the hospital did not intrude on my awareness or spoil things. I think this was because I did not have the stress of communicating with strangers.

Although this birth was personally satisfactory for me, and shows that with a mixture of research, determination, deviousness and luck, you can manage the system and survive intact, or even enhanced, unfortunately the system remains unchanged. Of course pregnant and labouring women are not well placed to battle against such odds, and nor should they have to. We need such drastic changes that they cannot be achieved in isolation.

That's why I think it is sad that although the influence of the women's movement can be seen in some of the organisations and publications of the last few years, in the newsletters and magazines of the movement itself childbirth is not a prominent theme, at least, not in Britain. I found AIMS and the local branch of the NCT more sympathetic and supportive than my women's group, some of whom seemed surprised that I could actually welcome a third child. Of the three collections of writing from the women's movement published so far in Britain, only one (Allen et al., 1974) has anything of substance on childbirth (Beels, 1974; Wallis, 1974). The *Spare Rib Reader* (1982) does not reflect the best of the sprinkling of articles over the years (e.g. Weare, 1979; Saunders and Walters, 1982). The potential illustrated by a special issue of *Scarlet Women* (1978) has not been explored elsewhere. Nor are the feminist publishers any more prominent. From Virago we had the important *Of Woman Born* (Rich, 1977), The Women's Press offer *Why Children?* (Dowrick and Grundberg, 1980), and Pandora has contributed *Your Body, Your Baby, Your Life* (Phillips, 1983).

Modern feminists have now had fifteen years' practice at challenging male domination and we are getting better at it; but we sometimes seem reluctant to contradict the patriarchal assumptions that, in our biological roles of childbearer, feeder and rearer, we are better unseen. For feminists to reject the centrality of the childbearing stage of many women's lives is to marginalise women with children even further. We need to reintegrate these aspects so that a woman's experience of herself as pregnant and giving birth does not seem irrelevant to her 'other life' as a feminist. Fighting for women-centred pregnancy and birth might be one way of starting.

## NOTE

1  For example, see the extraordinary reluctance to release figures on home and hospital births to a statistician doing a study on the safety of place of birth (Tew, 1983).

## REFERENCES

Allen, Sandra et al., eds. 1974. *Conditions of Illusion: Papers from the Women's Movement.* Feminist Books, Leeds.

Beels, Christine. 1974. 'Crisis in Childbirth.' In Allen, Sandra et al., eds. *Conditions of Illusion*, Feminist Books, Leeds: 8–18.

Beels, Christine. 1978. *The Childbirth Book*, Turnstone, London. 1980.

Boyd, Catherine and Lea Sellers. 1982. *The British Way of Birth*, Pan, London.

Brewer, Gail and Tom Brewer. 1977. *What every pregnant woman should know: the truth about diet and drugs in pregnancy*, Penguin, New York.

*British Medical Journal.* 1978. 'Hazards of amniocentesis,' 6153, 16 December: 1661.

Dowrick, Stephanie and Sibyl Grundberg, eds. 1980. *Why Children?* Women's Press, London.

Gaskin, Ina May. 1978. *Spiritual Midwifery.* Book Publishing Company, Tennessee.

Grierson, Linda. 1982–3. 'Living to give life.' *AIMS Quarterly Journal*, Winter: 9–10.

Inch, Sally. 1982. *Birthrights: a parents' guide to modern childbirth*, Hutchinson, London.

Jennings, Janet. 1982. 'Who controls childbirth?' *Radical Science Journal*, 12: 9–16.

*Journal of the American Medical Association.* 1982. vol. 247, no. 16, April: 2195–7.

Medical Research Council Working Party on Amniocentesis. 1978. *British Journal of Obstetrics and Gynaecology*, 85, suppl. 2.

*OPCS Monitors*. 1982. MB3 82/1 and 82/2. Office of Population Censuses and Surveys, London.

Paul, Ann. 1982. 'Birth Reborn.' *Listener*, 11 March: 5–6.

Phillips, Angela. 1983. *Your Body, your Baby, your Life*. Pandora Press, London.

Rakusen, Jill and Davidson, Nick. 1982. *Out of our hands: what technology does to pregnancy*. Pan, London.

Read, Grantly Dick. 1968. *Natural Childbirth*. Heinemann, London (fifth ed.).

Rich, Adrienne. 1977. *Of woman born: motherhood as experience and institution*, Norton, N.Y.; Virago, London, 1977.

Saunders, Leslie and Diane Walters. 1982. 'Who's birthing the baby?' *Spare Rib*, 118, May: 20–3.

*Scarlet Women* 6/7, April 1978.

*Spare Rib Reader*. 1982. Penguin, London.

Spinks, Jenny. 1978. 'Radical Midwives.' *Spare Rib*, 73, August: 6–8, 33.

Stanway, Penny and Andrew Stanway. 1978. *Breast is Best*. Pan, London.

Tew, Marjorie. 1983. Untitled article. In *AIMS Quarterly Journal*. Spring: 5–6.

Thorne, Angela. 1983. 'Just an ordinary birth.' *AIMS Quarterly Journal*. Spring: 5–6.

Wallis, Jan. 1974. 'Why I laughed when Anna was born.' In Allen, Sandra et al., eds. *Conditions of Illusion*. Feminist Books, Leeds: 19–26.

Weare, Tessa. 1979. 'Round in a flat world.' *Spare Rib*, 78, January 15–17.

Wynn, Arthur and Margaret Wynn. 1979. *Prevention of handicap and the health of women*. Routledge & Kegan Paul, London.

## ADDRESSES

Association of Breastfeeding Mothers, 71 Hall Drive, London SE26 6XL.

Association for Improvements in the Maternity Services, Hon. Sec. Christine Rogers, 163 Liverpool Road, London N1 0RF.

Association of Radical Midwives, 62 Greetby Hill, Ormskirk, Lancashire.

Birth Centre – contact: 14 Simpson Street, London SW11.

Foresight, Woodhurst, Hydestile, Godalming, Surrey.

La Leche League, BM 3424, London WC1V 6XX.

Maternity Alliance, 309 Kentish Town Road, London NW5 2TJ.

National Childbirth Trust, 9 Queensborough Terrace, London W2 3TB.

# REGAINING TRUST

Ruth Holland and Jill McKenna

Two midwives active in the Association of Radical Midwives in England raise questions about some of the technologies used during pregnancy and childbirth. They point out that these technologies have not been properly evaluated and that they undermine women's confidence in our ability to listen to our own selves and to give birth safely.

We are two midwives who met through the Association of Radical Midwives (ARM), having already begun to question many of the practices, procedures and ideas current within the institutions in which we work. We have seen women being given a very unbalanced view of pregnancy and child-birth without either the knowledge or self-confidence to question it. It is in the hope of changing this that we make this contribution.

We need to maintain a respect for the advances in obstetrics, as in some instances technology *has* reduced the infant and maternal mortality rates – for example, providing specialist care for very premature babies and hormonal infusions to accelerate truly prolonged and difficult labours. Also, we need to recognise that, at present, most of us work and give birth within a system which incorporates tech-nology, where policies are governed by the use of that tech-nology and where the obstetricians – invariably men – set the policies.

In this patriarchal society, technology has an unwhole-some appeal and is used extensively in pregnancy and child-birth *but has never been properly evaluated*. Its availability has been used to pressurise women into accepting many tests, investigations and interventions on the false assumption that they make pregnancy and childbirth safer. It also totally undermines women's confidence in their ability to give birth and midwives, once the skilled and trusted companions to the pregnant and labouring woman, have all too often become mere handmaidens to doctors and machinery.

ARM aims to restore the full role of the midwife – to help her regain confidence in her own skills and to be assertive in the face of inadequately evaluated medical technology and domineering obstetricians. Midwives can then encourage women to listen to their own selves, to trust in themselves and their ability to give birth and can help them make informed choices by giving more balanced information.

We can illustrate these points by briefly looking at some of the interventions now widely used – ultrasound scans, amniocentesis and electronic foetal monitoring.

Ultrasound scanning is based on the 'pulse-echo' principle, similar to that used in the navy's underwater sonar equipment. It is used to confirm the pregnancy and its gestation, thereby giving an apparently accurate expected date of delivery; to diagnose twins, placenta praevia (where the placenta lies over the cervix so preventing a normal birth); to exclude certain foetal abnormalities, e.g. hydrocephalus, and to give continuous assessment of foetal growth.

Most women feel reassured to see the outline of the baby, to watch it move and hear its heartbeat at a very early stage and to be told it is normal and growing well. However, this can give them a false sense of security. The information given by scans is seldom 100 per cent reliable. Possible long-term side effects are never mentioned, as the technology is relatively new, though animal studies have demonstrated:

(a) in rodents – delayed neuromuscular development; altered emotional behaviour, and foetal abnormalities
(b) in rabbits – blood changes, dilation of vessels and corneal erosion
(c) in monkeys – altered electro-encephalogram results. ('Research in Ultrasound Bioeffects', 1980)

Because of this, we feel that scans should only be used in clearly defined and limited circumstances. We need to encourage women to have confidence in their own estimation of delivery dates when they know them; perhaps even encourage them to keep a record of their monthly cycles before conceiving; to be aware of and trust in their baby's growth and movement and their own ability to produce a healthy and well-nourished child. As midwives, we need to regain our confidence in our skills of palpation and initial diagnosis, of which technology is depriving us.

Amniocentesis is done to detect sex-linked genetically transmitted abnormalities, e.g. muscular dystrophy; where there is a family history of these; and chromosomal abnormalities, e.g. Down syndrome, where there is a family history or the mother is at risk because of her age.

Obviously, these are important indications, but again women may be given a false sense of security that no other abnormality exists. Also the full implications of the test are not always explained, for example, if an abnormality is revealed, a woman may feel pressured into accepting a termination of pregnancy, even where this conflicts with her considered judgment or religious convictions. She may also not be warned of the possibility of spontaneously miscarrying a healthy foetus soon after the amniocentesis. A woman may even be swayed into undergoing this risky procedure simply in the knowledge that as well as its ability to detect certain abnormalities, the sex of the child can be determined.

Electronic foetal monitoring (EFM) is sometimes carried out in the antenatal period where there is concern about foetal growth or movement. An unsatisfactory tracing may lead to induction of labour or even emergency caesarean section, whereas an apparently healthy tracing may reassure the doctor that the pregnancy can safely be allowed to continue. EFM is more commonly used in labour to provide a continuous record of the baby's heartbeat and the frequency and length of contractions.

Many women are yet again offered the illusion of safety through the use of this technology. In reality there have been very few scientific studies; (i.e. random controlled trials) of EFM. Those that do exist have only shown increased rates of caesarean section with no significant improvement in foetal outcome. (Banta and Thacker, 1979)

There are also other disadvantages. The woman is

invariably confined to bed, and her movements severely restricted by the connecting leads to the machine. She therefore becomes a passive recipient of 'care', rather than an active collaborator in the birth of her child. She is denied all the well-documented advantages of mobility and an upright position, i.e. the assistance of gravity, less painful, more effective contractions, less need for analgesic drugs and a shorter labour. (Caldeyo-Barcia et al., 1960; Caldeyo-Barcia, 1979; Williams et al., 1980) In our experience as many women are frightened by monitors as are reassured by them.

Our conclusion both from the research we have read and from our own experience as midwives is that we urgently need to regain our trust in, and respect for, the natural process of childbirth. Where a woman is fit, well nourished and well prepared, physically and psychologically, for birth with good antenatal care, routine high technology mechanical intervention carries no benefit and may impair the delicately balanced body mechanisms which are involved. Where conditions are less favourable, the woman and her partner must be fully involved in the decision as to which choice or course of action is right to be taken.

As midwives, we aim to guide, to help her to take full account of her feelings, of her life situation, and to try to assess the relative advantages and disadvantages of the available technology. In contrast, the medical profession has sought not to guide, but to control, by means of technology. As women, and as midwives, we say 'No More'!

## REFERENCES

'Research in Ultrasound Bioeffects; – A Public Health View'. 1980. *Birth and the Family Journal*, vol. 7, no. 2, Summer.

Banta, David and Steven Thacker. 1979. *Birth and the Family Journal*, vol. 6, no. 4, Winter.

Caldeyo-Barcia, Roberto et al. 1960. 'The Effect of Position Changes on the Intensity and Frequency of Uterine Contractions During Labour'. *American Journal of Obstetrics and Gynecology*, no. 80: 284–90.

Caldeyo-Barcia, Roberto. 1979. 'The Influence of Maternal

# 418  RUTH HOLLAND AND JILL McKENNA

Position on Time of Spontaneous Rupture of Membranes, Progress of Labour and Foetal Head Compression'. *Birth and the Family Journal*, vol. 6, no. 1: 9–15.

Williams, R. M. et al. 1980. 'A Study of the Benefits and Acceptability of Ambulation in Spontaneous Labour.' *British Journal of Obstetrics and Gynaecology*, vol. 87, no. 2: 122–6.

# THROUGH THE SPECULUM [1]

Carol Downer

In this article, one of the founders of the Feminist Women's Health Center in Los Angeles describes the participation of the Self-Help Movement in the Women's Health Movement. Challenging the social control of women's sexuality and reproduction through the use of techniques like self-examination and information-sharing has led to a redefinition of the clitoris and the development of the technology of 'menstrual extraction.'

On April 7, 1971, a group of women met in a small women's bookstore in Venice, California. I had acquired a plastic vaginal speculum and wanted to share what I had seen with the group. After I demonstrated its use, several other women also took off their pants, climbed up on the table and inserted a speculum. In one amazing instant, each of us had liberated a part of our bodies which had formerly been the sole province of our gynecologists. Afterwards, in a consciousness-raising discussion, we observed that in this supportive, non-sexist setting, feelings of shame fell away and we acknowledged the beginnings of feelings of power from being able to look into our own vaginas and see where our menstrual blood, secretions and babies came from.

This meeting was the genesis of activities that spread and connected country-wide with other women engaged in similar pursuits, which became known as the 'Women's Health Movement.' Collectively we worked to reclaim a huge body of knowledge which had been coopted by the medical establishment; and, through research and observation, regained the technology for safe abortion and birth, self-insemination and redefined our sexual anatomy which had

419

been distorted, put down or simply ignored by mainstream sex educators and therapists.

Some women from this first group began to meet regularly to do self-examination with our own plastic speculums. These meetings provided an ongoing process of self-discovery and a growing body of vital information on vaginal conditions and our own reproductive anatomy.

Soon, we began doing referrals to illegal abortion clinics. Then we worked as assistants to physicians who were willing to do safe abortion procedures. By assisting at many abortions, we learned that the uterus is not such a remote, mysterious, inaccessible place and that early termination abortions by the suction method were far less technical and complicated than we had been led to believe. We planned to learn to do abortions ourselves, but the 1973 Supreme Court Decision on abortion made the procedure legal to twenty-four weeks of pregnancy. Fifty-three days after that decision, we borrowed $1200, rented a small house, hired a physician and opened up the first woman-owned, woman-controlled abortion clinic in the United States.

This clinic became the Los Angeles Feminist Women's Health Center. Within three years, similar clinics had started in Santa Ana, San Diego and Chico, California, and in Atlanta, Georgia. Because of similarities in philosophy and goals, these clinics decided to join together, to pool woman-power and resources to become the Federation of Feminist Women's Health Centers (FFWHCs). Later, clinics in Portland, Oregon and Yakima, Washington, joined us on an affiliate basis. All of these clinics are collectively woman-controlled and provide woman-centered abortion care (including later abortions), birth control (including cervical caps), and ongoing weekly Self-Help Clinics. At times, different clinics have offered lesbian health groups, birth programs and the Los Angeles FWHC started a donor insemination program in 1979.

At annual political education meetings, usually held in remote mountain retreats, we began developing a global consciousness and interest in women's issues and liberation struggles around the world. As a result of these discussions, we have traveled to Mexico, Canada, New Zealand, Europe,

Cuba, Iran and China, sharing the ideas of self-help and learning of the priorities of feminists in other cultures.

The underlying principle of all of the work of the Feminist Women's Health Centers is the strategy of undermining the patriarchal structure of society and male dominance by challenging the social control of women's sexuality and reproduction. The institutions of marriage and the laws which regulate divorce, abortion, prostitution, birth control and homosexuality isolate women from each other and brutally repress their sexuality and reproductive rights. The FWHCs have worked in national coalitions to support the women's movement's impressive campaigns against these laws.

As we progressed in our understanding of the patriarchy, we saw that in addition to laws which maintain the patriarchal family, all institutions of a sexist society function to reinforce women's inferior status, but the male-dominated medical institutions have the special role of enforcing women's sexual and reproductive compliance. Further, we realized that the external oppressive controls and exploitation of women's sexuality has a subjective expression – intense shame – which deprives us of the strength and vigor to assert our most basic rights. This universal shame, felt by all classes of women, causes us to feel extremely humiliated when we expose our genitals, except in situations which we define as medical or sexually intimate. Even in such situations, women frequently need special surroundings, props or rituals to allow another person (nearly always a male) to see or to touch her genitals. In our clinics, we have directly confronted the medical practice, peculiar to the United States, of draping women for exams, by dispensing with the drape altogether. The drape reinforces the feelings of shame we are supposed to feel and inhibits the free flow of information between a woman and her practitioner.

Indeed, these feelings of shame dictate and control many of our everyday decisions. Women are socialized to feel that their vaginal secretions are dirty and many feel the need to use vaginal deodorant sprays which have been found to be irritating and destructive to the natural ecology of the vagina. Many women shave their pubic hair so it won't show while wearing a bathing suit, or they are embarrassed to buy menstrual products in a market or are hesitant to do self-examination while menstruating.

In the past twelve years, we have held thousands and thousands of Self-Help Clinics and have repeatedly observed the immediate release of energy and the joy we experienced that first night in Venice. At the same moment the Self-Help Clinic breaks down the barriers between women and strips away repression and inhibition, it also provides us with a realistic alternative to total dependence on the medical profession. Women can take direct control of their own bodies from the simplest ability to check an IUD string directly by *looking*, instead of blindly by feeling, to identifying and treating common vaginal conditions with safe, inexpensive home remedies. No one would dream of running to the doctor for every sore throat, yet women are expected to regard each vaginal infection as a problem only a doctor can know anything about.

Through information gained in early Self-Help Clinics in Los Angeles, we were liberated from the oppression of misconceptions and misinformation. We learned that the structure of the cervix is beautifully simple. And by observing ourselves and each other on a regular basis, we learned that the medical definition of 'the range of normal' is impossibly narrow and restrictive. Such notions as 'tipped uteruses,' 'eroded cervixes,' 'irregular menstruation,' and 'vaginal discharge,' *all* considered 'health problems' by our doctors, became obviously absurd. We found that everyone's uterus is 'tipped' some way or other and that this term has no medical significance whatsoever. We realized that 'eroded cervix' merely means irritated, although the medical term connotes actual disintegration. We soon discovered that very few women have 'ideal' twenty-eight-day menstrual cycles. Unless noticeable signs of ill health are present, a woman's cycle can range normally from less than twenty days to six months, nine months, or even longer.

The first technology self-helpers gained was the ability to perform safe, early abortions in a procedure we called 'menstrual extraction.' We chose this term deliberately to blur the distinction between removing a menstrual period and terminating a pregnancy. In our society, abortion is used solely as a means to control women's reproduction, but to a woman faced with the possibility of terminating a pregnancy, the important thing is to have her period on time. Lorraine Rothman, a member of our group, invented a simple suction device which we called a 'Del-em' to extract the contents of the uterus. A Del-em is simply and inexpensively made from a glass jar, large syringe, a two-way automatic valve (to prevent air from accidentally getting into the uterus), acquarium tubing and stoppers. Through our observations of abortion procedures, we learned that a sterile plastic tube, about the circumference of a pencil, could be inserted into the uterus and that the uterine contents, menstrual blood or an early pregnancy, could be suctioned out. Women in other countries have likewise learned sterile techniques and have developed various methods of suction, such as converting used refrigerator motors, bicycle pumps or vacuum cleaners, with excellent results. Because menstrual extraction has traditionally been practiced in the watchful, caring environment of small groups of women, the experiences of women having extractions have been profoundly positive, and few serious problems have been reported.

Medical domination and control of pregnancy and childbirth has been more subtle than oppressive abortion laws, but is virtually complete in Western countries. The normal human experience of childbirth has been entirely removed from daily life, so that most of us have no direct knowledge of it, and it has been transformed into a dangerous, pathological event, so much so that normal birth is no longer even taught in medical schools. Lay midwives in the United States have been driven underground and have been replaced by Nurse Midwives, whose training is highly medical and who must operate under the direct supervision of physicians.

Self-helpers, other feminists and home-birth advocates have fought a monumental battle against the medical and legal establishments in the US to retain the right to choose birth attendants and settings. Lay midwives have been repeatedly arrested for murder and home-birth physicians have had their licenses revoked, while hospital-based physicians have remained beyond the law for even the most flagrant cases of excess and ineptitude.

In the face of increasing medical control, rising cesarean rates and a bewildering onslaught of technology, we have supported midwives and home-birth physicians and have opened our own birthing centers. In San Diego, Womancare operated a birth program for two years which supported women to have home or hospital births with lay birth attendants and physician back-up. Ultimately, the program closed because the back-up physician was openly threatened with the loss of his hospital privileges and medical society membership if he continued to attend home births. We have seen this to be a pattern nation-wide in the battle for control of birthing options.

Through using the techniques of self-examination and information-sharing, we reclaimed important and long-ignored information in the realm of women's sexuality. When we began to write about sex, we discovered a vast disparity between the way medical books and popular sex literature treated the sexual anatomy of men and women. The clitoris has always been considered to be the glands alone, while the penis is described as having many parts which function together to produce orgasm. We studied anatomical illustrations in both European and US medical texts and took off our pants and compared our genitals to these illustrations, some of which date back to the nineteenth century. Our group, comprised of both heterosexual and lesbian women, shared experiences and made photographs and movies of masturbation. Putting all of this information together, we *rediscovered* the entire clitoris, which encompasses structures of erectile tissue, blood vessels, glands, nerves and muscles. We learned that both visible and hidden structures of the clitoris undergo remarkable changes during sexual response including erection. The goal of the redefinition of the clitoris is to give women a concrete understanding of what actually occurs during sexual response and to offer clear explanations for various sexual phenomena.

After running clinics for a few years, we began to see this strategy as a limited solution to the monumental problems women faced in seeking medical care or in having control over their reproduction and sexuality. If we wanted to reach large numbers of women, we decided we needed to spread our ideas in written form. So far, this decision has resulted in four books, each focused on a different aspect of women's health.

*A New View of A Woman's Body* (1981) differs from all other women's health books in that it was researched and written by lay health-workers involved in day-to-day health care, and draws on the cumulative experience of more than 100,000 women who have visited our clinics over the past ten years. *A New View* also includes clear and detailed illustrations of women's anatomy, especially the redefinition of the clitoris, and the first color photographs of women's vaginas and cervixes to appear outside of a medical text. (Published by Simon & Schuster, New York.)

*How to Stay Out of the Gynecologist's Office* discusses in-depth problems that every woman is likely to encounter at some time in her life. We evaluated home remedies, over-the-counter preparations and medical remedies for effectiveness and possible harmful effects and compiled a glossary of over 1000 terms used by gynecologists. We also included information women might use when seeking to equalize the very unequal power relationship encountered in a gynecologist's office. (Published in 1981, by Peace Press, Culver City, California.)

Most recently, we completed *Woman-centered Pregnancy and Birth*, a book designed to give women more power and control over their birth experience. We included very detailed information to help women evaluate both the multitude of technological interventions they can be faced with in a medical setting and the designation of 'high risk,' which, once invoked, is the justification for *any* intervention the physician chooses. We also discuss self-defense techniques in the hospital, donor insemination and resources on how to work for political change in childbirth. (Published by Cleis Press, Pittsburgh, Pennsylvania, forthcoming.)

In 1979, in response to a request from Chilean women who were being raped while they were imprisoned, Suzann Gage and other women compiled information on self-abortion techniques. In 1979, we published this manuscript as *When Birth Control Fails . . . (How to Abort Ourselves Safely)*

(Speculum Press, Hollywood, California). This book became the object of a heated public debate, both within the women's community and in the mainstream press. Nevertheless, feminists from around the world, especially in countries where abortion is illegal or difficult to obtain, ordered copies and the entire edition was sold in a very short time. We hope that a future edition will include the experiences and research of many more women.

In researching and writing our books, we has found that our early belief in the power of self-examination have been reinforced and validated. Vaginal self-examination with a plastic speculum, when performed in a group setting, is a direct assault on the shame that has been inculcated in us regarding our genitals and is a powerful, positive act of trust and mutual support between women. After this barrier is broken, the information flows rapidly and voluminously. Myth after myth falls away. Using the format of the Self-Help Clinic, women could rediscover all of the old knowledge which has been ripped away from us. Combining this knowledge with a group study of medical texts, we could question existing medical information and put it on a more sound empirical basis.

In the 1980s, the Feminist Women's Health Centers face new challenges around the reproductive technologies mentioned in this book. We are confident that our philosophy of health care and our recognition and validation of women's experiences will allow us to play a significant role in developing a women-centered perspective of the new technologies.

## NOTE

1  This chapter was edited by Rebecca Chalker.

# FEMINIST ETHICS, ECOLOGY, AND VISION

## Janice Raymond

This article asserts the necessity for women to recognize the complexity of the issues surrounding reproductive technologies from an ecological vision. This means re-defining ecology so that the whole context in which a woman may 'choose' a particular technology, such as in vitro fertilization, is highlighted. It emphasizes the threat that such technologies pose to women's health and well-being, as well as the immense amount of bio-medical manipulation and experimentation to which women are subject.

Thoughtful women will have a variety of thoughtful responses to the technologies discussed in this book. However, one imperative – certainly not the only response, but perhaps the least discussed – is the necessity for *vision*. This essay considers the vision of a woman-centered health ethic.

At first glance, reproductive technologies seem to offer a positive vision to women, that is they appear to give so-called infertile women the ability to reproduce. At second glance, however, another not-so-positive vision looms large, and this is the persistent *medicalization* of women's lives. But many women accept only the first vision as truth and dismiss the second as reactionary.

To talk about the medicalization of life means that more and more areas of living have been colonized by medical intervention, and staked out as medical territory. Nowhere do we witness this medicalization more than in the establishment of the specialities of gynecology and obstetrics beginning in the nineteenth century in America. The medicalization of female existence rests on the availability of female bodies to be analyzed, quantified, qualified, and integrated into the sphere of medical practice on the grounds of a male-perceived pathology said to be intrinsic to women, that is, ability to reproduce.

The enormous increase in Caesarean sections and other birthing technologies, as well as the engineering of human reproduction made possible by sex preselection, test-tube fertilization, and the like, as discussed in this volume, cannot but add to the chronic medicalization of women's bodies, and thus to the bio-medical management of women's lives. Obscured and submerged in all the recent accounts of the 'miracles' of reproductive technologies is the immense amount of bio-medical probing, manipulation, and experimentation to which women who seek out such 'wonders' of technological fertility and birthing are subject.

The therapeutic rationale is inherent in the bio-medical vision and put forward as the primary rationale in all discussions of reproductive technologies. For example, in most discussions about in vitro fertilization, the desperation of women who are unable to have children in the natural biological way is highlighted. (What is not discussed is that many so-called infertile women are in this condition due to past technological and medical 'mistakes.') In this vision, test-tube pregnancies are touted as curative and humane. The therapeutic emphasis focuses the discussion away from the feminist and political dimensions of the technologies onto their more personal and supposedly benevolent aspects. All is envisioned in the light of technology as salvation.

Because the mainstream medical perspective of reproductive technologies depicts them as therapeutic, much of the public, and, most important, many of the women involved, have accepted them as benevolent. A feminist critique that emphasizes the medicalization of women by such technologies seems paranoid at worst and heartless at best. This is upsetting to those of us who are concerned with the disastrous consequences for women to which such technologies point.

Visionary thinking has always been suspect but today more so, when the truly real issues of health, education, and welfare are further removed from the majority of women. One economist has stated the female situation quite bluntly: 'We don't have male poverty in the United States any more. We only have female poverty.' (Thurow, 1982) Combine this fact with the not-so-dry statistics that:

Two-thirds of the world's illiterates are women. (United Nations, 1980a)

Women in the US earn 59 percent of what men earn. (US Department of Commerce, 1980)

Women are vastly more underemployed than men. While women represent over half of the world adult population and one-third of the official labor force, women perform for nearly two-thirds of all working hours and receive only one-tenth of the world income. Women also own less than 1 percent of world property. (United Nations, 1980b)

Every seven minutes, a woman in the United States is raped. (US Dept of Justice, 1980)

Every eighteen seconds, a woman in the United States is battered. (Moore, 1979)

And now, the medicalization of women's lives brought about by reproductive technologies produces further debilitation to women's bodies and spirits.

In facing all these 'real' issues, women cannot afford to dismiss the visionary task, for it is just as real. Nor can we allow despair at the overwhelming character of the state of female oppression to paralyze us in the man-made world. Commenting on the narrow vision of much materialist feminist theory, Lise Weil states: 'Within the materialist analysis . . . the system has allowed us just enough of our reasoning faculties to "decode the mechanisms of oppression," to analyze oppression "in order to fight it." ' However, if women have no vision of how things can be different, Weil asks, 'whence comes women's will to change?' One might add, whence comes women's determination to take action for change?

I am not trying to drive a wedge between the necessity for women to understand and act against the many forms of female oppression, and the necessity for feminist vision. Rather, I am saying that it is impossible to understand and act against the many kinds of assaults on women if women do not have a vision of how things could be different and develop some solutions for actualizing that vision. Vision ensures that our conflicts with and struggles against male supremacy do not become one-dimensional. For this reason, my vision of a woman-centered health ethic is *ecological*.

Much reproductive technology is dangerous to female health and well-being. Any vision which counters the one offered to women by this technology must therefore be based on a fundamental concern for female health and well-being. And any vision of female health and well-being must be ecological in the sense that it considers the *whole context* in which, for example, a woman may 'choose' a particular reproductive technology, such as a Caesarean section or in vitro fertilization. Just as we recognize the necessity for an ecological perspective on the physical environment of nature, that is, the ecosystem, so we must employ the same environmental standards to what I would call the female ecosystem.

Social and environmental dimensions are important to any consideration of what enhances health. Health certainly has a physical base, and is always manifested through the body, but the physical base is always surrounded by events external to the individual. Thus it is imperative to ask how healthy are the social milieux and environments of most women? How do most women live their lives? In particular, how do women who supposedly elect a particular reproductive technology live their lives? Another way of phrasing the question is to what must many women adapt?

Rene Dubos and others have seen *adaptation* as a positive indicator of health.

> The concept of perfect and positive health is a utopian creation of the mind. It cannot become reality because man will never be so perfectly adapted to his environment that his life will not involve struggles, failures, and sufferings. . . . The less pleasant reality is that in an ever-changing world each period and each type of civilization will continue to have its burden of disease created by the

unavoidable failure of adaptation to the new environment.
(Dubos, 1965)

Because Dubos is using adaptation in a restricted sense here,
he can define health as maximum adaptability to the unavoidable course of disease. Anyone seeking a more expan-
sive definition of health must view adaptation in a wider
sense. I would argue that Dubos and other adaptationists
overlook in their emphasis on 'man' adapting, that woman
over-adapts. Failure to adapt is disease-producing and not
healthy, but so is over-adaptation!

Woman adapts to a self and a world she never created.
Simone de Beauvoir's description of woman as 'the Other,'
existing through man's fabrication of her, describes the social
construction of feminine reality. Initially, women adapt to
the man-made construction of female behavior, roles, and life
'choices.' A host of functional adaptations follow: channeling
energy and creativity to others (mainly men); learning modes
of indirect discourse; assuming the body language of an
inferior; wearing immobile and constraining clothing;
cosmeticizing the body; and bearing the burden and 'side
effects' of male-directed femininity, such as birth control.

Indeed in the realm of reproductive technologies, women
adapt to very debilitating situations. Take the case of in vitro
fertilization. Most of the women who seek this kind of technology are branded 'infertile women.' They therefore have
undergone multiple medical tests and exploratory procedures to determine the cause of their infertility, as well as
treatments to remedy their conditions. Obstruction or other
irregularities of the Fallopian tubes are said to produce 45
percent of female infertility in those women who are tested.
Such obstruction may be caused by scar tissue which results
from infection or endometriosis, a condition in which the
uterine lining sloughs off into the pelvic cavity, grows, and
scars the tubes, thus closing them off. The tests for detecting
tubal obstruction or irregularities are intrusive and painful.
In one test, carbon dioxide gas is injected into the uterus.

With many infertile women, doctors 'blow out the tubes'
every four to eight weeks for a considerable period of time.
This is a procedure in which pressurized liquid is forced

through the tubes in order to maintain a limited opening. One woman, interviewed in *People* magazine, who had undergone this treatment and who considered in vitro fertilization her last hope of conceiving and bearing a child, was quoted as saying: 'When I have the therapy, I put a towel over my head and cry.' (Witt, 1978)

For those women who seek salvation through further bio-medical monitoring and technique, the pain and probing continues. Having been subjected to a whole series of infertility 'work-ups,' the eschatological remedy becomes test-tube fertilization. The first step in this process is extraction of an egg from the woman at ovulation. The doctor uses a laparoscope equipped with lens and light, and inserted through the navel, to look for a mature egg. The egg is then removed by suction from a needle. During laparoscopy and needle puncture, the ovaries are traumatized.

The egg is transferred to a culture dish containing nutrients and sperm. After fertilization and development to the blastocyst stage, the egg is implanted into the uterus of the woman. Trauma to the uterus can also occur when a cannula, or small tube, is inserted to introduce the embryo. Furthermore, when the ovaries are surgically manipulated, as in the laparoscopy and suction procedures, they may not secrete the proper amounts of estrogen or progesterone that are required. The woman is then given hormones, in some combination, so that her uterus is better able to accept the implanted embryo. (Kolata, 1978)

In addition to extraction and implantation, a number of other bio-medical procedures are performed on the woman. Amniocentesis is often done to determine the chromosomal normality of the fetus. The risks of amniocentesis include hemorrhage, perforation of the viscera, and infection. Some women who have had amniocentesis also reported cramps and discomfort lasting from a few hours to a few days. In addition, amnioscopy is often done to gauge the structural normality of the fetus. Finally, ultrasound is frequently used to gain information and certitude about normal fetal growth. The dangers of ultrasound have been chronicled by many sources. And as the final bio-medical intervention, a Caesarian section may be performed.

Much of the pain and debilitation that women who undergo these procedures assume was attested to by John Brown, father of Louise Brown, the world's first test-tube baby. On the television special aired after Louise Brown was born, John Brown spoke of his wife's tremendous pain and profuse bleeding spells which followed her multiple visits to the doctor.

Any woman-centered health ethic focusing on reproductive technologies emphasizes the ecology in which women supposedly 'choose' such debilitating procedures. A feminist vision of health does not encourage the adaptation to manmade femininity that is reified by such technologies. Instead it points out that the environment in which women make such choices is designed to make women adapt to the offerings at hand.

Reproductive technologies are being urged on women at a rapid rate. In 1981 alone, 702,000 Caesareans were performed in the United States. A 1981 survey done by the National Center for Health Statistics confirmed that the Caesarean rate is still rising, and that the number of Caesareans accounts for 17.9 percent of all 1981 births. In vitro clinics are opening their doors at a rapidly growing rate. At the time of this writing, there are forty-two clinics in the US that, as one newspaper account phrased it, 'offer an estimated 600,000 infertile women their only chance to give birth.' (*Providence Journal*, 1983) While forty-two clinics may not seem like an extraordinarily high number, it must be remembered that these clinics have been established only in the last three years, when they were given the go-ahead by a ruling of the Ethics Advisory Board convened by the Department of Health, Education and Welfare. This ruling paved the way for medical institutions to initiate in vitro clinics under guidelines that, among other stipulations, limited the technology to married couples.

Pat Hynes, a writer and environmental engineer, has compared conditions of women under patriarchy with those of natural ecosystems under the stress of extreme pollution. She has noted that polluted or stressed environments are identified by their low species and occupational diversity:

Now imagine a graph of the number of women in various
occupations: large numbers of women are concentrated in
few occupations: housewife, secretary, and service
professions. In other words, women may be characterized
by low occupational diversity. (Hynes, 1980)

Hynes cites Howard Odum, a noted ecologist, who states:
'When ecological systems must adapt their function and
organs to survive in conditions which are physically severe
for life . . . energy is required for the process of adaptation and
less energy remains to support complex network specializ-
ations.' (Odum, 1971) Reproductive technologies are indeed
energy-draining!

A feminist ecological vision notes that the technological
ethic is simplifying the complexity of the issues that
surround these technologies. Using Odum's point about
ecological systems that are forced to adapt, we might say
about infertile women who go the route of in vitro technology
that they adapt their 'function and organs to survive in conditions which are physically severe for life.' A remarkable
amount of these women's energy is required for the process of
adapting to the debilitating effects of the technologies themselves. However, more than this, women adapt to the patriarchal ideology that reproduction is a woman's prime
commodity, no matter what the cost to herself. Women, of
course, have always adapted to environments that are
unhealthy. What the new reproductive technologies do is to
give a scientific and therapeutic boost to female adaptation,
thereby reinforcing women's oppression.

It is nothing new to state that environmental factors are
a major determinant of health. Even the World Health
Organization defines health as 'A state of complete physical
and mental and social well-being and not merely the absence
of disease or infirmity.' What is new in a feminist ecological
vision is to expand the definition of environment so that it
means more than ecologists or environmentalists currently
define it. Environment is more than clean air, clean water,
and the like. It encompasses the whole personal and social
milieu in which a woman lives, including clean air, water,
proper nutrition, light, sleep – but, more expansively, it also

includes economic independence, ability to make choices, motivation and opportunities to choose, and friendship, among others. In other words, health is the constant process to recreate a female environment that is Self-defined,[1] on the boundary of an environment that has been man-made. The first imperative for female health is mythic, in the sense that women must reverse the patriarchal creation myths and live Self-defined lives. This is not a mere individual act. It is a political reality that undergirds other political realities of our lives. And it is, of course, a spiritual reality.

With the advent of the new reproductive technologies, the myth of patriarchal creation is re-fabricated. Once more, man fashions woman in his own image.

In the midst of such a man-made environment, it is important for women not only to see the whole picture, but to persist in asking woman-centered ecological questions. Why do these fabulous medical techniques require that women adapt to the most painful and debilitating circumstances? Why do such technologies eminently reinforce the bio-medical 'fact' that a woman's reproductive system is pathological and requires an enormous amount of bio-intervention? Why do these techniques reduce the totality of a woman's being to that which is medically manipulatable? Under the cover of a new science of reproduction, how is the female body being fashioned into the biological laboratory of the future? And finally, will the ultimate feat of these technologies be to remove not only the control of reproduction, but reproduction itself, from women? It is my contention that the engineering of human reproduction, and the forms it has taken, could only occur in a society where the anti-feminist dimensions of the technologies run far deeper than is apparent at first glance.

Faced with the reality of these technologies, women must ask ecological questions and assert our own ecological vision. When accused of being callous toward women who desperately desire to have children, we must respond by raising the spectre of the real inhumanity that reproductive technologies force upon women. It is not callous or inhumane to ask why women are channeled, at such a cost to themselves, into reproducing. An ecological sensitivity should examine the *why – and the how –* behind the supposed therapeutic goals of the reproductive counselors and technologists. These technologies cannot be abstracted from the total environment in which women live our lives.

## NOTE

1 I use Mary Daly's device of capitalizing *Self* here to distinguish between the man-made feminine self, the 'imposed/internalized false "self"' of women, and the authentic Self that women are beginning to re-create. See Daly, 1978.

## REFERENCES

Daly, Mary. 1978. *Gyn/Ecology: The Metaethics of Radical Feminism.* Boston, Beacon Press.

Dubos, Rene. 1965. *Man Adapting.* Yale University Press, New Haven.

Hynes, Patricia. 1980. 'The Survivors: Women and Nature.' Paper presented at the Women and Science Colloquia, Boston College. April.

Kolata, Gina Bari. 1978. '*In Vitro* Fertilization: Is It Safe and Repeatable?' *Science*, 201, August 25: 698–9.

Moore, D. 1979. *Battered Women.* Sage Publications, Beverly Hills.

Odum, Howard. 1971. *Environment, Power, and Society.* Wiley-Interscience, New York: 80.

*Providence Journal.* 1983. June 12, 1.

Thurow, Lester. 1982. As quoted in *Second Century Radcliffe News.* April.

United Nations, 1980a. 'Review and Evaluation of Progress Made and Obstacles Encountered at the National Level in Attaining the Objectives of the World Plan of Action,' Item 8a of the Provisional Agenda 80-14909, World Conference of the United Nations Decade for Women: Equality, Development, and Peace. Copenhagen, Denmark.

United Nations, 1980b. 'Program of Action for the 2nd Half of the U.N. Decade for Women: Equality, Development, and Peace,' Item 9 of the Provisional Agenda 80-12383, World Conference of the United Nations Decade for Women: Equality, Development, and Peace. Copenhagen, Denmark.

United States Department of Commerce. 1980. Table 12: Comparison of Median Earnings of Year Round Full Time

Workers by Sex, 1955–1978, in *Money Income of Families and Persons in the U.S., Current Population Reports, 1957–1977; Money Income and Poverty Status of Families and Persons in the U.S.;* 1980 Census.

United States Department of Justice. 1980. *F.B.I. Uniform Crime Reports.* Crime in the United States: 1979 (release date, September 24).

Weil, Lise. 'Patriarchal Realism and Female Reality.' Doctoral Dissertation in Comparative Literature, unpublished and in progress, Brown University: chapter 1.

Witt, L. 1978. 'Two Nashville Doctors May Help An American Mother Have Her Own Test-Tube Baby.' *People*, 10, August 14: 28–30.

# A WOMB OF ONE'S OWN

Jalna Hanmer

This article seeks to unveil and contest dominant ideology about the new reproductive technologies. Examples from the British press and the work of major medical and scientific experimenters are used to illustrate how dominant ideology is reinforced and utilized. The claim to produce 'perfect babies' and of meeting the needs of 'unfulfilled women' is presented as resolving all the ethical issues raised by the new technologies. But the interests of women, as women, remain subterranean. The author suggests ways in which actions around the demand of the Womens' Liberation Movement for 'control over our bodies' can evolve and thereby challenge men's 'right' to determine what is 'best' for women.

'Perfect' babies, 'unfulfilled' women – these are the stories with which the mass media has introduced the public to the phenomena of test-tube babies and other new reproductive technologies. We are given admiring views of modern man's (sic) technology, and are reminded that all of this is done 'for the good' of individual women. The justification for reproductive experiments on women is always couched in terms of a woman's 'right' to have a baby, or of every baby's 'right' to be 'perfect.' The cost, however, in terms of women who endure hormonal injections and surgery, and who frequently do not conceive or carry a pregnancy to term despite prolonged and painful interventions, is steadfastly ignored. And the question of whether these technologies are really in the interest of women as a group is never asked.

The justifications put forward for these experiments have not altered over the last decade but there has been a gradual

438

increase of reports in the British press (which I use as an example) about the new technologies. One strand has been a steady trickle on research into sex selection, ranging from accounts of new methods for pre- and post-conception determination of sex to a limited discussion of moral and ethical issues and results of studies on sex preference. In addition, there has been a growing public awareness of female infanticide in China and India.

Were we to summarise press coverage of the last decade, it could be said that the 1970s saw a fascination with cloning, (assisted by Rorvik's undoubtedly fictional account of a man who cloned himself, 1978; see also Genoveffa Corea's and Jane Murphy's papers in this collection). By 1980, while animal experiments on cloning continued to be reported, two years after the birth of the world's first test-tube baby, Louise Brown, there was one report after the other on in vitro fertilisation. In 1981 we saw the championing and questioning of surrogate motherhood, and by 1982 'egg donating' became a news topic. The major controversy of that year was the ethical question of experimenting on embryos that were not intended for implantation. In Britain, in vitro fertilisation was officially taken up by the National Health Service (NHS) which started to run its own fertilisation programmes.

In 1983 these two areas of press interest merged with reports of the ability to divide embryos before implantation. The technique is to split an embryo at its four-cell stage, when each cell is genetically identical and capable of growing into a child. It was developed on non-humans to determine sex and to produce more than one offspring and also to permit easy analysis of chromosomes. While this form of cloning has yet to be seized upon as a possibility for human reproduction by the in vitro fertilisers, we should anticipate that it will be soon (see, for instance the British report on in vitro fertilisation of the RCOG Ethics Committee, 1983: 12).

We also saw in 1983 an intensification of the publicity about embryo transfer, the genetic manipulation of embryos, and the freezing of embryos – most successfully undertaken so far in Australia. The implicit message in these media accounts is that embryos are being perfected, which no woman, of course, would be able to do unaided by male medical and scientific experts. In 1983 we also saw the start of stories about how man alone could gestate babies with some embryos beginning development outside a woman's uterus (up to 7 days!) and increased interest in the development of 'artificial wombs' (see also Robyn Rowland's chapter in this collection). Dr Robert Edwards was hailed as 'father of the century' – Louise Brown indeed is seen as *his* product. We also saw accounts of how sub-fertile men could become fathers through in vitro fertilisation, as in the controlled environment of a Petri dish only a few sperms are needed. And, finally, another round started in the competition between the boys to control the market by eliminating potential competitors, described as 'cowboys': private gynaecologists who could set up practices as in vitro fertilisation specialists by paying centralised laboratories to do the actual fertilisations (*Guardian*, 6 July 1983).

What we have *not* seen over the decade is a discussion of what has been going on in terms of experimentation. Largely untested techniques are presented as scientific breakthroughs. As far as I know there has been no questioning of the success rate until very recently, when it began, of course, to improve. In 1982, Mr Robert Winston, the surgeon in charge of the infertility clinic at Hammersmith Hospital in London, backtracked on his use of the phrase 'confidence trick' to describe the publicity surrounding so-called test-tube babies, but he did go on to say that claims of a 25 per cent success rate were questionable (*Guardian*, 14 October 1982). He found that 50 per cent of the women who came to his infertility clinic were medically unsuitable, which for a large percentage was due to previous surgery (not always necessary) causing irreparable damage (*Guardian*, 16 August 1983).

Press publicity can thus be seen as encouraging women to become human guinea pigs. The under- and *de*valuation of women as people, our valuation only as wives and mothers, makes women vulnerable to social pressures to reproduce and to go through any torture to be able to do so. As Winston said,

Virtually every infertile patient now has the fantasy that if she is able to save up the money and get herself into the hands of somebody practising in vitro fertilisation, that she is going to have a baby. . . . The real problem is that at least half the patients referred to me are medically unsuitable for IVF and their hopes are dashed. (*Guardian*, 14 October 1982.)

The very limited questioning of the desirability of these developments also takes place on the individual level. For example, the issues are phrased as:

Is choice (of the sex of the offspring, in vitro fertilisation, etc.) a 'right' every woman should have?
Would government restriction, say of amniocentesis for sex choice or egg donation, be likely to lead to general restriction of reproductive rights?
What is the motivation of those involved in this research?

Discussion based on 'rights' and 'choice' assumes a society without differential distribution of power and authority, or at least without *serious* differentials. But 'rights' and 'choice' gradually fade as coercion increases. The notion of power imbalance in society implies structural inequalities with a supporting ideology. In other words, do you have a 'choice' if there are no viable options? (See also Barbara Katz Rothman in this volume.)

In reality we live in a world dominated by men and the interests of men; every aspect of women's reproduction is controlled in a very collective way in the interest of their continuing power domination over women. This type of thinking gives rise to a very different set of priorities; for example, a need to explore the interpenetration of professional and scientific groups with state, political, and financial support. We need to know how dominant ideology is used to further scientific and medical control over women. We need to understand how women are silenced, our complicity and collusion assured, and how our challenges are undercut.

One frequently met pattern is for the experimenter to also assume the position of the ethicist who defines the terms of the debate and offers the solution to the problem. Ordinary women, including the experimented upon, are relegated into the back wings of the stage, unseen and silenced. For example, Britain at the present moment has a Governmental Committee investigating the ethical issues involved in in vitro experimentation on women.[1] This is a culmination of a process that began a number of years ago with the work of Patrick Steptoe, a gynaecologist at Oldham General Hospital, and Robert Edwards, a physiologist at Cambridge University. Both these institutions are funded by the tax payments of British citizens, and the facilities of both were used until eventually Louise Brown was born. Steptoe and Edwards's research received support from the Ford Foundation as well, but its experimental nature led to a refusal of funding by the British Medical Research Council, a semi-private agency. They voiced serious doubts about the ethical aspects of in vitro fertilisation, given the lack of preliminary studies, possible hazards, and the use of laparoscopy (see Glossary, p. 459) for purely experimental purposes. (Edwards and Steptoe, 1980: 106) Financial support continued, however, from sources which Edwards and Steptoe described as 'private' and mainly American. Moreover, once Louise Brown was born, opposition to in vitro programmes melted in Britain. National Health Service hospitals began experimenting with the technique. Steptoe and Edwards established a private clinic at Bourn Hall near Cambridge, where fees are, of course, payable whether or not the experiment is a success.

But even before Louise Brown was born, Edwards reported, after the Medical Research Council's refusal to fund their research and attacks from colleagues during a major professional meeting:

> I would not wish the reader to imagine that we were overly vulnerable. I had been a member of a small committee for some years now that had been formed to clarify ethical issues arising from advances in biology. (Edwards and Steptoe, 1980: 115)

This committee, chaired by an influential scientist at Oxford University, included major Labour politicians, a theologian who comments on science, and the editor of a widely read scientific publication. Through this committee Edwards was able to gain considerable powerful support for his and

Steptoe's in vitro experiments. By 1983 their confidence to occupy all the relevant positions had been made fully public in the *Guardian* (25 June 1983): 'It's like nuclear weapons. The people who know what they can do have got to lead and stimulate the debate.' Further, readers are assured that he (Edwards) welcomes the debate, 'as long as it is conducted rationally without people shouting at each other.' Steptoe and Edwards are portrayed as 'experts' who 'help' women. But it is not made evident that simultaneously they continue to function as part of the very establishment that decides what 'true' womanhood is all about. Anyway – with true *noblesse oblige*, they will permit us to speak as long as we do it gently and are good-mannered!

In the promotion of reproductive technologies, relations between professional groups, the state, and the media are not limited solely to scientists and medical men. Social scientists are also implicated. For example, the rationale for research on sex preferences is to explore the relation of preference to fertility, and thereby the potential contribution of sex selection to population control. There have been a relatively large number of studies on sex preference (for a review see Williamson, 1976). They are dominated by assumptions that methods of determining sex before conception will be used as soon as they are introduced, although some account is taken of the large number of respondents who express no interest in determining the sex of their children. The questioning of social scientists implies that sex pre-determination is an accepted idea. It is just a matter of finding out which method is preferred and when and how many children are desired. The question *why* people want to determine the sex of their children or why *males* are thought more desirable by both men and women is not explored in any depth. The disparity between the percentage of women and men who prefer males has not been systematically explored, although the greater preference of men for male children is a major consistent finding. In short the area is treated as unproblematic (Hanmer, 1981). Social scientists also live, by and large, off government money and, by and large, the researchers are men (or male-identified women). However unconscious the process, dominant interests are purveyed through research that does not question the ideology it is based on.

We live in a culture dominated by men and, therefore, we should expect that these technological developments will be used to maintain and probably reinforce male dominance, even if, for example, the occasional woman benefits by having the sex of the child *she* and not her husband, father, or some other male wants. We women must break into their cosy world. As feminists we have an ethical position to make that differs from the medical and scientific communities' 'concern' for the unborn, or to 'improve' the gene pool. In examining the so-called ethical literature produced by men, no one so far has spoken for the rights and concerns of women. The women who are being researched and experimented upon, *and all of us*, present and future, who will be affected by a greater control by men over women's bodies, must be heard.

A major demand, maybe *the* major demand of the Women's Liberation Movement is control over our own bodies. One of the ways women have demanded this control is by taking part in many local and national campaigns, for example, around contraception, abortion, sterilisation, home versus hospital births. Women for the last fifteen years have continually made demands for less alienating uses of reproductive technologies. Further, self-help attempts to provide health-care services, from pregnancy-testing to abortion and self-insemination groups, are examples of women actually taking control of these technologies (as reported by various authors in this collection). Whether women will remain the researched upon – the 'nature' to be controlled – will depend upon the success of these and future challenges. Challenging the way so-called 'services' are organised for women also challenges the dominant social interests that lie behind the mobilisation of research, funding, and state and public support for present and future developments in reproductive technologies. The struggle over who shall control female biological reproductive processes involves major restructuring that has profound implications for women, as a class, whether or not we personally use these technologies (Hanmer, 1983). We do not know exactly how these implications will be expressed, but the greater the asymmetry, the greater the potential abuse of the less powerful group. And this, to repeat myself, has implications for *all* women, whether we 'choose' to have children (see Barbara Katz Rothman) or whether we are being used as 'egg providers' (see Genoveffa Corea and Jane Murphy in this volume).

As feminists have pointed out, it is not inevitable that women have to have children, or particular types of children. Motherhood is not so much a biological 'urge' as a social response. Ideas do not 'free float' in culture divorced from the actual life conditions of women. In families, men and women occupy different positions. Families (of whatever 'type') are groups with differential distribution of power and authority among its members. Women, like men, often prefer males because they are the favoured sex within their marriage and family, as well as the culture generally. Women frequently believe they must have children to be 'real' and 'full' women because they are not valued as autonomous human beings but only as servicers to men, primarily as wives and mothers. Indeed, given the world as it is, women may need children because at least children love you if only for those few short years before they become yet another male-preferring person identifying with fathers, valuing men highly, and eventually looking for another primary relationship in which this can be expressed; for daughters, of course, with a man. These insights are crucial: we need to voice them in our protests about the intensifying control over women's reproductive potential.

How do our ideas about material life interact with women's actual life conditions? Looked at negatively, separating women from the naturalness of conception, pregnancy, and birth by intensifying the control over these processes by a largely male medical and scientific community, undermines women's confidence as biological reproducers of new life. While it is now inevitable that biological reproduction will become a more conscious decision (and process) for women, is it inevitable that control of reproduction will continue to remain with or progressively pass even more into male hands?

One place to begin the struggle against a worsening of

women's positions *vis-à-vis* men as a social group is to challenge the consistently 'good press' of the male medical and scientific communities involved in these developments; that is, to unveil and contest dominant ideology. We need a demystification of reproductive technologies, an exposure of what their politics really are: the continued oppression of women.

We need supporting research; the kind that breaks into the closed logic of greater male control of women. For example, it is imperative to study the differential preference of men and women for male children. While son preference is common to virtually all societies, the degree varies between countries and groups within each, and between men and women. The basis exists for serious policy-oriented research. We must help tell the stories of the silenced women who do *not* prefer boys over girls, and explore how to enlarge their numbers. We must ask ourselves *why* men pursue developments in reproductive technologies and to what lengths they are prepared to go to implement them. And above all we must ask: who benefits?

We need to organise. As major experimentation occurs, women's health groups must take up this issue. We must gather information on powerful medical empires. When male scientific bodies hold conferences on in vitro fertilisation or on any of the new reproductive technologies, we need to be there too. The information we obtain in such ways, we must share. We need an international feminist network to monitor developments, to expose links between the state, professional groups, profits, the media and the pervasiveness of worldwide woman-hating. We should call for an International Tribunal on Medical Crimes Against Women on the 'old' as well as the 'new' reproductive technologies. We need a series of meetings within the feminist movements around the world on what action to take, as major experimentation is taking place in many countries. We must develop and share a critique that can successfully challenge men's 'right' to define what is best for women.

We must begin all this immediately. For such is the pace of developments in the reproductive engineering field that by the time, a few months only from this writing, when this book is published, significant further advances in controlling women's bodies are highly likely to have been made. We must act on our own behalf. Quickly. Better today than tomorrow – for it might soon be too late.

## ACKNOWLEDGMENT

I am grateful to Genoveffa Corea for her suggestions about strategies to form an international feminist network and for her help with the final draft of this article.

## NOTE

1  The Government Inquiry into Human Fertilisation and Embryology, chaired by Mrs Mary Warnock, is due to report in 1984. The above-mentioned report of the RCOG Ethics Committee on in vitro fertilisation is publicly available and highly recommended reading for its bone-jarring use of technological language to describe women and ethical and legal questions of reproductive technologies. Available at £1 from The Royal College of Obstetricians and Gynaecologists, 27 Sussex Place, Regent's Park, London NW1 4RG.

## REFERENCES

Edwards, Robert and Patrick Steptoe. 1980. *A Matter of Life*. Hutchinson, London.

*Guardian*. 1982. ' "False Hope" Charge Over Fertility Claim'. 14 October.

*Guardian*. 1983. 'Father of the Century'. 25 June.

*Guardian*. 1983. 'The Fertile Spin-off'. 6 July.

*Guardian*. 1983. 'Surgeon Condemns Operating Errors'. 16 August.

Hanmer, Jalna. 1981. 'Sex Predetermination, Artificial Insemination and the Maintenance of Male-dominated Culture.' In Roberts, Helen, ed. *Women, Health and Reproduction*. Routledge & Kegan Paul, London and Boston.

Hanmer, Jalna. 1983. 'Reproductive Technology: The Future for Women?' in Rothschild, Joan, ed. *Machina Ex Dea*. Pergamon Press, New York and Oxford.

'Report of the RCOG Ethics Committee on In Vitro Fertilisation and

Embryo Replacement or Transfer'. 1983. Royal College of Obstetricians and Gynaecologists, London. March.

Rorvik, David. 1978. *In His Image*. Hamish Hamilton, London.

Williamson, Nancy. 1976. *Sons or Daughters: A Cross-Cultural Survey of Parental Preferences,* Sage Library of Social Research, Russell Sage, New York.

# THE COURAGE OF SISTERS

Cris Newport

This story was written specifically for this anthology. It grew out of the question 'what if?' as many stories do. What if the government decided whose children could be carried to term? What if you loved your husband, but he worked for the department that would decree the death of your unborn child? What if the child you were carrying was the 'wrong' sex?

Kira poured herself a finger of brandy and went again to the window. The sun had just set and the western sky was still dappled with pink and orange clouds. Through the dome of the city above her, she could see the deep blue, the color she had always loved. A knock on the door interrupted her reverie.

It was Kam, her older sister. Kira opened the door to admit her quietly, knowing she didn't have to say anything, that Kam probably already knew.

'It's a girl, then?' Kam asked, when she, too, had a glass of brandy in hand. Kira just nodded. 'I thought it would be, or you would have been at my door hours ago.' Kam turned to refill her glass. Kira noticed her sister seemed even more bent and frail today than she had recently. She had never been the same since her child, also a girl, had been taken from her by a government-ordered abortion a year ago.

'Why do they have those stupid laws, Kam? Why must they take all our girl children from us as if they were just toys?'

Kam sighed. 'I don't know. I mean, I know what the Decree says.'

'So do I, they read it to me when they told me I was

449

carrying a girl. Something like, "since the nuclear attacks of the nineties, it has been recorded that too many healthy girl children are being born. The proportionate rate of male children being much lower, the Department of Health does hereby decree that only women carrying boy children will be allowed to carry them to term." ' Kira broke off, too hurt and angry to continue. 'It isn't fair, dammit. It's my child! What right do they have to take it from me, regardless?' Kam looked at her younger sister, seeing the rage reflected in her face, the familiar pain she had felt herself, once. She could think of nothing to say. She had wanted to hear nothing at that time, because no words would change that reality.

'How was it for you Kam? When you found out?'

'Like my worst nightmare come true.' She paused and looked out the window, 'How long have you lived in this city now, Kira?'

David and I moved here two years ago. It was because of his job, you know, with the Health Department. We had to be in New Hope because that's where the government is now,' she hesitated, 'since the war.'

'I'm glad it ended when it did,' Kam replied, very softly, remembering the two strikes and the months of terror that followed.

'Yes, but is this cold war any better?' Kira asked, sipping from her glass. Kam only shrugged.

'What difference does it make anymore? This whole way of life is right out of Orwell's books. Maybe it would be better to be dead. At least I'd be with my baby.'

'Kam! Don't say that.'

'Kira,' Kam began, suddenly agitated, 'they took my child, and fucked it up so badly that I can't have another one. What have I to live for? They won't publish my books, Karl won't even touch me anymore. . . .' She trailed off, tears welling up in her eyes. 'I'd better go, all I'm doing is getting you depressed.' Kira only nodded, knowing her sister's moods and needing herself to be alone. They stood silently at the door, neither wanting to say goodby. From the pocket of her battered smock, Kam took out a worn pamphlet. Wordlessly, she handed it to Kira. 'I don't even know if they're in existence anymore,' she said, before shuffling out the door and down the hall to the elevators that would take her home. Kira watched the dwindling figure of her sister for a moment before she even glanced down at the paper in her hands. But as she began to comprehend the printed words on the page, her hands began to tremble. She shut and locked the door quickly.

'Fight the Patriarchal Government's Slaughter! Women carrying girl children escape to the Barrens, have your child in peace,' the pamphlet read. Could this be true? Kira asked herself. It had to be, Kam wouldn't have given it to her if it was a lie.

She sank into a chair, absorbed in the words of those angry women who were not going to let the government kill their children. She was suddenly startled when she heard David's key in the lock. Stuffing the pamphlet quickly inside her pant's pocket, she rose to meet him.

He came in smiling, the blond-haired golden boy of the Health Department, the very office that had issued the decree about aborting girl children. At first, she had convinced herself he had had no part in it, as he had told her himself, but now, for the first time, she wasn't so sure. He embraced her affectionately and kissed her cheek. Then, pulling back, he looked expectantly into her eyes. 'Well?' he demanded. She was immediately angry with him. Couldn't he see it? Couldn't he tell by now, after five years of marriage, that she was angry and afraid. She said nothing. After a moment, he drew her into the protective circle of his arms again.

They held each other for a long time, Kira finally releasing her tears and David joining with her. She held him tighter as he began to cry, loving the part of him that felt with her, his gentle sensitivity that made him so astute when he wanted to be.

After a while, he drew back. 'Did you make the appointment?'

'No,' she replied, bristling at him for being so clinical. 'I couldn't handle it right then. I'll make it in the morning,' she lied. He smiled a thin smile, but said nothing. Loosening his tie, he headed for the bedroom to change.

All through dinner, they were quiet. Kira immersed in the information the pamphlet had told her, and David perhaps thinking about his job, or his weekend plans, she didn't know. After dinner, she drifted into the living room again. She had cooked, he had to clean up. As she gazed once more at the colorful cityscape spread below her, she could hear in the background the clanking of pots and the softer sound of dishes being washed and dried.

They went to bed early, David wanting to make love, acting as if he believed that would take care of everything, Kira refusing, gently but firmly. 'I want one night to myself with my baby, if they're going to take her tomorrow.' David only nodded, disappointed and a little frustrated that there was nothing he could do. He sat propped on his pillow, golden hair tousled, barechested, the muscles rippling as he turned the pages of his book. He glanced over at her from time to time, touching her leg as she lay staring at the ceiling, catching her green eyes with his sky blue ones and smiling.

'It's going to be ok, honey,' he said.

'Kam wasn't ok.'

'I'll get you the best. I can pull rank, hon, really. I want you to have the best. I can even take time off from work to be there. Would you want me to?' Kira smiled.

'Let me think about it, ok? I'll tell you in the morning.' David nodded, but did not go back to his reading. Instead, he closed the book and lay beside her, touching her gently, trying his best to reassure his frightened and bitter wife.

Moonlight spilled into the bedroom from the uncurtained windows. Kira looked at the clock, it was 1 a.m. David slept heavily beside her, she had been long awake. She kept thinking about the women in the Barrens keeping their children, for hours she had been considering escaping the city, now she chided herself on her foolishness.

She watched the second hand of the clock whiz by. The swift passage of time frightened her, she knew she must make a decision soon. The night guards at the city gates would not question her, but, by tomorrow, her name would be on the gatehouse roster of pregnant women who were to be aborted. None of those women would be allowed to leave the city. Kira had never understood why that was before, now she began to suspect it was because they were afraid too many good 'breeding women' would try to defect to the Barrens, if such a place existed.

She rose from her shared bed and went into the other room to dress. Automatically, she pulled on travelling clothes, all the while telling herself she hadn't really even made the decision yet. But fifteen minutes later, she stood before a half-packed knapsack, saved from her schooldays, trying to decide what else to put in it.

She threw it down suddenly, feeling outraged at having to make the choice, yet at the same time torn. But the moment passed swiftly like clouds across the moon, and, almost automatically, she picked up the knapsack and finished filling it. Then she went into the kitchen and packed some fruit, nuts and water. Standing in the eerie glow of the open refrigerator's light, she decided to call Kam.

'Who the hell is this?' It was Karl's angry voice on the line. Kira had forgotten the phone was on his side of the bed.

'Kira, I have talk to Kam.'

'Kam's asleep.'

'Well wake her up, dammit,' Kira replied annoyed. Karl grumbled on the other end, but a moment later Kam's endlessly weary voice said hello.

'Kam, this is Kira. I'm going.' She paused. 'And I want you to come with me.' There was dead silence on the other end of the phone. 'Kam?'

'You're sick, Kira, and David's not there?'

'Yes,' Kira replied, suddenly understanding, 'come quickly, and bring a bag.'

'Ok, calm down, Kira. I'll be right there.'

'Kam, where should I meet you, you can't come here.'

'Meet me in front of the Pit,' Kam whispered into the phone.

'The bar?'

'Yes, you know, on the corner.' Kira could not understand her whisperings, but she knew the building.

'Ok, Kam, ten minutes.'

'Yes. Bye.'

'Bye.' Kira held the receiver for a moment before it went dead. The bar was just a block from Kam's house, but it was a good ten minutes walk from hers.

Picking up the knapsack, she went to the door, then hesitated. Didn't she owe David something? A note or at least one last kiss? She knew he would try to find her, or she thought he would. Taking the pamphlet from her pocket, she went to the ashtray. Lighting a match, she let the paper burn carefully so a clue was left. She hesitated again. What if David did find her and brought all his New Hope buddies with him? Would they destroy the village Kira hoped to find? She could not risk it. She let the pamphlet burn until it was nothing more than ashes in the tray. Then she slipped out the door, locking it and dropping her keys back through the mail slot, knowing if she made it, she would never have use for them again.

Kam was waiting for her outside the dark-windowed bar. People milled around them in groups or in couples, all races, all types mingling together in the teeming section of New Hope. Kam took her arm and smiled into her eyes. 'The West Entrance,' she whispered. 'Take my hand, I don't want to lose you.' Kira only nodded, her heart pounding.

As they climbed onto the moving sidewalk, people wove about them. Neon flashed and pleaded against the dark night while screaming and laughter filled the air. Kira's head spun with the fast-moving colors and life. She'd never been in the bar section after dark before.

They reached the West gate. Only one guard was there. 'Passports,' he said sullenly. Each handed a thin leather book to the man. He glanced at them, then at the passport pictures and wrote their names on a clipboard. 'Destination.'

'Am'ert,' Kam replied smoothly. Kira fought to control the violent shaking that swept over her body. Her stomach rolled over as it occurred to her he might not let them through. She swallowed audibly and tried to cover it with a cough. The guard looked up suspiciously.

'Reason for the visit?' he queried staring directly at Kira. She noticed his grey eyes and sharp, pointed nose seemed to accent his mood, making his long and sallow face even more unpleasant. She unstuck her tongue from the roof of her mouth.

'Our mother is dying. We received a 'gram requesting we

go to Am'ert to make the final arrangements for her personal –'

'What's her name?' he demanded turning to a computer console.

'Her name?' Kira stammered.

'Yes, are you deaf? Don't think I'm stupid. People aren't allowed to leave the city for no reason. I'm going to check the records to see if you even have a mother in Am'ert. "My dying mother" stories got worn out in the lower school. Now give me her name or I'll call the border patrol.'

'Cory Jochild,' Kam put in impatiently, 'If you take all night, she really will be dead before we get there.'

Ignoring her, the guard turned on the console. Kira watched as the green letters spilled onto the screen. He halted the rolling scroll in the Js.

'Street.'

'Maple,' Kam said. He looked at them with utter disgust. Kira tried to keep her face blank, but a smile began to play about the corners of her mouth.

'You may proceed,' he said haughtily, returning their passports to them, 'but I'm informing the border patrol in Am'ert that you're coming.'

'Sure you will,' Kam said under her breath. 'Am'ert doesn't even have a border patrol.' Laughing silently as the gates opened with a whoosh, they walked through.

The night around them was suddenly silent as the gates slid shut. The great glasslike bubble that encased the city prevented noise from traveling outside its walls. Kira felt suddenly weak, she stumbled.

'Are you ok?'

'What are we doing?' Kira asked, wishing very much to be back in her warm bed with David.

'Going to find our freedom,' Kam answered softly, confidently. Kira looked over at her. She seemed to glow with a radiance she had not had since they had been children together. Kira smiled even as she began to cry.

'David, I left David. I never even said goodby.' In her mind, she could see him sleeping, his face relaxed, his mind untroubled. There was such a contradiction between his compliant attitude towards life and her struggle to find a balance that, in reality, did not exist. As much as she hated all that he had come to stand for in the last hours, she knew she would always love David, the man. She broke down into long silent sobs. Kam held her gently, stroking her honey-colored hair.

'Say goodby now,' Kam said, turning her sister to face the domed city. Kira stared up at it, a structure miles high and miles wide, a vast oasis on the otherwise desertlike earth. She spoke with her mind, softly, caressingly, she said farewell to the man she had known for ten years, loved and lived with for five. Then she turned away, toward the vast darkness, the unknown. Kam touched her shoulder as they began walking westward towards the Barrens and the gathering of women who had chosen to keep the children growing in their wombs.

# GLOSSARY

*Alpha-fetoprotein test. AFP test.* The test is carried out on a woman's blood between sixteen–twenty weeks of pregnancy. It helps to detect a fetus with NTD. However, it will fail to diagnose about 10 percent of 'open' NTDs (the most serious ones) and 95 percent of closed NTDs (less serious ones). Also a number of positive tests are 'false positives,' due to twins or wrong dates in the calculation of pregnancy. A positive AFP is further checked by taking another blood sample, by ultrasound and by amniocentesis.

*Amniocentesis.* Under a local anesthetic, a needle is inserted in the abdomen of a pregnant woman and a sample of the fluid surrounding the fetus (amniotic fluid) is removed. Usually performed around the sixteenth week of pregnancy. The extracted cells are then artificially cultured and analyzed. It can be used to identify the sex of the fetus.

*Artificial insemination. AI.* A very simple procedure by which sperm is deposited in a woman's vagina, as close to the cervix as possible. AIH: when the sperm comes from the husband. AID: when the sperm comes from an anonymous donor. (See also *Self insemination.*)

*Cloning.* The development of an organism bypassing sexual reproduction. Popularly called 'Xeroxing' or 'carbon-copying,' it offers the possibility to create a population of genetically identical organisms. Not yet achieved in humans. (See also *Embryo division.*)

*Chorionic villi sampling. CVS.* A new experimental procedure, originally developed in China during early 1970s, which can be used to detect a variety of genetic abnormalities in a fetus and can be performed in the first trimester of pregnancy (eight–fourteen weeks). Like amniocentesis it can be used for sex-determination. Results can be evaluated overnight.

*Depo-Provera.* A long-lasting injectable contraceptive, designed to be administered to women once every three months. Manufactured by the Upjohn Corporation, it has never been approved as a contraceptive in the US (and under medical supervision only in the UK), but it has been widely promoted by international 'aid' agencies in the Third World.

*DES (Diethylstilbesterol).* An estrogen frequently given to pregnant women twenty to thirty years ago to prevent miscarriage. It has been found to cause cancer and other severe deformities and was apparently not effective in preventing miscarriage.

*Down syndrome.* A genetic abnormality due to the presence of an extra (third) chromosome 21. There is a significant but not yet fully understood link between the age of the parents and this condition. In the past, Western doctors called Down syndrome babies 'Mongoloid Idiots,' a term that reflects not only an incredible insensitivity to mentally disabled people, but also the racist assumption that these children resembled 'inferior' Eastern people.

*Egg fusion.* Fertilization of an egg with another egg. Procedure not yet developed for humans. Would allow procreation without sperm.

*Electronic fetal monitoring. EFM.* A method that monitors the fetus's heartbeat reaction to movement, either its own movement or the movement due to contractions of the womb in late pregnancy. A machine uses ultrasound to detect the heartbeat of the fetus or picks up electrical activity from the heart and then prints these out on a piece of paper or it shows as a trace on a TVscreen.

*Embryo division.* This procedure consists of dividing the developing fertilized egg (usually in its four-cell stage called blastula) into individual cells which potentially can then develop into four identical human beings (one form of cloning). These developing embryos could be investigated to determine their chromosomal composition and subjected to genetic manipulations.

*Embryo replacement.* In IVF, when the developing embryo is placed in the womb of the same woman who donated the egg.

*Embryo transfer.* A technique by which an embryo (from a woman's womb or through IVF) is transferred into a second woman's womb.

*Epidural anesthesia.* Anesthetic injected through a tube in the outer portion of the spinal canal. It allows for continuous medication and literally 'knocks out' a birthing woman by removing pains and all sensation from her womb and genitals while she gives birth.

*Episiotomy.* An incision to enlarge the vaginal opening, in the US, now commonly practised at childbirth.

*Fetoscopy.* The direct examination of the fetus through a fetoscope (a fine fibre-optic telescope) with attachments that allow the removal of samples of fetal blood or tissue. Usually carried out between the sixteenth–twentieth weeks of pregnancy.

*Frozen embryo.* Also called cryostorage. A technique by which embryos are frozen in liquid nitrogen at a temperature of $-200$ F. The frozen embryo can later be thawed and put into a womb. Currently at the experimental stage in Australia.

*Gene therapy.* The replacement of a 'bad' gene with a 'good' one; a technology which has not yet been developed but which some geneticists predict will be used in the future to treat genetic disorders resulting from a single gene.

*Intrauterine device. IUD.* Plastic or metal device that is inserted into the uterus in order to prevent pregnancy.

*In vitro fertilization. IVF.* Fertilization of a human egg by a sperm out of the womb. Currently, after fertilization, the egg is implanted in a woman's uterus. It involves a number of new procedures whose risks we know very little about as yet.

*Laparoscopy.* Surgical procedure requiring general anesthesia in which the abdomen is distended by inserting a tube and pumping in carbon dioxide. Then the laparoscope, a long tube with a fibre-optic telescope, can be inserted to take a look at the pelvic organs and to remove egg(s) from a woman's ovaries.

*Neural tube defects. NTD.* Neural tube defects include anencephaly (severe deformity of the brain) and spina bifida (where some vertebrae might be missing and some spinal chord tissue may protrude outside the body). Very little is known about its causes.

*Parthenogenesis.* Development of the egg into a complete organism without fertilization from the sperm. It occurs in some species, but has not yet been achieved in humans. It would produce only female offspring.

*Self insemination. SI.* Artificial insemination without the involvement of an official donor organization.

*Surrogate mother.* A woman who 'carries' the pregnancy for another woman. She might furnish the egg and the womb and be artificially inseminated with the semen of the partner of another woman. Or she might provide the womb to an embryo obtained by IVF, in which case, both the egg and sperm will be furnished by donors. This last possibility has not yet been done but there is no reason to believe that it is not feasible.

*Ultrasound.* High frequency sound waves used to make on a TV screen a picture of the fetus inside the womb. It is now widely used in prenatal 'care' and assumed to be safe, though no long-term studies have been made on its effects. Also called sonogram, sonography, or ultrasound visualization.

# RESOURCES

*National organizations*

Anti-Depo-Provera Campaign. 62 Regent Street, Chippendale 2008, Sydney Area, Australia.

Association of Radical Midwives. 8a The Drive, Wimbledon, London SW20, Great Britain.

Committee for Abortion Rights and Against Sterilization Abuse (CARASA). 17 Murray St, 5th Floor, New York, NY 10007, USA.

Committee for Responsible Genetics. P.O. Box 759, Cambridge, MA, 02138, USA.

Federation of Feminist Women's Health Centers. 6411 Hollywood Blvd, Los Angeles, California, 90028, USA.

Health Alternatives For Women (THAW). P.O. Box 884, Christchurch, New Zealand.

National Women's Health Network. 224 Seventh St, SE Washington, DC, 20003, USA.

National Abortion Campaign. 374 Grays Inn Road, London WC1, Great Britain.

Reproductive Rights National Network (R2N2). 17 Murray St, 5th floor, New York, NY 10007, USA.

Science for the People. 897 Main Street, Cambridge, Ma, 02139, USA.

Women's Abortion Action Campaign. 62 Regent Street, Chippendale 2008, Sydney Area, Australia.

Women's Health Information Centre (WHIC). 12 Ufton Rd, London N1, Great Britain.

*International*

International Contraception, Abortion and Sterilization Campaign (ICASC). 374 Grays Inn Road, London WC1, Great Britain.

*Periodicals*

*Broadsheet*. P.O. Box 5799, Wellesley Street, Auckland, New
   Zealand.

*Connexions*. Peoples Translation Service, 4228 Telegraph
   Avenue, Oakland, Ca 94609, USA.

*ISIS*. P.O. Box 50 (Cornavin), 1211 Geneva 2, Switzerland.

*Off Our Backs*. 1841 Columbia Road, No. 212, Washington,
   DC, 20009, USA.

*Outwrite*. Oxford House, Derbyshire Street, London E2,
   Great Britain.

*Spare Rib*. 27 Clerkenwell Close, London EC1R 0AT, Great
   Britain.

*Manushi*. C1/202 Lajpat Nagar, New Delhi 110024, India.

*Filmguides*

*Guide to Films on Reproductive Rights*. Produced by US
   Media Network and the Reproductive Rights National
   Network, in cooperation with the Film Fund. Describes
   sixty of the best films, videotapes and slideshows on:
   abortion, teen pregnancy and parenthood, sterilization,
   sexuality and aging, birth control, hazards to reproductive
   health, childcare, lesbian and gay issues, sexuality and the
   disabled, midwifery, etc. Order from Reproductive Rights
   National Network, 17 Murray Street, New York, NY,
   10007, USA.

*Pamphlets*

Two excellent US pamphlets published by CARASA, 17
   Murray St, New York, N.Y. 10007, USA are : *Sterilization:
   It's Not as Simple as Tying your Tubes* and *Women Under
   Attack*. Order from CARASA or from the R2N2.

Local Women's Health Centers worldwide can be contacted
   for information/counselling on the old and new reproductive technologies. Local family planning associations
   may be useful too, but vary greatly in their feminist
   attitudes.

# FURTHER READING

## A SELECTED BIBLIOGRAPHY ON WOMEN, SCIENCE, AND TECHNOLOGY

Alic, Margaret. Forthcoming. *Hypatia's Heritage. The History of Women's Science*. The Women's Press, London. A thorough look at lost and forgotten women scientists from ancient Egypt to the present and a celebration of women's achievements in science.

Arditti, Rita, Pat Brennan, and Steve Cavrak. 1980. *Science and Liberation*. South End Press, Boston. A collection of essays that draws attention to the many connections between scientific work and the social context from which it emerges.

Bleier, Ruth. 1984. *Science and Gender. A Critique of Biology and its Theories on Women*. Athene Series. Pergamon, New York and Oxford. A thorough critique of patriarchal research on female biology looking at hormonal, brain and sexuality research and exposing the misogynist nature of sociobiology and theories of cultural evolution.

The Brighton Science Collective. 1980. *Alice Through the Microscope. The Power of Science over Women's Lives*. Virago, London. A collection looking at various ways in which science affects the lives of women, particularly in educational settings and in conditioning us to a male world view.

Cockburn, Cynthia. 1982. *Brothers. Male Dominance and the New Technology*. Pluto Press, London. A feminist exploration of the development of computer software.

Gornick, Vivian. 1983. *Women Scientists*. Simon & Schuster, New York. An exploration of women scientists' lives and careers, revealing clearly the sexist, misogynist practices that a woman scientist has to put up with.

Holmes, Helen B., Betty B. Hoskins, and Michael Gross, eds. 1980. *Birth Control and Controlling Birth – Women-Centered Perspectives*. Humana Press, New Jersey.

Holmes, Helen B., Betty B. Hoskins, and Michael Gross, 1981. *The Custom-Made Child? – Women-Centered Perspectives*. Humana Press, New Jersey. These two pioneering volumes contain the papers presented at the Conference on Ethical Issues in Human Reproductive Technology: Analysis by Women, held in June 1979 at Hampshire College in Amherst, Massachusetts.

Hubbard, Ruth, Mary Sue Henifin and Barbara Fried, eds. 1982. *Biological Woman – The Convenient Myth*. Schenkman, Cambridge, MA. An anthology (the updated version of *Women Look at Biology Looking at Women*, 1979) questioning the validity of traditional descriptions of women's biology. Especially valuable is the excellent eighty-page bibliography with books on women and science.

Huws, Ursula. 1982. *Your Job in the Eighties. A Woman's Guide to New Technology*. Pluto Press, London. A practical guide to the effects of new technology on women's jobs.

Lowe, Marian, and Ruth Hubbard. 1983. *Woman's Nature. Rationalizations of Inequality*. Athene Series. Pergamon, New York and Oxford. A collection that critiques theories of biology that have been used to justify the oppression of women.

Merchant, Carolyn. 1980. *The Death of Nature*. Harper & Row, San Francisco. A critical reassessment of the Scientific Revolution during the sixteenth and seventeenth centuries from a feminist perspective.

Rothschild, Joan. 1983. *Machina Ex Dea. Feminist Perspectives on Technology*. Athene Series. Pergamon, New York and Oxford. An exploration of the exclusion of women from technological history and culture by providing feminist perspectives on the social context and the nature of technology.

Sayers, Janet. 1982. *Biological Politics*. A discussion of feminist and anti-feminist perspectives on biological accounts of sex differences. Tavistock, London.

Sayre, Ann. 1980. *Rosalind Franklin and DNA*. W. W. Norton, New York. The dramatic story of how Rosalind Franklin came to discover the structure of DNA, and how the sexist traditions of science allowed two men, Watson and Crick, to receive the credit.

SPRU Women and Technology Studies. 1982. *Microelectronics and Women's Employment*. University of Sussex, Brighton. An investigation into the implications of new technology for women's jobs by looking at women's contribution to many occupations and their expulsion from them by means of the new technology.

Trescott, Martha Moore. 1979. *Dynamos and Virgins Revisited. Women and Technological Change in History*. Scarescrow Press, Metuchen NY. A collection of eleven essays on the interactions between women and technology, both contemporary and historical, European and American.

Zimmerman, Jan, ed. 1983. *The Technological Woman: Interfacing with Tomorrow*. Praeger, New York. A collection of articles on household technologies, technologies in the workplace, and health care technologies.

For an excellent and thorough bibliography on women, science and health, see Ruth Hubbard et al., eds. *Biological Woman – The Convenient Myth*, cited above.

# NOTES ON CONTRIBUTORS

**Rebecca M. Albury** has had a continuing involvement with theoretical and practical aspects of female sexuality, fertility control, reproduction, mother-daughter relations and women's health care for the past sixteen years. She currently lives in Sydney, New South Wales, Australia, and teaches politics at Macquarie University.

**Vimal Balasubrahmanyan** is a freelance journalist writing mainly on feminist and socio-medical issues for a number of Indian newspapers and periodicals. She is married and has two teenage children, a daughter and a son.

**Nancy Breeze** is glad to have traded in forty years of Michigan winters and summers for a St Augustine beach home. When she is not at her typesetting job, she can be found sunbathing, disco-dancing, arguing, sunset-watching, bike-riding or listening to classical music.

**Phillida Bunkle,** an active feminist, was raised in England and educated at girls' schools, Keele University, and St Anne's College, Oxford, before going to American graduate schools at Smith College and Harvard University. In 1972 she came to New Zealand, after a year of teaching women's studies at the University of Massachusetts, because as a woman she was at that time not allowed to take her New Zealand-born partner to England. Sharing a university position teaching history enabled them both to care for their two children. Phillida is now co-ordinator of women's studies at Victoria University, Wellington, New Zealand, and a regular contributor to *Broadsheet; New Zealand's Feminist Magazine.*

**Adele Clarke,** doctoral candidate at the University of California, San Francisco, was co-ordinator of the women's studies program at Sonoma State University, specializing in women's health. Her doctoral research in the sociology of science examines the emergence and implications of the modern division of labor in reproductive biology.

**The Coalition to Fight Infant Mortality** is an Oakland-based action group made up of concerned citizens, including health workers, educators and representatives of other community groups. It was formed in 1978 and it publishes a quarterly newsletter describing its activities. Its address is P.O. Box 10436, Oakland, CA, 94610.

**Genoveffa (Gena) Corea** is a journalist and author of *The Hidden Malpractice*, 1977, William Morrow, New York (reprint forthcoming, 1984, Harper & Row, New York). For the past four years, she has been writing a book on the new reproductive technologies, *The Mother Machine*.

**Carol Downer** is a founder and administrator of the Feminist Women's Health Center in Los Angeles. She has written articles and spoken widely on self-help and on women's health.

**Anne Finger** is a writer whose work has appeared in *Thirteenth Moon, Off Our Backs, Plexus* and *Antioch Review*. She lives in San Francisco, where she works as a secretary and is active in the Committee to Defend Reproductive Rights.

**Jalna Hanmer** studied sociology at the University of California in Berkeley and began her employed life as a community worker in England in the East End of London. Later, when teaching community work at the London School of Economics, she became active in Women's Aid (shelter movement). Moving North, where she lives in a collective household with her son, she now co-ordinates the Diploma/MA in Women's Studies (Applied) at the University of Bradford, West Yorkshire. She researches and writes on violence to women and reproductive technology and is part of a group producing a new radical feminist magazine, *Trouble and Strife*.

**Ruth Holland** is a hospital-based midwife, working in East Sussex, England, with some experience of practising in the community and abroad.

**Helen Bequaert 'Becky' Holmes** is a biologist with special interests in population genetics, human biology, and bioethics. She edited (with Betty B. Hoskins and Michael Gross) the books, *Birth Control and Controlling Birth: Women-Centered Perspectives* (1980, Humana Press, Clifton, NJ) and *The Custom-Made Child? Women-Centered Perspectives* (1981, Humana Press, Clifton, NJ). She has taught biology at several colleges, spent a year as a Visiting Scholar in the philosophy department at Spelman College in Atlanta, Georgia, and now works independently as a researcher and writer on ethical and social issues raised by the new reproductive technologies.

**Francie Hornstein's** interest in women's health issues has spanned a fifteen-year period, from doing illegal abortion referrals in Iowa in the late 1960s to working at the Feminist Women's Health Center in Los Angeles from 1972 to 1979. Her working for reproductive choices for women was a direct result of her friends who found themselves pregnant when they did not want to be and her own experience of being a lesbian who has always wanted to have children. She is currently working with the National Health Law Program on a project to lower infant death rates among poor and minority communities.

**Betty B. Hoskins** supports herself, her family, and her feminist activities as a senior technical editor at a computer company. Educated as a developmental and molecular biologist, she has taught at community, liberal arts and engineering colleges. She established a bioethics program for undergraduate science students at Worcester Polytechnic Institute. She later became a textbook editor, and now she works in women's studies as an independent scholar. She edited two volumes with Becky Holmes (*q.v.*), chairs a national liberal religious group of scholars (mostly Unitarian Universalist), and folkdances.

**Ruth Hubbard** is a professor of biology at Harvard University, where she teaches courses dealing with the interactions of science and society, particularly as they affect women. She has written numerous articles and co-edited several books, the most recent of which are *Biological Woman – The Convenient Myth* (Schenkman, 1982), with Mary Sue Henifin and Barbara Fried, and *Woman's Nature: Rationalizations of Inequality* (Pergamon Press, 1983), with Marian Lowe. She is a member of Science for the People and of the National Women's Health Network and has worked with the Boston Women's Health Book Collective on the 1984 edition of *Our Bodies, Ourselves*.

**Susan Ince** is a feminist activist and a freelance writer based in New York. Trained in medical genetics, she has worked in urban neighborhood health clinics to provide information and support for women's reproductive choices.

**K. Kaufmann** has x-ray vision, walks through walls and is learning to live with her limitations. She is a writer working and living in the San Francisco Bay Area and is Calendar editor for *Plexus, West Coast Women's Press*.

**Jill McKenna** is a Community midwife working in Mid-Sussex.

**Jane Murphy** received a BA from Hampshire College in 1981 and was supported in her study of cloning research by a grant from the Threshhold Fund, associated with Hampshire College, Amherst, Massachusetts. She presently lives and works on Cape Cod and plans to study environmental health hazards in a masters program in Public Health.

**Julie Murphy** is an assistant professor of philosophy at the University of Santa Clara. Her research interests are ethics, the history of philosophy, and feminist theory. She is active in research on issues of abortion, pregnancy and reproductive technologies.

**BarbaraNeely** is an African of American slave descent. She is the founder of The Third World Women Writers Workshop and Yenga Productions. She is currently working on a novel about working-class black women, a series of radio tapes on the literary works of women of color and a book on the socio-political roots of black male sexism. *A Yenga Tale* is one of a series of prehistory myths Neely is developing.

**Cris Newport** is a writer looking to create a genre of fantasy written for women. Recently she became a member of the web of women who will publish a new magazine called *Women of Power: A Magazine of Feminism, Spirituality and Politics*. She lives in Boston and can be written to through the magazine.

**Scarlet Pollock** is a Jewish lesbian feminist whose interests include farming, women's health, sexuality, fatherhood and feminist theory. She lives in Yorkshire in constant negotiation with ten cats, one dog, five cows, twenty-three hens, five ducks, a carthorse and one lover. She is co-editor (as Friedman) with Elizabeth Sarah of *On the Problem of Men*, 1982, The Women's Press, London and author of *Women, Sexuality and Contraception*, forthcoming, Routledge & Kegan Paul.

**Rayna Rapp** teaches anthropology at the New School for Social Research, helps to edit *Feminist Studies*, serves on the *Ms.* magazine Board of Academic Advisers, and has been an activist in the reproductive freedom movement for over fifteen years. A version of her article appeared in *Ms.* magazine in April 1984.

**Janice Raymond** is associate professor of women's studies and medical ethics in the Women's Studies Program at the University of Massachusetts in Amherst. She is the author of *The Transsexual Empire: The Making of the She-Male*

(Beacon, Boston, 1979), and is currently working on a book on female friendship, to be published in 1985.

**Maureen Ritchie** is a bibliographer, who has worked on various bibliometric research projects on social science and humanities information provision, before specialising in women's studies information and bibliography. She now lives in Whitstable, Kent, with her husband and three children, and is working on a guide to information sources for women's studies.

**Viola Roggencamp**, born in Hamburg, Germany, has been a freelance journalist for the past seven years. For the last four years she has spent four to six months each year in Asia, with India as her headquarters. She is a regular contributor to *Emma*, a German feminist magazine for women by women and *Die Zeit*, a German weekly, published in Hamburg.

**Barbara Katz Rothman** is assistant professor of sociology, Baruch College of the City University of New York. She is the author of *In Labor: Women and Power in the Birthplace* (published in the USA by W. W. Norton and in Great Britain by Junction Books, 1982; published in paperback by Penguin as *Giving Birth: Alternatives in Childbirth*). Her current work is on reproductive and genetic technology, *The Products of Conception: The Genetic Tie* (working title, Viking Press, forthcoming).

**Robyn Rowland** is lecturer in social psychology and women's studies at Deakin University, Australia. She has researched the childfree lifestyle and is currently working on research into the social and psychological consequences of human artificial insemination. She has published in both psychology and women's studies. She edited *Women Who Do and Women Who Don't, join the women's movement,* (Routledge & Kegan Paul, 1984), and has written a women's studies interdisciplinary textbook, *Woman Herself: A Women's Studies Perspective on Self-Identity* (Oxford University Press, Melbourne, 1984). Robyn has also written two books of poetry: *Filigree in Blood* (Longman Cheshire, Melbourne, 1982) and *Rainbow Warrior* (in press).

**Kumkum Sangari** is a lecturer of English in Indraprastha College, University of Delhi. She has a doctoral dissertation in American literature from the University of Leeds and has written several articles on literature and on women in contemporary India.

**Marsha Saxton** is consultant to healthcare agencies, employers and schools about disability issues. She currently directs a conjoint project of the Feminist Press and Boston Self Help Center on disabled women. She is author of articles on women, peer counseling and mental health.

**Eleanor Trawick** has worked as a teenager in organizing for reproductive rights at Cleveland Heights High School, a public high school in the Cleveland area. She is now a freshman at Columbia University and is working with the Barnard Abortion and Reproductive Rights Network and the International Socialist Organization.

# INDEX

# WOMEN AND THE AIDS CRISIS

Diane Richardson

*The book of the year, if not the decade'* – *Angela Carter*

In this fully revised, up-dated and enlarged New Edition of *Women and the AIDS Crisis*, Diane Richardson gives us the latest figures and research findings, recent developments in policy on AIDS and a fully up-dated Resources Section for Britain and Australia. She provides an extended section on safer sex and racism, and she includes further interviews with HIV positive women and with carers of people who have AIDS, illuminating how women today are coping with the challenge of AIDS.

This brand new edition also explores those issues that AIDS raises for pregnant women, for lesbians, for women who use drugs and for prostitutes.

'This is the first well-documented book on women and AIDS to appear in a form accessible to the non-professional public. Diane Richardson's approach is candid and her research excellent. It is original, thought-provoking and timely. Any reader who does not emerge with a warmer compassion and understanding of the problems must be a harsh individual indeed.'
– *Janet Green, Counselling Administrator, Terrence Higgins Trust*

'. . .this is the one you should be reading – it may turn out to be the only one you ever need to read.' – *Rose Collis, City Limits*

'A strong counterblast to all the misinformation.'
– *Anna Raeburn*

'. . . her politics are inherent to her approach, her feminism intrinsic and her style of writing accessible to readers of all political persuasions.' – *Amanda Hopkinson, New Statesman*

004 440357 7

£3.95

# THE POLITICS OF BREASTFEEDING

Gabrielle Palmer

- As publicity about the benefits of breastfeeding increases, so too do the worldwide sales of artificial baby milk and feeding bottles
- Over-population and child malnutrition are the direct results of the decline in breastfeeding
- Every year, in USA alone, 70,000 tons of tin plate are used up in discarded baby milk tins
- For the first time in recorded history, the impotent female breast has become a mass sexual fetish

Gabrielle Palmer's powerful and provocative book shows that breastfeeding is much more than a matter of personal inclination. Women all over the world are being pressurised into feeding their babies artificially and this affects us all: our health, our environment and the global economy.

Gabrielle Palmer questions whether bottlefeeding really frees women to lead more fulfilling lives, and examines social attitudes in a world where a woman who does breastfeed her child risks losing what little income she earns. She traces the commercial reasons behind medical recommendations, and alerts us to basic nutritional facts and the controversy over breastfeeding in the light of AIDS, radiation and breast cancer.

0 86358 219 2

£6.95 pbk

# THE TENTATIVE PREGNANCY

*Prenatal Diagnosis and the Future of Motherhood*

Barbara Katz Rothman

'Anyone who thinks that prenatal diagnosis is liberating for women should read this book.' – *Ruth Hubbard, Harvard University*

More and more women are having children when they are over 30 and amniocentesis, primarily used as a test for Down's Syndrome, is becoming an automatic and routine part of prenatal care.

In this groundbreaking book, Barbara Katz Rothman draws on the experience of over 120 women and a wealth of expert testimony to show how one simple procedure can radically alter the way we think about childbirth and becoming a parent. The results of amniocentesis, and the more recently developed chorion villus sampling, force us to confront agonising dilemmas. What do you do if there is a 'problem' with the foetus? What kind of support can you expect if you decide to raise a handicapped child? How can you come to terms with the termination of a wanted pregnancy?

Passionate, sympathetic and at times heartbreaking, Barbara Katz Rothman's book is a must for anyone thinking of having a child.

'. . . makes women's experience of the technology visible for the first time . . . an immensely intelligent, sensitive and passionate book. No one can read it and remain unmoved.' – *Gena Corea*

'Wise, sensitive and disturbing – it should be obligatory reading for all health professionals working in this field, and for everyone who wants to understand the increasingly complex face of childbearing in today's world.' – *Ann Oakley*

0 86358 255 9

£5.95 pbk

# THE HEROIN USERS

Tam Stewart

What do you think of heroin? Pushers? Junkies? If you know someone taking heroin and panic is gripping you, put down that newspaper, turn off the TV and stop and think for a moment or two. Is your son or daughter, your husband or sister really a lost cause? Is he or she a deranged deviant who can never hope to quit drugs alive or re-enter the society which will shun him or her if it finds out? If you can separate the person you know from the deluge of declamatory articles, and the notion of a 'devil drug', you may perceive that all is not lost.

This book tells the inside story of the heroin users. It sets out to reveal who takes heroin, why they do it, and how their lives change once heroin has become a part of them. But it also provides informed and realistic hope and encouragement, not just for addicts, but for all those trying to help them.

0  86358  111  0

£5.95

## Also Available from Pandora Press